Perinatal HIV

Editors

AVY VIOLARI
ANN CHAHROUDI

CLINICS IN PERINATOLOGY

www.perinatology.theclinics.com

Consulting Editor
LUCKY JAIN

December 2024 • Volume 51 • Number 4

ELSEVIER

1600 John F. Kennedy Boulevard • Suite 1800 • Philadelphia, Pennsylvania, 19103-2899

http://www.theclinics.com

CLINICS IN PERINATOLOGY Volume 51, Number 4
December 2024 ISSN 0095-5108, ISBN-13: 978-0-443-12913-1

Editor: Kerry Holland
Developmental Editor: Nitesh Barthwal

Clinics in Perinatology (ISSN 0095-5108) is published quarterly by Elsevier Inc., 360 Park Avenue South, New York, NY 10010-1710. Months of issue are March, June, September, and December. Business and Editorial Offices: 1600 John F. Kennedy Blvd., Ste. 1800, Philadelphia, PA 19103-2899. Customer Service Office: 3251 Riverport Lane, Maryland Heights, MO 63043. Periodicals postage paid at New York, NY and additional mailing offices. Subscription prices are $351.00 per year (US individuals), $398.00 per year (Canadian individuals), $475.00 per year (international individuals), $100.00 per year (US and Canadian students), and $195.00 per year (International students). For institutional access pricing please contact Customer Service via the contact information below. International air speed delivery is included in all Clinics subscription prices. All prices are subject to change without notice. Orders, claims, and journal inquiries: Please visit our Support Hub page https://service.elsevier.com for assistance.

Reprints. For copies of 100 or more, of articles in this publication, please contact the Commercial Reprints Department, Elsevier Inc., 360 Park Avenue South, New York, NY 10010-1710. Tel. 212-633-3874; Fax: 212-633-3820; E-mail: reprints@elsevier.com.

Clinics in Perinatology is also published in Spanish by McGraw-Hill Interamericana Editores S.A., P.O. Box 5-237, 06500 Mexico D.F., Mexico.

Clinics in Perinatology is covered in *MEDLINE/PubMed (Index Medicus) Current Contents, Excepta Medica, BIOSIS and ISI/BIOMED.*

Contributors

CONSULTING EDITOR

LUCKY JAIN, MD, MBA
George W. Brumley Jr. Professor and Chair, Department of Pediatrics, Emory University School of Medicine, Pediatrician-in-Chief, Children's Healthcare of Atlanta, Executive Director, Emory+Children's Pediatric Institute Atlanta, Georgia, USA

EDITORS

AVY VIOLARI, FCPaed (SA)
Director, Paediatric Research and Care, Perinatal HIV Research Unit, Faculty of Health Sciences, University of the Witwatersrand, Johannesburg, South Africa

ANN CHAHROUDI, MD, PhD
Professor and Vice Chair for Basic Science, Department of Pediatrics, Emory University School of Medicine, Children's Healthcare of Atlanta, Atlanta, Georgia, USA

AUTHORS

MOHERNDRAN ARCHARY, MBChB, DCH(SA), FCPaeds(SA), Paeds ID (SA), PhD(UKZN)
Professor, Department of Paediatrics and Child Health, Nelson R Mandela School of Medicine, Berea; Department of Paediatrics, Victoria Mxenge Hospital (Previously King Edward VIII Hospital), Durban, South Africa

SOUMIA BEKKA, BS
PhD Candidate, Department of Molecular Microbiology and Immunology, Johns Hopkins Bloomberg School of Public Health, Baltimore, Maryland, USA

ADRIE BEKKER, MBChB, DCH(SA), MMed (SU), FCPaeds(SA), Cert Neo(SA), PhD(SU)
Professor, Department of Paediatrics and Child Health, Department of Medicine, University of Stellenbosch, Cape Town, South Africa

SCARLETT BERGAM, MPH
Medical Student, Department of Behavioral and Social Sciences, George Washington University of Medicine and Health Sciences, Washington, DC, USA

CHRISTIAN BINUYA, BS
Research Technician, Department of Pediatrics, Weill Cornell Medicine, New York, New York, USA

KRISTINA BROOKS, PharmD
Assistant Professor, Department of Pharmaceutical Sciences, Skaggs School of Pharmacy and Pharmaceutical Sciences, University of Colorado Anschutz Medical Campus, Aurora, Colorado, USA

LISA MARIE CRANMER, MD, MPH
Associate Professor, Departments of Pediatrics and Epidemiology, Emory University, Atlanta, Georgia, USA

AHIZECHUKWU C. EKE, MD, PhD, MPH
Associate Professor, Division of Maternal Fetal Medicine, Department of Gynecology and Obstetrics, Johns Hopkins University School of Medicine, Baltimore, Maryland, USA

CARLO GIAQUINTO, PhD
Professor, Department of Pediatrics, University of Padova, Head of Penta Foundation, Padova, Padova, Italy

MARIELLE S. GROSS, MD, MBE
Affiliate Professor, Johns Hopkins Berman Institute of Bioethics, Baltimore, Maryland, USA

KRITHIKA P. KARTHIGEYAN, PhD
Postdoctoral Associate, Department of Pediatrics, Weill Cornell Medicine, New York, New York, USA

KRISTEN KELLY, BS
PhD Candidate, Department of Molecular Microbiology and Immunology, Johns Hopkins Bloomberg School of Public Health, Baltimore, Maryland, USA

MEDRINE KIHANGA, BS
Baccalaureate Student, Earlham College, Richmond, Indiana, USA

AARTI KINIKAR, MD, MRCP
Professor, Department of Pediatrics, BJ Government Medical College and Sassoon General Hospital, Pune, India

ELIZABETH D. LOWENTHAL, MD, MSCE
Associate Professor, Department of Pediatrics, University of Pennsylvania School of Medicine, Children's Hospital of Philadelphia, Department of Biostatistics, Epidemiology, and Informatics, University of Pennsylvania School of Medicine, Philadelphia, Pennsylvania, USA

KATHLEEN M. MALEE, PhD
Professor, Department of Psychiatry and Behavioral Science, Northwestern University Feinberg School of Medicine, Chicago, Illinois, USA

MEGAN S. MCHENRY, MS, MD, FAPP
Associate Professor, Department of Pediatrics, Ryan White Center for Pediatric Infectious Disease and Global Health, Indiana University School of Medicine, Indianapolis, Indiana, USA

CHARLES D. MITCHELL, MD, MS
Professor, Division of Pediatric Infectious Diseases and Immunology, Batchelor Childrens Research Institute, University of Miami Miller School of Medicine, Miami, Florida, USA

KAGISO MOCHANKANA, MBBS, FCPaeds(SA), MMeD(UB)
Pediatric Infectious Diseases Fellow, Department of Paediatrics, Victoria Mxenge Hospital (Previously King Edward VIII Hospital), Durban, South Africa

CINTA MORALEDA, PhD
Researcher, Department of Pediatrics, Pediatric Infectious Diseases Unit, Madrid, Spain

GRACE M. MUSIIME, MBBCh, MSc, MMed, FC Paed (SA), DTM&H, Cert Neonatology
Neonatologist, Kenya Paediatric Association, Nairobi, Kenya

SHARON NACHMAN, MD
Distingished Professor, Pediatric Infectious Disease, Department of Pediatrics, Renaissance School of Medicine, State University of New York at Stony Brook, Stony Brook, New York, USA

ASHLEY N. NELSON, PhD
Assistant Professor of Immunology Research, Department of Pediatrics, Weill Cornell Medicine, Drukier Institute for Children's Health, New York, New York, USA

SHARON L. NICHOLS, PhD
Research Scientist, Department of Neurosciences, University of California, San Diego, La Jolla, California, USA

KIRA J. NIGHTINGALE, MS, MBA
PhD Candidate, Department of Biostatistics, Epidemiology, and Informatics, University of Pennsylvania School of Medicine, Philadelphia, Pennsylvania, USA

SALLIE R. PERMAR, MD, PhD
Chair and Professor, Department of Pediatrics, Weill Cornell Medicine, Drukier Institute for Children's Health, New York, New York, USA

DEBORAH PERSAUD, MD
Director of Pediatric Infectious Diseases, Professor, Division of Infectious Diseases, Department of Pediatrics, Johns Hopkins University School of Medicine, Department of Molecular Microbiology and Immunology, Johns Hopkins Bloomberg School of Public Health, Baltimore, Maryland, USA

JENNA S. POWERS, MD
Medical Student, Emory School of Medicine, Emory University, Atlanta, Georgia, USA

WHITNEY PUETZ, MPH
Student, Department of Behavioral, Social and Health Education Sciences, Emory University Rollins School of Public Health, Atlanta, Georgia, USA

SHATHANI RAMPA, MSc
PhD Student, Department of Psychology, Queens College, The Graduate Center, CUNY, New York; Department of Psychology, Queens College, Flushing, New York, USA

REUBEN N. ROBBINS, PhD
Associate Professor of Clinical Medical Psychology, Department of Psychiatry, Columbia University Vagelos College of Physicians and Surgeons, New York State Psychiatric Institute, New York, New York, USA

PABLO ROJO, PhD
Professor, Department of Pediatrics, Pediatric Infectious Diseases Unit, Universidad Complutense, Madrid, Spain

ANNETTE H. SOHN, MD, PhD
Director, TREAT Asia, amfAR - The Foundation for AIDS Research, Bangkok, Thailand

LYNDA STRANIX-CHIBANDA, MBChB, MMed (Paeds)
Adjunct Researcher, Lecturer, Child, Adolescent and Women's Health Department, Faculty of Medicine and Health Sciences, University of Zimbabwe, Belgravia, Harare, Zimbabwe

TAVITIYA SUDJARITRUK, MD, PhD
Associate Professor, Division of Infectious Diseases, Department of Pediatrics, Faculty of Medicine, Chiang Mai University, and Clinical and Molecular Epidemiology of Emerging and Re-emerging Infectious Diseases Research Cluster, Faculty of Medicine, Chiang Mai University, Chiang Mai, Thailand

KENNETH VUONG, BS
Research Technician, Department of Pediatrics, Weill Cornell Medicine, New York, New York, USA

CATHERINE J. WEDDERBURN, MBChB, MA, MSc, DTM&H, MRCPCH
Chief Research Officer, Department of Paediatrics and Child Health, Neuroscience Institute, University of Cape Town, Cape Town, South Africa

BRIAN C. ZANONI, MD, MPH
Associate Professor, Emory University Rollins School of Public Health, Departments of Medicine and Pediatric Infectious Diseases, Emory University School of Medicine, Children's Healthcare of Atlanta, Atlanta, Georgia, USA

Contents

Foreword: Can We Eliminate Perinatal HIV? **xv**

Lucky Jain

Preface: Perinatal HIV: Past, Present, and Future **xix**

Avy Violari and Ann Chahroudi

Care of Pregnant Women Living with Human Immunodeficiency Virus **749**

Lynda Stranix-Chibanda, Kristina Brooks, and Ahizechukwu C. Eke

Managing human immunodeficiency virus (HIV) during pregnancy requires attention to psychosocial aspects of maternal health in addition to providing medical and obstetric care. Ideal care plans promote sustained HIV suppression and optimize maternal health prior to conception. Engagement with maternity services creates opportunities to support women with HIV to remain engaged in life-long care, monitor their health frequently, screen for co-morbid conditions, and develop a personalized antiretroviral therapy adherence strategy. This article summarizes antiretroviral drug use in pregnancy, pregnancy outcomes in women with HIV, and the key elements of providing holistic care.

Research on Maternal Vaccination for HIV Prevention **769**

Krithika P. Karthigeyan, Christian Binuya, Kenneth Vuong, Sallie R. Permar, and Ashley N. Nelson

Despite increased uptake of antiretroviral therapy (ART) among pregnant people living with human immunodeficiency virus (HIV), vertical transmission remains the most important route of pediatric HIV acquisition. The numbers of HIV acquisitions in infancy have remained alarmingly stagnant in recent years. It is evident that additional strategies that can synergize with ART will be required to end the pediatric HIV epidemic. In this review, we discuss the potential for immune-based interventions that can be administered in conjunction with current ART-based strategies to the birthing parent for prevention of vertical transmission of HIV-1, and the potential challenges associated with each approach.

Considerations and Mechanisms of Transmission in the Modern Era of Combined Antiretroviral Therapy (cART) **783**

Jenna S. Powers, Medrine Kihanga, and Lisa Marie Cranmer

Combined antiretroviral therapy has significantly reduced perinatal human immunodeficiency virus (HIV) transmission risk through breastfeeding, prompting shifts in clinical guidance to support breastfeeding for women with HIV who have sustained viral suppression. This review examines the current evidence on HIV transmission via breast milk, including risk factors, mechanisms, and risk reduction strategies to inform patient-centered and evidence-driven clinical care.

When Black and White Turns Gray: Navigating the Ethical Challenges of Implementing Shared Infant Feeding Decisions for Persons Living with Human Immunodeficiency Virus in the United States 801

Kira J. Nightingale, Elizabeth D. Lowenthal, and Marielle S. Gross

In 2023, US guidelines for feeding perinatally human immunodeficiency virus (HIV)-exposed infants were revised to encourage collaborative decision-making in lieu of categorical proscription of breastfeeding. This change advances autonomy and health equity for persons living with HIV in the United States, for the first time supporting those who prioritize the maternal and infant benefits of breastfeeding in the setting of effective, well-established HIV risk mitigation. The authors review key moral dilemmas facing clinicians and patients who must navigate the reversal of long-standing dogma against breastfeeding and provide recommendations for implementation of a new ethical paradigm.

Treatment of HIV Infection in Children Across the Age Spectrum: Achievements and New Prospects 817

Moherndran Archary, Kagiso Mochankana, and Adrie Bekker

Despite advances in human immunodeficiency virus (HIV) prevention, new pediatric HIV infections continue, necessitating optimized and simplified antiretroviral treatment (ART) regimens tailored for children. Advances in treatment options have been made possible by the availability of child-friendly fixed-dose formulations with decreased dosing frequency, especially in low- and middle-income countries. Ongoing work to improve ART options for neonates and supporting the shift toward long-acting ART for children and adolescents remains a priority. Achieving the UNAIDS goal of 95:95:95 for children will require a comprehensive and holistic approach that addresses both the biomedical and social challenges of managing children with HIV.

Prevention, Diagnosis, and Treatment of Tuberculosis in Children with Human Immunodeficiency Virus 833

Charles D. Mitchell

While tuberculosis (TB) is an ancient disease, its global prevalence and concomitant human immunodeficiency virus (HIV)-1 infection have hampered efforts at effectively controlling TB in children in many countries where these 2 pandemics coexist. This review briefly discusses the current status of TB prevention strategies including preventative regimens designed to prevent the progression of latent TB infection to active disease, current recommendations regarding treatment of TB disease, and the problematic nature of diagnosing TB in children living with HIV. Promising recent data regarding novel diagnostic techniques that rely upon detecting *Mycobacterium tuberculosis* molecular components in blood will be reviewed.

The Long-Term Health Outcomes of People Living with Perinatal Human Immunodeficiency Virus: A Scoping Review 849

Scarlett Bergam, Whitney Puetz, and Brian C. Zanoni

Since the first reported cases of perinatally acquired human immunodeficiency virus (HIV) in 1982, a generation born with HIV has reached adulthood. The authors conducted a scoping review of PubMed and Google Scholar for articles published between January 2000 and June 2023 to assess the long-term, multisystem health outcomes of this population. Long-term health outcomes studied in this population pertain to the effects of perinatal HIV (PHIV) infection and life-long antiretroviral therapy on the endocrine, reproductive, psychosocial, neurobehavioral, immunologic, and cardiovascular systems. Holistic health of all body systems should be considered in the long-term care of people with PHIV.

Neurocognitive Outcomes Following Perinatal Human Immunodeficiency Virus Infection **865**

Sharon L. Nichols, Reuben N. Robbins, Shathani Rampa, and Kathleen M. Malee

Perinatally acquired human immunodeficiency virus (HIV) has the potential to affect neurodevelopment and long-term cognitive and behavioral outcomes. Early, consistent viral suppression through antiretroviral therapy is a priority for protection of neurodevelopment. Monitoring of neurodevelopment and cognitive functioning, referral for appropriate interventions, caregiver/family support, and assessment of mental health, socioeconomic, and environmental risks are important to optimize health and well-being. Support for medication and health care adherence may be necessary to sustain best outcomes.

Care of the Child Perinatally Exposed to Human Immunodeficiency Virus **881**

Catherine J. Wedderburn, Grace M. Musiime, and Megan S. McHenry

Substantial progress in preventing vertical human immunodeficiency virus (HIV) transmission has led to a dramatic decline in new pediatric HIV infections. Alongside this success, a growing population of children who are HIV-exposed but uninfected face unique health challenges due to a variety of risk factors. Recommendations for healthcare providers caring for this population include optimizing and integrating general and HIV-related care for both mother and child through comprehensive care packages. Further research and multidisciplinary approaches are needed to address the long-term health implications for this vulnerable population.

Research Toward a Cure for Perinatal HIV **895**

Kristen Kelly, Soumia Bekka, and Deborah Persaud

In virtually all people living with HIV-1 (PLWH), including children, HIV-1 integrates and becomes latent in $CD4^+$ T cells, forming a latent HIV-1 reservoir that current antiretroviral drugs and immune surveillance mechanisms cannot target. This latent infection in $CD4^+$ T cells renders HIV-1 infection lifelong and incurable. Consequently, there is intense research focused on identifying therapeutic strategies to reduce and control the latent reservoir, aiming to avert a lifetime of antiretroviral therapy for PLWH. This review discusses the global efforts for children and adolescents living with HIV-1.

Research on Perinatal HIV in Asia: Data on Treatment Outcomes and Emerging Co-Morbidities from the TREAT Asia Network **911**

Tavitiya Sudjaritruk, Aarti Kinikar, and Annette H. Sohn

Although new pediatric human immunodeficiency virus (HIV) infections have declined in the Asia-Pacific region, coverage of interventions to prevent vertical HIV transmission remains inconsistent. The TREAT Asia pediatric HIV cohort includes data from ~7700 children and adolescents with HIV (90% perinatally acquired) who have been under care at 18 centers in six Asian countries. Research on their HIV treatment outcomes has been complemented by studies on coinfections and comorbidities. These studies have shown that greater attention is needed to support and sustain clinical and social outcomes as children with perinatal HIV age into adulthood and transition to adult HIV care.

Penta Network: State-of-the-Art Research in Pediatric Human Immunodeficiency Virus **925**

Pablo Rojo, Cinta Moraleda, and Carlo Giaquinto

The Penta Network has made significant strides in pediatric human immunodeficiency virus (HIV) research, initially focusing on clinical trials for children in Europe, before expanding globally to countries with high HIV prevalence. Key contributions include the ODYSSEY trial, which established dolutegravir as a superior treatment for children and the Early-treated Perinatally HIV-infected Individuals: Improving Children's Actual Life with Novel Immunotherapeutic Strategies consortium, aimed at developing strategies for HIV remission. The ongoing empirical and thrive projects address advanced HIV disease, particularly severe pneumonia and post-discharge mortality in children. Going beyond clinical trials, the Penta Network also plays a key role in bringing stakeholders and industry together to achieve better antiretroviral formulations for children.

Maternal–Child Human Immunodeficiency Virus Clinical Trials Networks across the Ages **935**

Sharon Nachman

The clinical trial networks that included a maternal–child focus have evolved since first funded by NIH in the 1990s. Since then, US domestic and international sites were combined into one network, with a focused agenda on therapeutics (for both prevention and treatment), human immunodeficiency virus (HIV) cure, tuberculosis, and complications of HIV, largely specific to the brain. Key to the success of the network has been a strong partnership with the community, collaborations with industry and other strategic partners, and recognition that one size does not fit all when it comes to antiretrovirals, diagnosing and treating TB, and other treatments for our populations.

JOURNAL TITLE: Clinics in Perinatology
ISSUE: 51.4

PROGRAM OBJECTIVE

The goal of *Clinics in Perinatology* is to keep practicing perinatologists, neonatologists, obstetricians, practicing physicians and residents up to date with current clinical practice in perinatology by providing timely articles reviewing the state of the art in patient care.

TARGET AUDIENCE

Perinatologists, neonatologists, obstetricians, practicing physicians, residents and healthcare professionals who provide patient care utilizing findings from *Clinics in Perinatology*.

LEARNING OBJECTIVES

Upon completion of this activity, participants will be able to:

1. Recognize holistic care of women living with HIV during pregnancy spans multiple disciplines.
2. Discuss current evidence on HIV transmission via breast milk, including risk factors, mechanisms, and risk reduction strategies.
3. Review prevention, diagnosis, and treatment of tuberculosis in children with HIV.

ACCREDITATION

The Elsevier Office of Continuing Medical Education (EOCME) is accredited by the Accreditation Council for Continuing Medical Education (ACCME) to provide continuing medical education for physicians.

The EOCME designates this journal-based CME activity for a maximum of 13 *AMA PRA Category 1 Credit*(s)™. Physicians should claim only the credit commensurate with the extent of their participation in the activity.

All other health care professionals requesting continuing education credit for this enduring material will be issued a certificate of participation.

DISCLOSURE OF RELEVANT FINANCIAL RELATIONSHIPS

The EOCME assesses conflict of interest with its instructors, faculty, planners, and other individuals who are in a position to control the content of CME activities. All relevant conflicts of interest that are identified are thoroughly vetted by EOCME for fair balance, scientific objectivity, and patient care recommendations. EOCME is committed to providing its learners with CME activities that promote improvements or quality in healthcare and not a specific proprietary business or a commercial interest.

The authors and editors listed below have identified no financial relationships or relationships to products or devices they have with ineligible companies related to the content of this CME activity:
Moherndran Archary, MBChB. DCH(SA), FCPaeds(SA), Paeds ID (SA), PhD (UKZN); Soumia Bekka, BS; Adrie Bekker, MBChB, DCH(SA), MMed (PAED), FCPaeds(SA), Cert Neo(SA), PhD (SU); Scarlett Bergam, MPH; Christian Binuya, BS; Kristina Brooks, PharmD; Ann Chahroudi, MD, PhD; Lisa Marie Cranmer, MD, MPH; Ahizechukwu C. Eke, MD, PhD, MPH; Carlo Giaquinto, PhD; Marielle S. Gross, MD, MBE; Lucky Jain, MD, MBA; Krithika P. Karthigeyan, PhD; Kristen Kelly, BS; Medrine Kihanga, BS; Aarti Kinikar, MD, MRCP; Elizabeth D. Lowenthal, MD, MSCE; Kathleen M. Malee, PhD; Megan S. McHenry, MS, MD, FAPP; Charles D. Mitchell, MD, MS; Kagiso Mochankana, MBBS. FCPaeds (SA). MMED (UB); Cinta Moraleda, PhD; Grace M. Musiime, MBBCh, MSc, MMed, FC Paed (SA), DTM&H, Cert Neonatology; Sharon Nachman, MD; Ashley N. Nelson, PhD; Sharon L. Nichols, PhD; Kira J. Nightingale, MS, MBA; Sallie R. Permar MD, PhD; Deborah Persaud, MD; Jenna S. Powers, MD; Whitney Puetz, MPH; Shathani Rampa, MSc; Reuben N. Robbins, PhD; Pablo Rojo, PhD; Annette H. Sohn, MD, PhD; Lynda Stranix-Chibanda, MBChB, MMed (Paeds); Tavitiya Sudjaritruk, MD, ScM, PhD; Avy Violari, FCPaed(SA); Kenneth Vuong, BS; Catherine J. Wedderburn, MBChB, MA, MSc, DTM&H, MRCPCH; Brian C. Zanoni, MD, MPH

The authors and editors listed below have identified financial relationships or relationships to products or devices they have with ineligible companies related to the content of this CME activity:
Ann Chahroudi, MD, PhD: *Advisor*: ViiV Healthcare, Inc.

Sallie R. Permar, MD, PhD: *Consultant*: Moderna, Inc., Merck & Co., Inc., Pfizer Inc., Dynavax Technologies, GSK plc; Researcher: Moderna, Inc., Dynavax Technologies, and Pfizer Inc.

Deborah Persaud, MD: *Advisor*: ViiV Healthcare, Inc.

The planning committee and staff listed below have identified no financial relationships or relationships to products or devices they have with ineligible companies related to the content of this CME activity:
Nitesh Barthwal; Kerry Holland; Michelle Littlejohn; Patrick Manley; Jeyanthi Surendrakumar

UNAPPROVED/OFF-LABEL USE DISCLOSURE
The EOCME requires CME faculty to disclose to the participants:
1. When products or procedures being discussed are off-label, unlabelled, experimental, and/or investigational (not US Food and Drug Administration [FDA] approved); and
2. Any limitations on the information presented, such as data that are preliminary or that represent ongoing research, interim analyses, and/or unsupported opinions. Faculty may discuss information about pharmaceutical agents that is outside of FDA-approved labelling. This information is intended solely for CME and is not intended to promote off-label use of these medications. If you have any questions, contact the medical affairs department of the manufacturer for the most recent prescribing information.

TO ENROLL
To enroll in the *Clinics in Perinatology* Continuing Medical Education program, call customer service at 1-800-654-2452 or sign up online at http://www.theclinics.com/home/cme. The CME program is available to subscribers for an additional annual fee of USD 254.00.

METHOD OF PARTICIPATION
In order to claim credit, participants must complete the following:
1. Complete enrolment as indicated above.
2. Read the activity.
3. Complete the CME Test and Evaluation. Participants must achieve a score of 70% on the test. All CME Tests and Evaluations must be completed online.

CME INQUIRIES/SPECIAL NEEDS
For all CME inquiries or special needs, please contact elsevierCME@elsevier.com.

CLINICS IN PERINATOLOGY

Foreword

Can We Eliminate Perinatal HIV?

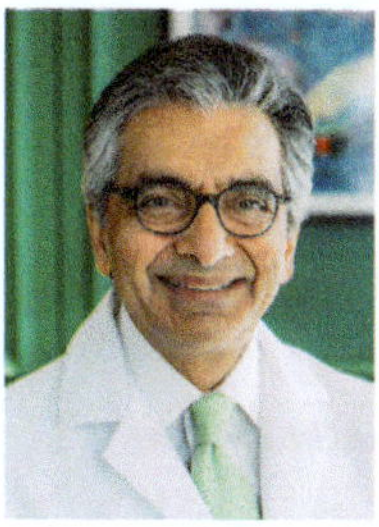

Lucky Jain, MD, MBA
Consulting Editor

Reduction of perinatal HIV transmission over the past three decades is a modern-day success story. From a high of 1630 annual infections due to perinatal transmission in the United States in 1993, only 53 cases of mother-to-baby transmission were reported in 2015.[1] Indeed, there is true optimism fueling the aspiration of perinatal HIV elimination, at least in nations like the United States, where prophylaxis and data tracking are such a public health priority. Recent data show that at least 15 countries have eliminated the vertical transmission of HIV, while others continue to march toward that goal (**Fig. 1**).[2] Elimination of vertical transmission would require infection rates to drop below 1 per 100,000 impacted live births.[2] Those who are less enthusiastic about such goals recognize the impediments encountered in any multistep public health program, which includes routine HIV testing of all pregnant women, initiation of combination antiretroviral treatment (ART) during pregnancy, elective cesarean delivery for women with a high plasma viral load, and avoidance of breast feeding.[3] There is an added layer of complexity due to wide variations in public health policies from region to region, and the interplay of maternal, placental, and fetal conditions that may impact transmission rates. This is particularly true in parts of the world that still lack universal ART availability.

As is the case with most perinatally acquired infections, there are three time zones for actions that can disrupt vertical transmission: during gestation, during delivery, and postnatally (**Fig. 2**).[2] In each of these time periods, appropriate ART and reduction in viral load directly impact vertical transmission rates. Intrapartum transmission is generally secondary to infected blood and secretions from the mother, and such exposure continues to account for the maximum number of infections passed on to babies worldwide. Prolonged rupture of membranes, not surprisingly, increases the risk of infection, prompting the widespread use of cesarean sections to prevent transmission.

More recently, experts have been evaluating additional strategies that may decrease the risk of transmission further. These include universal third-trimester HIV retesting of

Clin Perinatol 51 (2024) xv–xviii
https://doi.org/10.1016/j.clp.2024.09.002
0095-5108/24/© 2024 Published by Elsevier Inc.

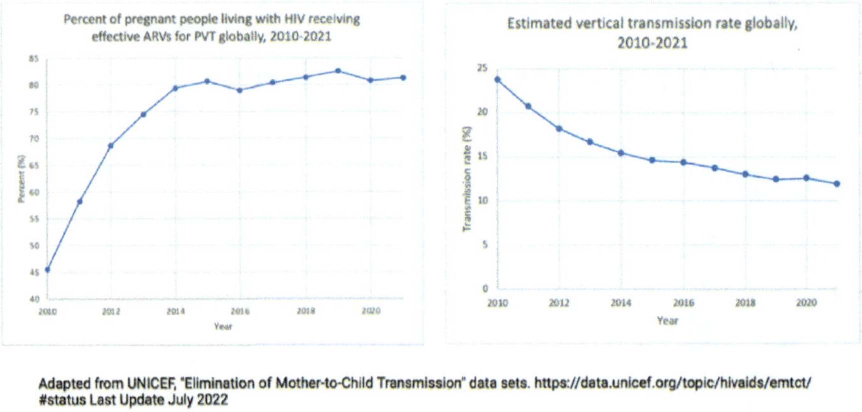

Fig. 1. The percentage of HIV-positive people on antiretroviral medication in terms of the prevention of VT from 2010 to 2021 (*left*) and the estimated vertical transmission rate globally from 2010–2021 (*right*). ARVs, antiretrovirals; PVT, prevention of vertical transmission; VT, vertical transmission. (*Data from* Cardenas MC, Farnan S, Hamel BL, et. al. Prevention of the Vertical Transmission of HIV; A Recap of the Journey so Far. Viruses 2023;15:849. http://doi.org/10.3390/v15040849.[2])

the mother and her partner, treatment with integrase inhibitors such as dolutegravir in women who present late for ART, and preexposure prophylaxis during pregnancy to prevent acquisition of HIV.[2]

On July 22, 2024, the Joint United Nations Programme on HIV/AIDS released a new report at the culmination of the 25th International AIDS Conference in Munich,

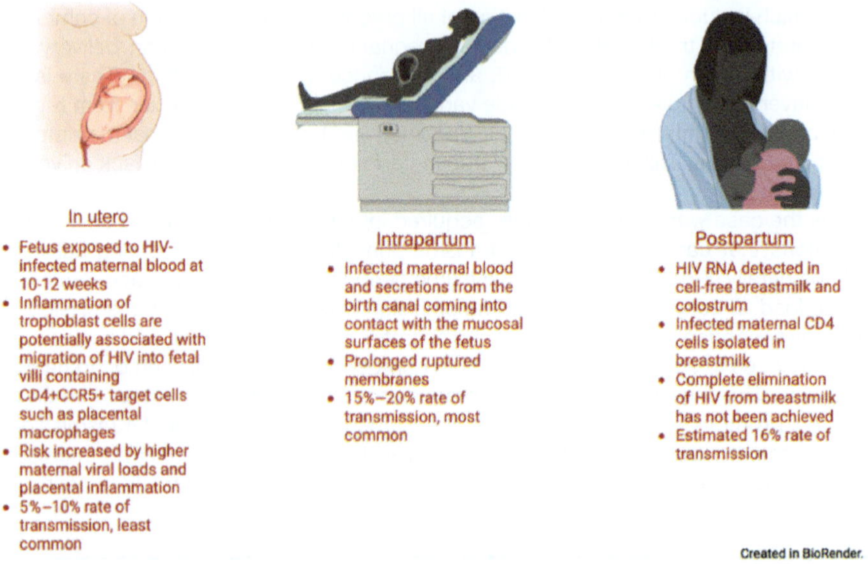

In utero
• Fetus exposed to HIV-infected maternal blood at 10-12 weeks
• Inflammation of trophoblast cells are potentially associated with migration of HIV into fetal villi containing CD4+CCR5+ target cells such as placental macrophages
• Risk increased by higher maternal viral loads and placental inflammation
• 5%–10% rate of transmission, least common
Intrapartum
• Infected maternal blood and secretions from the birth canal coming into contact with the mucosal surfaces of the fetus
• Prolonged ruptured membranes
• 15%–20% rate of transmission, most common
Postpartum
• HIV RNA detected in cell-free breastmilk and colostrum
• Infected maternal CD4 cells isolated in breastmilk
• Complete elimination of HIV from breastmilk has not been achieved
• Estimated 16% rate of transmission
Created in BioRender.

Fig. 2. Mechanisms of vertical HIV transmission. (*Adapted from* Cardenas MC, Farnan S, Hamel BL, et. al. Prevention of the Vertical Transmission of HIV; A Recap of the Journey so Far. Viruses 2023;15:849. http://doi.org/10.3390/v15040849.[2])

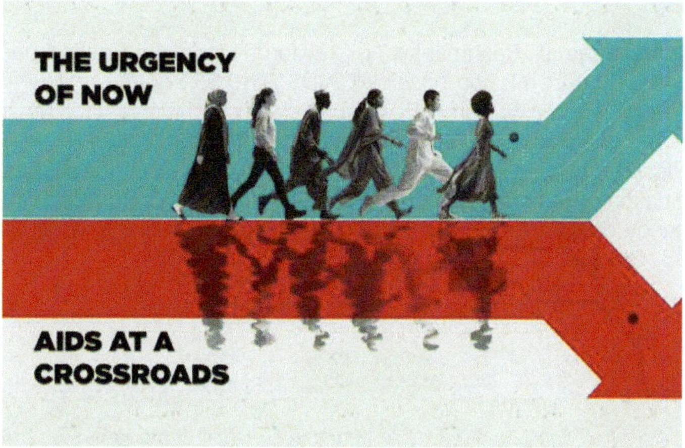

Fig. 3. 2024 global AIDS report—The urgency of now: AIDS at a crossroads. (With permission from UNAIDS. The urgency of now: AIDS at a crossroads. Geneva: Joint United Nations Programme on HIV/AIDS; 2024.)

Germany.[4] The report highlights the fact that for the first time in history, the majority of new HIV acquisitions occurred outside of sub-Saharan Africa (**Fig. 3**).[4] The UNAIDS 2024 report is the most up-to-date compilation of new data and case studies from all across the globe. This report points out that *"world leaders can fulfil their promise to end AIDS as a public health threat by 2030, and in so doing prevent millions of AIDS-related deaths, prevent millions of new HIV infections, and ensure the almost 40 million people living with HIV have healthy, full lives."*

As Drs Chahroudi, Violari, and the many esteemed authors in this issue of the *Clinics in Perinatology* point out, high rates of HIV in women in the reproductive age group point to the need for newer strategies to eliminate vertical HIV transmission. As a neonatologist, I am encouraged to see how collaborative work between multiple subspecialties (obstetrics, infectious diseases, pediatrics) has brought hope to what was a dismal situation just a few decades ago.

I want to congratulate Drs Chahroudi and Violari for assembling a true state-of-the-art offering on this subject. As always, I am grateful to the authors for their contributions, and to my publishing partners at Elsevier (Kerry Holland and Nitesh Barthwal) for their help in bringing this valuable resource to you. While infections continue to evolve and create new challenges for health care providers worldwide, tackling vertical transmission of serious infections such as HIV truly amplifies the benefits of public health efforts everywhere!

Lucky Jain, MD, MBA
Department of Pediatrics
Emory University School of Medicine
Children's Healthcare of Atlanta
2015 Uppergate Drive Northeast
Atlanta, GA 30322, USA

E-mail address:
ljain@emory.edu

REFERENCES

1. Gnanashanmugam D, Rakhmanina N, Crawford K, et al. Eliminating perinatal HIV in the United States: mission possible? AIDS 2019;33:377–85.
2. Cardenas MC, Farnan S, Hamel BL, et al. Prevention of the vertical transmission of HIV: a recap of the journey so far. Viruses 2023;15:849.
3. Yang L, Cambou MC, Nielsen-Saines K. The end is in sight: current strategies for the elimination of HIV vertical transmission. Curr HIV/AIDS Rep 2023;20:121–30.
4. The urgency of now: AIDS at a crossroads. Joint United Nations Programme on HIV/AIDS. Geneva: 2024. License: CC BY-NC-SA 3.0 IGO.

Preface

Perinatal HIV: Past, Present, and Future

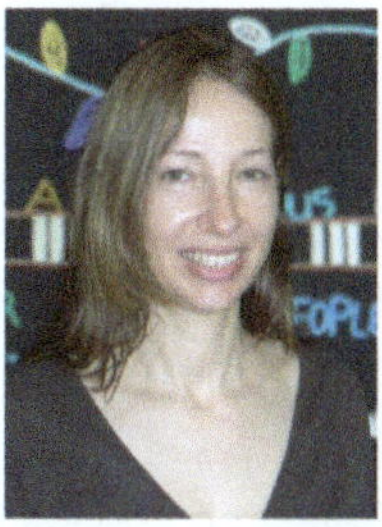
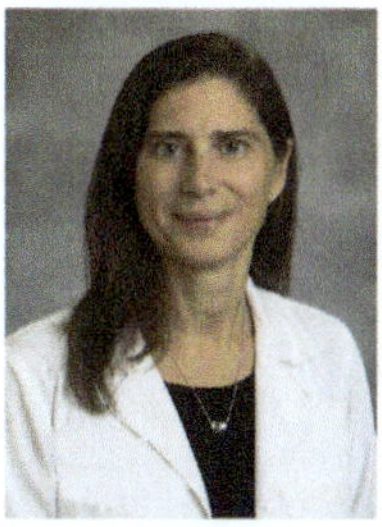

Avy Violari, FCPaed (SA)   Ann Chahroudi, MD, PhD
Editors

Thirty years since the 1994 discovery that antepartum and intrapartum zidovudine could prevent transmission of HIV-1 from pregnant mothers to their infants, the successes in treatment and prevention of HIV have been monumental. Despite the prevailing sentiment that HIV is no longer front-page news, the actual number of pregnant people living with the disease has only slightly declined, meaning that efforts to prevent vertical transmission are consistently in demand. The prospects for a cure are under intense research and remain a priority for people living with HIV, as is the search for an HIV vaccine that can impact both vertical and horizontal transmission.

This issue of *Clinics in Perinatology* provides a review of the current standards of care and state-of-the-art research to assist in clinical decision making when caring for pregnant people and children living with or exposed to HIV. The articles are written by expert researchers who are also health care providers and carry out their work in different parts of the world. We start with the care of those living with HIV during pregnancy, research on maternal vaccination for HIV prevention, and two reviews of breastfeeding-specific topics. Much of this issue focuses on infants and children living with HIV—the status of current treatments and what novel agents are in the pipeline, the common coinfection with *Mycobacterium tuberculosis*, as well as neurocognitive and other long-term outcomes of living with perinatally acquired HIV. We have not forgotten about the many children perinatally exposed to HIV that remain uninfected, with an article outlining the complexities and effects of that exposure and the tailored care these children require. Ultimately, an HIV cure is what is needed, and the steps and advances made to date are reviewed here. We close this issue with a look back at the guideline-changing clinical trials conducted across the worldwide networks, TREAT Asia, Penta, and IMPAACT, and preview the next horizons for these research groups.

Clin Perinatol 51 (2024) xix–xx
https://doi.org/10.1016/j.clp.2024.09.001

In summary, in this issue we take stock of the incredible advances made in pediatric HIV, while being cognizant of the challenges that still exist and highlighting future areas of development. We hope that the broad readership of *Clinics in Perinatology* finds this issue helpful for their clinical practice and finds inspiration from the incredible talent and tenacity of pediatric HIV providers and scientists. Appreciation of the ongoing stigma attached to an HIV diagnosis can help us to educate communities and advocate for centering individuals' needs in the contexts of research and health care.

We would like to express our gratitude to all the authors for their outstanding work and contributions.

DISCLOSURES

A. Chahroudi reports no conflicts of interest but receives funding from the NIH (UM1 AI164566, P01 HD112217). A. Violari reports no conflicts of interest but receives funding from the NIH (RO1 MH119878), IMPAACT, PENTA, and HVTN Networks.

Avy Violari, FCPaed (SA)
Paediatric Research and Care
Perinatal HIV Research Unit
Faculty of Health Sciences
University of the Witwatersrand
26 Chris Hani Road
Diepkloof 1864
Johannesburg, South Africa

Ann Chahroudi, MD, PhD
Department of Pediatrics
Emory University School of Medicine
Children's Healthcare of Atlanta
HSRB II N447
1750 Haygood Drive
Atlanta, GA 30322, USA

E-mail addresses:
violaria@phru.co.za; violari@mweb.co.za (A. Violari)
ann.m.chahroudi@emory.edu (A. Chahroudi)

Care of Pregnant Women Living with Human Immunodeficiency Virus

Lynda Stranix-Chibanda, MMed[a,*], Kristina Brooks, PharmD[b], Ahizechukwu C. Eke, MD, PhD, MPH[c]

KEYWORDS

• HIV • Women • Pregnancy • ART

KEY POINTS

- Holistic care of women living with human immunodeficiency virus (HIV) during pregnancy spans multiple disciplines, at a minimum, including obstetric, medical, and psychological as well as HIV management.
- Several antiretroviral agents are safe to use in pregnancy, with dosage adjustment in the third trimester only required for a small selection of agents.
- Women living with HIV face increased risk of adverse pregnancy outcomes, such as preterm delivery, and have higher rates of co-morbid conditions which may complicate the clinical course of pregnancy, such as tuberculosis, hypertension, obesity, and diabetes.
- Retention in care throughout pregnancy is important for optimal monitoring and prompt access to treatment, when necessary.

BACKGROUND

General Epidemiology and History of Care

About half the global population of people living with HIV are women, mainly living in Africa (**Fig. 1**),[1] where women experience an average of 4 pregnancies during their reproductive years.[2] After the World Health Organization (WHO) revised the guidelines for antiretroviral drug (ARV) use in pregnancy in 2016, the cornerstone of HIV care for pregnant and lactating persons has been life-long antiretroviral therapy (ART) regardless of immune or clinical disease status.[3] Consequently, ART coverage during

[a] c/o University of Zimbabwe Clinical Trials Research Centre, 15 Phillips Avenue, Belgravia, Harare, Zimbabwe; [b] Department of Pharmaceutical Sciences, Skaggs School of Pharmacy and Pharmaceutical Sciences, University of Colorado Anschutz Medical Campus, 12850 E. Montview Boulevard, Mail Stop C238, Aurora, CO, USA; [c] Division of Maternal Fetal Medicine, Department of Gynecology & Obstetrics, School of Medicine, Johns Hopkins University, 600 N Wolfe Street, Phipps 228, Baltimore, MD, USA

* Corresponding author.

E-mail address: lstranix@uz-ctrc.org

Twitter: @Stranchi2 (L.S.-C.); @KMB_PharmD (K.B.); @AhizechukwuEke (A.C.E.)

Clin Perinatol 51 (2024) 749–767

https://doi.org/10.1016/j.clp.2024.08.010 **perinatology.theclinics.com**

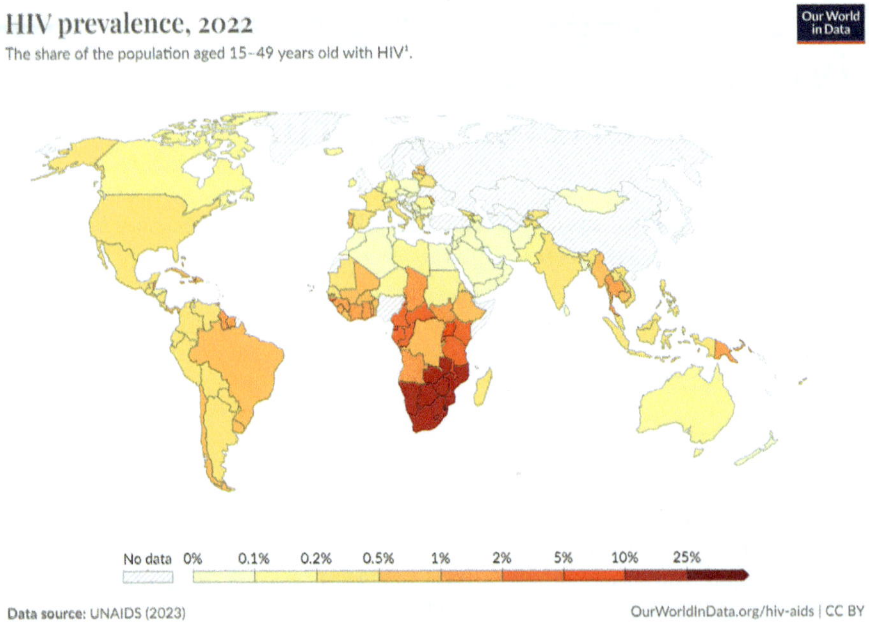

Fig. 1. Human immunodeficiency virus (HIV) prevalence, 2022: The share of the population aged 15 to 49 years old with HIV (Joint United Nations Programme on HIV/AIDS (2023) - with minor processing by Our World in Data. "HIV prevalence" [dataset]. Joint United Nations Programme on HIV/AIDS, "Global AIDS Update" [original data]. Retrieved September 11, 2024 from https://ourworldindata.org/grapher/share-of-the-population-infected-with-hiv).

pregnancy almost doubled and rates of vertical HIV transmission decreased by 58% between 2010 and 2022.[1] However, delivery of care falls short in many settings, with too many women remaining undiagnosed or not being served with appropriate HIV services; among mothers of children who acquired HIV in 2022, 49% had not received ART and 22% had dropped off ART, whereas 20% acquired HIV during pregnancy and lactation. Evidently, a significant shift in HIV program delivery is called for, so that women who are living with HIV but not receiving ART are identified and linked with care for their own health, as well as to attain the global target of eliminating pediatric HIV.[4]

Treatment Goals

The goal of HIV treatment in pregnancy is to promote maternal health through achieving viral suppression with ART, thus limiting disease progression while also reducing the risk of vertical transmission to the fetus *in utero* and to the infant during labor and delivery or via breastmilk. Historically, licensure of novel ARVs for use in pregnancy was delayed by inadequate pharmacokinetic and safety data for pregnant women, although there is a recent shift in consensus toward their earlier involvement in research (**Fig. 2**).[5–7] Achieving optimal health for people living with HIV requires a holistic approach, especially in the perinatal period when psychosocial stressors related to childbirth and HIV add complexity to HIV treatment and may pose new challenges to regular ART dosing.[8] In communities affected by HIV, routine maternity services should include integrated HIV care, ensuring that all women have a known HIV status throughout pregnancy and lactation and receive quality, respectful services that are client-centered and address psychosocial needs that could influence care outcomes.

This article presents considerations for selecting ART regimens for use in pregnancy, HIV-related adverse pregnancy outcomes and co-morbidities, and outlines the key elements of holistic care for pregnant women living with HIV. We use "women" and "mother" to reflect people in all their diversity who may become pregnant and require HIV care.

ANTIRETROVIRAL USE IN PREGNANCY

Overview

HIV treatment requires at least 2 active ARV medications with different mechanisms of action to achieve sustained virologic suppression. In pregnancy, ART also reduces the risk of perinatal HIV transmission from ~25% without treatment to <1% in the setting of virologic suppression.[9] Recommended oral ART options in pregnancy include the use of an integrase strand transfer inhibitor, boosted protease inhibitor, or non-nucleoside reverse transcriptase inhibitor (NNRTI) in combination with a nucleos(t)ide reverse transcriptase inhibitor (N(t)RTI) backbone,[10,11] with varying levels of evidence supporting certain combinations over others based on available pharmacokinetic (PK), safety, and efficacy data.[11,12] Several of these are available as once-daily, fixed dose combination pills, which help confer improved ART adherence comparatively to regimens that require more frequent administration or multiple tablets.

Physiologic Changes During Pregnancy

Key considerations regarding ARV use during pregnancy generally include (1) whether ARV exposures are reduced, which could increase risk of virologic failure and perinatal HIV transmission; (2) the extent to which drug crosses the placenta; and (3) associations with pregnancy outcomes and maternal/infant safety. The concern over adequate ARV exposures stems from several physiologic changes that occur during pregnancy and later recover postpartum.[13,14] These changes include increases in cardiac output, glomerular filtration rate, and blood volume; alterations in the expression of cytochrome P450 enzymes and transporters; and reduced drug binding to plasma proteins. Though these changes are known to occur and potentially impact drug safety and efficacy, there is still a median delay of 6 years between regulatory approval of a drug and availability of PK data supporting the appropriate dosing of therapies in pregnancy.[15]

Oral Antiretroviral Options

Net effects of pregnancy-induced physiologic changes on ARV exposures, recommended dosing, and other clinical pearls are outlined in **Table 1**. Though several drugs have altered PK during pregnancy, only a few are either recommended against or require dose adjustments to offset the decreases that occur. Plasma exposures of INSTIs are reduced during pregnancy due in part to increased expression of CYP3A4 and UGT1A1. Despite these decreases, raltegravir,[16] dolutegravir,[17–19] and bictegravir[20,21] exposures were still above minimum concentrations associated with virologic efficacy, and thus no dose adjustments are needed. Some of the N(t)RTIs, notably those that are cleared renally, are decreased by ~20%-30% during pregnancy,[22,23] but also do not require dose adjustment. Tenofovir alafenamide (TAF) is a newer prodrug formulation of tenofovir that results in ~10-fold lower plasma

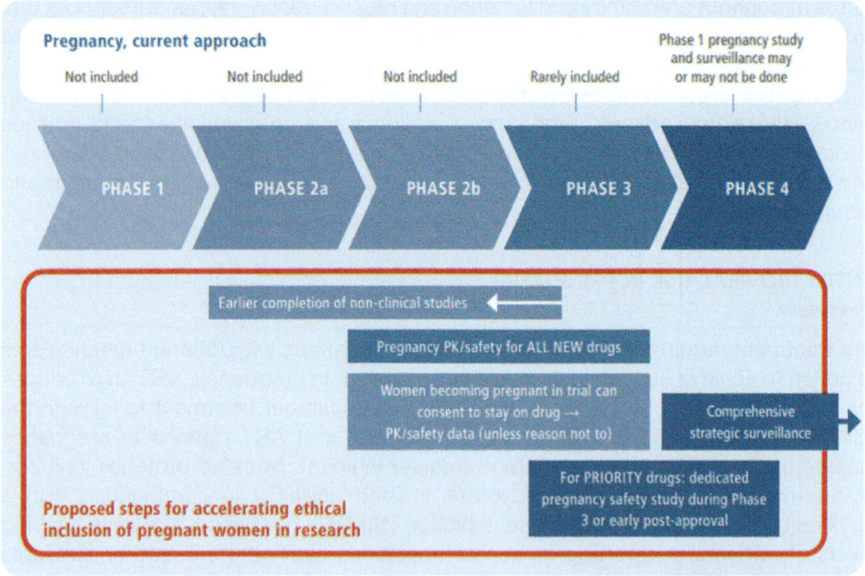

Fig. 2. Framework for accelerated inclusion of pregnant women in pre-licensure clinical trials. (Approaches to enhance and accelerate study of new drugs for HIV and associated infections in pregnant women: meeting report. Geneva: World Health Organization; 2021.)

tenofovir concentrations in comparison to tenofovir disoproxil fumarate (TDF). PK differences with TAF during pregnancy vary depending on whether coadministered with a pharmacoenhancer,[24–26] but overall exposures are comparable to historical data in non-pregnant adults, and thus no dose adjustments are required.

The NNRTIs have shown variable PK differences in pregnancy. Efavirenz is primarily metabolized by CYP2B6 and studies have shown either no or modest decreases in exposures during pregnancy.[27,28] Rilpivirine is decreased by ~30% to 50%, and unbound concentrations are decreased by ~25%.[29,30] Etravirine is typically only used in treatment-experienced individuals, but exposures during pregnancy were shown to be 30% to 90% higher due to decreased CYP2C19 activity, while unbound concentrations were unchanged.[31] There are no PK data reported in pregnant populations yet, but a physiologically-based PK model suggested exposures could potentially be decreased by 55%.[32] Additional data are needed to inform the appropriate dosing and use of this newer NNRTI.

Cobicistat-containing regimens are not recommended during pregnancy as drug exposures are significantly reduced and there is no viable alternative for adjusting doses.[33] Ritonavir-boosted protease inhibitors, such as atazanavir or darunavir, are options in cases where this drug class needs to be used. However, their exposures are decreased due to the increased expression of CYP3A4 during pregnancy, andthus do require dose adjustment to offset the decreased exposures that occur.

Entry inhibitors are generally used in cases where an individual is treatment-experienced. The only entry inhibitor with PK data during pregnancy is maraviroc.[34] Maraviroc exposures are reduced during pregnancy subsequent to increased CYP3A4 activity, but concentrations did still remain above minimum targets. Thus, no special dose adjustments during pregnancy are required, but providers should still

Table 1
Pharmacokinetic changes observed for preferred and alternative antiretroviral medications during pregnancy

Class	Antiretroviral	Change in Exposure during Pregnancy	Dose Recommendation in Pregnancy	Clinical Considerations
Integrase strand-transfer inhibitors	Bictegravir[21]	AUC ↓55%–60% Cmin ↓70%–73%	50 mg once daily	Only available as a coformulation with tenofovir alafenamide (TAF) and emtricitabine
	Dolutegravir[17–19]	AUC ↓14%–37% Cmin ↓20%–37%	50 mg once daily	Preferred/first-line antiretroviral option
	Raltegravir[16]	AUC ↓24%–53% Cmin ↔	400 mg twice daily	Once-daily dosing with 1200 mg not recommended
N(t)RTI	Abacavir[35,36]	AUC ↔	600 mg once daily or 300 mg twice daily	Metabolized by alcohol dehydrogenase and UGT1A1 Do not use in people with HLA*B-5701
	Emtricitabine[22]	AUC ↓18%–25% Cmin ↓3%–13%	200 mg once daily	Renally eliminated Considered interchangeable with lamivudine
	Lamivudine[23]	AUC ↓19%	300 mg once daily or 150 mg twice daily	Renally eliminated Considered interchangeable with emtricitabine
	TAF[24–26]	TAF AUC ↓20%–46% TFV AUC ↓33%	25 mg once daily or 10 mg once daily (with cobicistat)	Parent tenofovir component renally eliminated
	Tenofovir disoproxil fumarate (TDF)[37]	AUC ↓20%–23% Cmin ↓18%–21%	300 mg once daily	Parent tenofovir component renally eliminated

(*continued on next page*)

Table 1
(continued)

Class	Antiretroviral	Change in Exposure during Pregnancy	Dose Recommendation in Pregnancy	Clinical Considerations
NNRTI	Efavirenz[27,28]	AUC ↓16% Cmin ↓12%–14%	600 mg once daily	Reduced dosing with 400 mg not recommended
	Rilpivirine[29]	AUC ↓20%–25% Cmin ↓16%–30%	25 mg once daily	Should be taken with food Cannot be used if baseline viral load >100,000 copies/m: or CD4 count <200 cells/mm3 Increased frequency of viral load monitoring may be considered Requires an acidic environment for absorption so cannot be coadministered with PPIs and must be spaced from H2RAs and antacids
Boosted PIs	Atazanavir/ritonavir[38–40]	AUC ↓6% and Cmin ↓47% with 300 mg/100 mg once daily AUC and Cmin ↔	300 mg/100 mg once daily (standard) 400 mg/100 mg once daily (increased)	Can cause maternal hyperbilirubinemia due to inhibition of UGT1A1 Requires an acidic environment for absorption so cannot be coadministered with PPIs and must be spaced from H2RAs and antacids
	Darunavir/ritonavir	Cmin ↓42%–50% with 800/100 mg once daily Cmin ↓12%–42% with 600/100 mg twice daily	600 mg/100 mg twice daily (increased)	

Abbreviations: AUC, area under the concentration-time curve; Cmin, minimum concentration.

follow the dose adjustment recommendations depending on whether this medication is coadministered with other CYP3A4 inhibitors or inducers. There are no PK data for ibalizumab (monoclonal antibody administered via intravenous infusion) or fostemsavir (postattachment inhibitor) in pregnant populations; thus, these medications are not recommended to be used in this population.[11]

Long-Acting Antiretroviral Therapy & Future Directions

Key areas of future research in pregnant populations are the long-acting therapies and newer therapies that are in development. The combination of injectable cabotegravir with rilpivirine represented a significant advance in therapeutic options for HIV, as injections are only required every 1 to 2 months in virally suppressed non-pregnant adults. This combination was also recently shown to be superior to oral ART in adults at higher risk of non-adherence, which could be a significant breakthrough for this population.[41] Multiple studies have shown variable adherence during pregnancy and postpartum in women with HIV,[42–44] and thus therapeutic options that could help foster improved adherence could be a tremendous help. PK data with injectable cabotegravir/rilpivirine during pregnancy are limited,[45] but available data have shown comparable washout PK to non-pregnant women. A clinical study to evaluate the PK and safety of this combination when either continued or initiated during pregnancy is in the final stages of development by the IMPAACT network (https://www.impaactnetwork.org/studies/impaact2040). Lenacapavir is another long-acting injectable that is currently Food and Drug Administration (FDA)-approved for heavily treatment-resistant adults with HIV for administration every 6 months. However, it is also under investigation in treatment-naïve adults and as a potential option for HIV prevention. As other long-acting products and novel therapies progress through clinical development, for example, islatravir and monoclonal antibodies, collecting PK and safety data during pregnancy remains a priority.

HUMAN IMMUNODEFICIENCY VIRUS AND PREGNANCY OUTCOMES

Adverse pregnancy outcomes associated with ART are categorized as either maternal or fetal/neonatal/infant-related.[46,47] Maternal adverse effects linked to use of ART encompass ART-induced renal and liver complications, mental health disorders (including peripartum depression), gestational diabetes, hypertensive disorders unique to pregnancy (gestational hypertension; pre-eclampsia, HELLP syndrome (Hemolysis, Elevated Liver enzymes and Low Platelets)), anemia, weight gain, and other metabolic complications (**Table 2**). These adverse effects can significantly impact both maternal health and pregnancy outcomes, highlighting the importance of careful monitoring and management of ART during pregnancy to optimize maternal and fetal well-being.

ART regimens containing INSTIs such as dolutegravir (DTG) and raltegravir, when combined with TAF, have been associated with greater weight gain compared to regimens containing TDF or efavirenz.[48–50] This finding was demonstrated in the IMPAACT 2010 randomized trial,[48] and corroborated by other randomized trials in pregnancy, including the NICHD P1081[51] and DOLPHIN-2[52] trials. The observed weight change may be attributed to TDF suppressing weight gain, excess weight gain associated with INSTIs (augmented by TAF), or a combination of both factors, as inadequate weight gain was frequently observed in pregnant women with HIV in low-income and middle-income countries (LMICs) receiving TDF-based ART in the IMPAACT 2010 trial.[48] Nevertheless, it is reassuring that the mean weekly weight gain among women using DTG (specifically DTG + TAF/FTC regimens) during pregnancy in these trials still fell within the optimal weight gain recommended by the United States National Academy of Sciences, Engineering, and Medicine for pregnant women.[53]

Although there exists a significant body of literature addressing these maternal adverse events related to ART use, determining whether ART is causally related to these outcomes remains extremely challenging. One constraint is the limited availability of safety data from pregnancy studies, which are often either not conducted or completed in pregnancy years after these studies are completed in non-pregnant adults (see **Fig. 2**). Studies investigating the timing of ART initiation during pregnancy are susceptible to selection bias, while observational studies frequently do not optimally control for confounding. In addition, inconsistencies in endpoint definitions across HIV in pregnancy studies further complicate interpretation of these adverse effects and their relationship to ART.[46] Moreover, the wide variability in background rates of adverse pregnancy outcomes across different populations, timeframes, and contexts complicates the comparison with observational HIV-based research during pregnancy.[46]

It is crucial to highlight that pregnant women with HIV who are not on ART are more likely to experience more severe adverse fetal, neonatal, and infant outcomes, including intrauterine fetal growth restriction (IUGR), spontaneous preterm birth, small for gestational age (SGA), low birth weight (LBW), and neonatal demise compared to their HIV-negative women.[46,47,54] While maternal ART significantly reduces the risk of these unfavorable fetal outcomes, certain older ARVs, such as nevirapine and lopinavir/ritonavir, have been associated with a slightly higher risk of adverse fetal outcomes compared to more recent ART like dolutegravir-based regimens.[46,47] A 2022 study published in the New England Journal of Medicine found that a dolutegravir-based regimens resulted in lower rates of composite adverse birth outcomes compared to

Table 2
Pregnancy-related adverse effects linked to antiretroviral therapy

Adverse Effect	Antiretroviral Therapy
Spontaneous preterm birth	Protease inhibitors (lopinavir-ritonavir), tenofovir disoproxil fumarate (TDF)
Renal disease (acute kidney injury)	TDF
Excessive maternal weight gain (weight gain in excess of 18 kg or 0.5 kg/week during pregnancy)	Dolutegravir, TAF
Inadequate weight gain	TDF (when combined with efavirenz)
Gestational diabetes	Protease inhibitors (lopinavir-ritonavir)
Acute liver injury	Protease inhibitors, non-nucleoside reverse transcriptase inhibitors. Atazanavir is associated with indirect hyperbilirubinemia
Low birth weight, intrauterine fetal growth restriction, small for gestational age	Protease inhibitors (lopinavir-ritonavir), efavirenz-TDF based ART
Psychiatric and behavioral disorders	Efavirenz, dolutegravir, rilpivirine
Anemia	Zidovudine
Hypertensive disorders unique to pregnancy (gestational hypertension; pre-eclampsia, HELLP syndrome (Hemolysis, Elevated Liver enzymes and Low Platelets))	Not linked to any particular ART
Congenital anomalies	Not linked to any particular ART

other ART regimens, underscoring the importance of using newer regimens for preventing adverse outcomes in pregnant women with HIV.[55]

Congenital anomalies associated with the use of ART deserve special mention. Early results from the Tsepamo birth surveillance study in Botswana suggested that babies born to women who had taken dolutegravir during their conception would be at risk for neural tube abnormalities.[56] However, analysis of the final data of the Botswana cohort of pregnant women with HIV who started taking dolutegravir at conception showed no difference in the prevalence of neural tube defects between pregnant women with HIV in comparison to those without.[57] It is crucial to highlight that to establish causal relationships between ART and a rare adverse event like a neural tube defect, a sufficiently large sample size over 2,000 exposures is needed to reliably detect a 3-fold increase in malformations when the true prevalence of such anomaly is $\leq 0.1\%$.[58] Hence, it is unsurprising that congenital anomalies are infrequently used as outcome measures in HIV research, given their rarity and the limited statistical power to establish causal links between ART and congenital anomalies.[54]

Close monitoring of pregnant women with HIV is essential due to the potential for adverse effects related to ART. To improve pregnancy outcomes, it is crucial to identify fetuses at risk of intrauterine demise, IUGR, and SGA. This can be accomplished through fetal non-stress testing and ultrasound assessments. Antenatal fetal monitoring should be initiated to closely monitor at-risk fetuses. Additionally, it is important to establish optimal criteria for diagnosing gestational diabetes and differentiate hyperglycemic risk based on the type of ART regimen. Monitoring maternal mental health, weight gain, and blood pressure is also essential during pregnancy. Women with declining renal or hepatic function should undergo regular clinical and laboratory evaluations. Furthermore, the provision of noninvasive prenatal testing, such as cell-free fetal DNA or ultrasound imaging, can promptly detect congenital anomalies, enabling timely intervention.

HUMAN IMMUNODEFICIENCY VIRUS AND CO-MORBID CONDITIONS AFFECTING PREGNANCY

Pregnant women with HIV often face a myriad of medical co-morbidities that affect various organ systems, presenting complex challenges for both maternal and fetal health. Among the most common co-morbid conditions are infectious diseases (especially tuberculosis and hepatitis C), cardiovascular (chronic hypertension, cardiac disease), endocrine (pre-gestational diabetes, thyroid disorders), gastrointestinal (gastro-intestinal reflux, peptic ulcer), and mental health (depression, anxiety, bipolar) disorders.[59] These conditions can persist despite suppressive ART, and can exacerbate pregnancy-related symptoms and may require tailored management approaches to alleviate symptoms and prevent complications.

Co-infections

While research into the management of HIV/HCV[60] and HIV/TB[61] co-infections in pregnant women is advancing rapidly, the inclusion of syphilis and hepatitis B into the WHO triple elimination agenda represents a major advancement in the fight against infectious diseases that have a substantial impact on global maternal health.[4,62] As international initiatives and global efforts continue to eliminate these infectious diseases, there is growing focus on identifying the next targets for elimination. Cytomegalovirus (CMV) and human papillomavirus (HPV) emerge as potential candidates for future inclusion in elimination agendas, given their substantial global impact on maternal and infant health.

Both CMV[63] and HPV[64] represent significant public health challenges, and their inclusion in future elimination agendas could help focus attention and resources on reducing their global burden. Although both conditions typically cause mild or asymptomatic illness in healthy non-pregnant women, they can result to serious complications during pregnancy.[63,64] While there are currently no licensed vaccines to prevent CMV infection, there are highly effective HPV vaccines currently deployed globally in an attempt to eradicate HPV, but vaccine coverage remains sub-optimal in many regions, particularly in LMICs.[65] In addition to CMV and HPV, emerging infectious diseases, such as Zika virus and Ebola virus disease, may also pose significant threats to global health security and could benefit from targeted elimination efforts. Ultimately, the identification of the next frontier in disease elimination will require collaboration between policymakers, researchers, health care providers, and affected communities to assess the feasibility and impact of potential interventions and prioritize efforts to achieve global health goals.

Finally, prophylaxis for tuberculosis (TB) and opportunistic infections in the setting of HIV during pregnancy remain an integral part of HIV care in pregnant women with HIV. The IMPAACT P1078 (TB APPRISE) study provided reassuring data regarding the safety during pregnancy of tuberculosis prophylaxis with isoniazid (INH) for women with HIV, but raised concerns regarding potential adverse pregnancy outcomes associated with INH prophylaxis, such as spontaneous preterm birth, stillbirth, and low birth weight.[66] These findings underscore the need for further research to better understand the potential impact of TB prophylaxis on pregnancy outcomes in women with HIV. Weighing the risks and benefits of TB prophylaxis in pregnant women with HIV, and considering individual patient factors and the potential consequences for both maternal and fetal health, is critically important when making decisions about prophylaxis during pregnancy. In addition, close monitoring and ongoing evaluation are essential to ensure optimal management and outcomes in pregnant women with HIV.

Maternal Mental Health

The important issue of maternal mental health is gaining significant momentum worldwide, and concerns regarding maternal mental health issues in pregnant and postpartum women with HIV are now health priorities for international health agencies such as the World Health Organization (WHO)[67] and the President's Emergency Plan for AIDS Relief .[68] Pregnant women with HIV are at an increased risk of experiencing mental health disorders at any trimester of pregnancy or postpartum when compared to women without HIV.[69] Mental health disorders in women with HIV have been associated with several adverse pregnancy outcomes, including preterm birth, IUGR, SGA, and LBW, as well as neurodevelopmental and cognitive delays in children born to these mothers.[46] Furthermore, there is an increased risk of suicidal thoughts and self-harm among women with HIV experiencing perinatal depression.[69] Certain ARVs, such as efavirenz,[70] dolutegravir[71] and rilpivirine,[71] have been associated with an increased risk of depression and suicidal ideation in non-pregnant adults with pre-existing mental health conditions (see **Table 2**). Given these risks and relative lack of long-term data on contemporary ARVs, routine screening for depression is advised during and after pregnancy in pregnant women with HIV on ART. A comprehensive and integrated strategy that provides mental health promotion, prevention, treatment and care, and social support is needed to address maternal mental health issues in pregnant women with HIV. Indeed, maternal and child health services offer an ideal opportunity to support women's mental health. Early detection and treatment of mental health concerns during pregnancy and the postpartum period can be

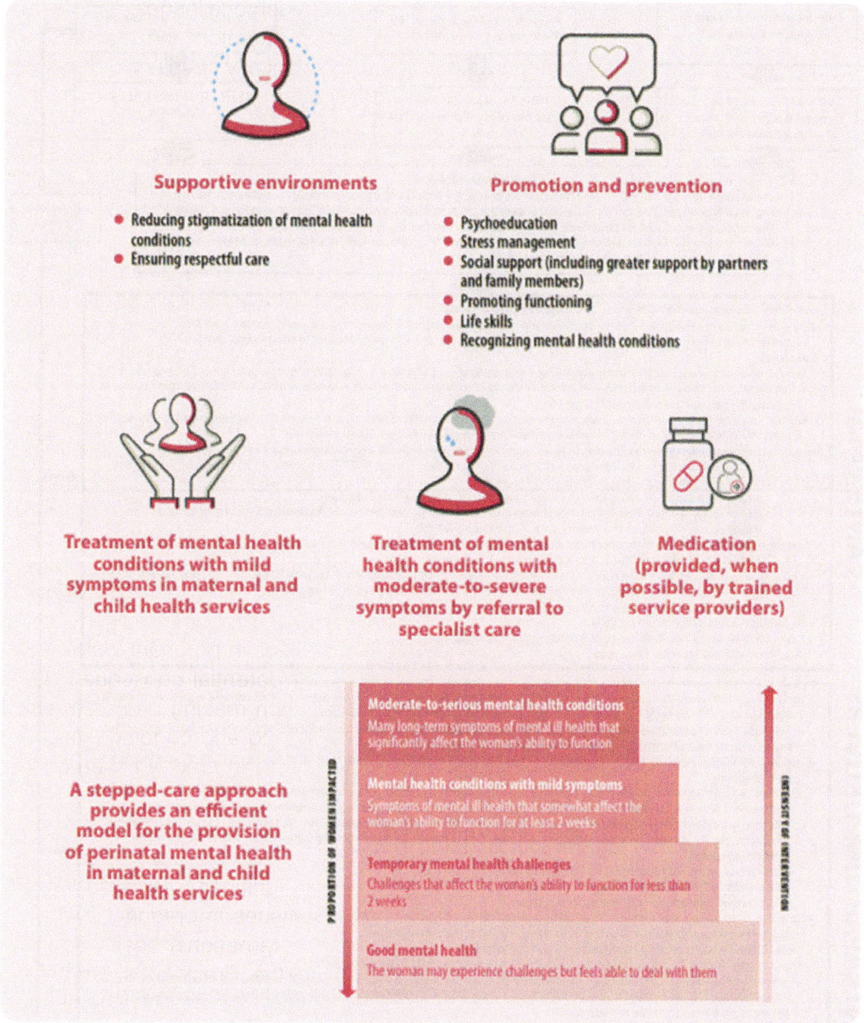

Fig. 3. Provision of Perinatal Mental Health Care (Guide for integration of perinatal mental health in maternal and child health services. Geneva: World Health Organization; 2022.)

achieved by creating a respectful and caring environment where women with HIV feel safe to speak about any difficulties they are experiencing without stigmatization (**Fig. 3**). Reducing HIV-related stigma and prejudice can lessen psychological suffering and enhance the mental health of pregnant women with HIV, potentially supporting better engagement in care.

DISCUSSION

Ongoing health system strengthening initiatives at local and global levels support ART delivery to increasing numbers of women living with HIV aiming to achieve sustained viral suppression, including while pregnant and breastfeeding. However, inequitable access to HIV care and disparities in pregnancy outcomes driven by social

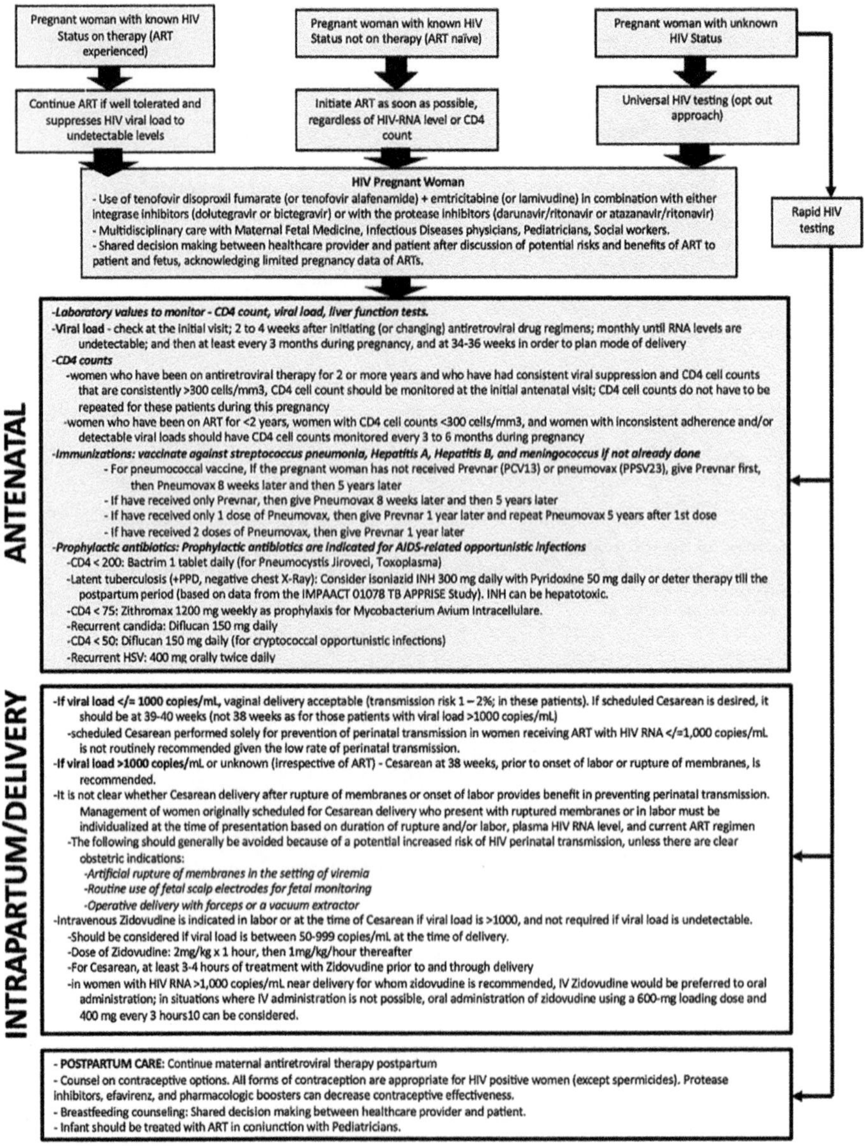

Fig. 4. HIV management algorithm in pregnant and postpartum women.

determinants of health undermine the well-being of women and children on a global scale. Of paramount importance for maternal and child health is the availability of essential and emergency obstetric care (EmOC) such as HIV care, prenatal care, and other accessible medications for pregnant women living with HIV, which requires further investment in infrastructure and strengthening the supply chain. Communities, especially those most affected by HIV, should lead the development and implementation of policies related to ARV use during pregnancy to ensure that HIV care is centered on the client, who is supported to make informed choices related to the use of ARVs during pregnancy. Finally, there remains a need for more robust monitoring and surveillance systems to track ARV use during pregnancy for continuous post-marketing evaluation of their impact on maternal and infant health outcomes. The WHO/IMPAACT task force for HIV, sexually transmitted infections (STIs), TB, and hepatitis created an online repository of documentation for research teams and regulators on the rationale for and ethics of including pregnant and breastfeeding women in research, and guidance on standardized measurements and definitions to promote robust data collection in the peripartum period. With time, such initiatives stand to improve the quantity and quality of data and post-marketing surveillance among pregnant and lactating people relating to ARV use, but also for newer, shorter, TB treatment regimens and medication for STIs and hepatitis.

SUMMARY

In summary, providing care during pregnancy for women living with HIV extends far beyond supporting them to achieve sustained viral suppression throughout the period of risk for vertical transmission. While some ARVs are associated with increased risk of maternal toxicity and adverse pregnancy outcomes, the risks associated with current first-line ART regimens are outweighed by the risk to the mother and the fetus/neonate/infant of untreated HIV. The growing momentum surrounding the earlier inclusion of pregnant and lactating people in research could shorten the delay between licensure of promising new therapeutic agents and their use in the peripartum period, allowing pregnant women with HIV to benefit from enhanced treatment success resulting from rapidly evolving technology. Screening for HIV-associated co-morbid medical conditions and infections is essential to optimizing maternal health, pregnancy outcomes, and infant survival. Maternal and child health services offer opportunities to support perinatal mental health for women with HIV, requiring health providers to actively create a conducive environment for respectful interactions with pregnant women. This article outlines best practice for a human-centered care approach to providing care during the peripartum period for women living with HIV (Best Practices Box).

Best Practices

What is the current practice for care of human immunodeficiency virus in pregnancy?

- Antiretroviral therapy (ART) for women living with HIV with standard first-line ART regimens initiated at the time of diagnosis and continued throughout pregnancy and for life.

Best Practice/Guideline/Care Path Objective(s):

- For every woman living with HIV to receive quality, respectful care during pregnancy and postpartum to promote optimal health outcomes for herself, the pregnancy, and her child. Specifically, that she be taken care with following:
  - Supported to achieve sustained HIV viral suppression;
  - Screened for other sexually transmitted infections, mental distress, and other co-morbidities often associated with HIV;
  - Provided with support to choose and initiate her preferred infant feeding method and contraception option; and
  - Assisted to overcome structural and psychosocial barriers to remaining engaged in life-long HIV care.

What changes in current practice are likely to improve outcomes?

- Investment and effort to provide quality and accessible health care for women with HIV
- Licensure of long-acting combination ART formulations that are safe and efficacious for use in pregnancy and lactation

Is there a Clinical Algorithm? If so, please include

- See **Fig. 4**. HIV Management Algorithm in Pregnant and Postpartum Women.

Pearls/Pitfalls at the point-of-care:

- Failure to deliver HIV care because the woman's diagnosis is not known by the health care provider or herself.
- Focusing on the ART aspects alone, ignoring the importance of psychosocial drivers of retention in care and ART adherence.
- Inadequate engagement and discussion to plan for long-term HIV care, specifically postpartum.

Major Recommendations:

Screening

- All pregnant women should be tested for HIV, syphilis, and HBsAg at least once and as early as possible in the pregnancy.
- In high-HIV-burden settings, women who initially test negative for HIV should be retested regularly throughout pregnancy and postpartum.
- Women with HIV should be screened in pregnancy and postpartum for the following:
  - TB with the 4-item verbal questionnaire
  - Common mental disorders with a locally validated tool, such as the Patient Health Questionnaire (PHQ-9) or Edinburgh Postnatal Depression Scale (EPDS).
- Weight gain and blood pressure should be monitored closely.

Human Immunodeficiency Virus Treatment

- ART should be initiated urgently among all pregnant and breastfeeding women living with HIV, even if they are identified late in pregnancy or postpartum.
- Pregnant women are a priority population for viral load monitoring which should be frequent enough to mark the progress toward achieving sustained viral suppression (undetectable HIV RNA polymerase chain reaction [PCR]) throughout pregnancy and lactation.

Planning for Postpartum Period

- Women living with HIV should be supported to choose an appropriate infant feeding method and contraception option prior to delivery.
  - Women who breastfeed should be fully supported for ART adherence.
  - Breastfeeding should last for at least 12 months and may continue breastfeeding for up to 24 months or longer.
  - Dual contraception including barrier method and hormonal method protects against STIs as well as supporting family planning decisions.
- Routine cervical cancer screening should be done postpartum for women living with HIV aged 25 years and older.

Bibliographic Source(s)

Geneva, World Health Organization. Consolidated guidelines on HIV prevention, testing, treatment, service delivery, and monitoring: recommendations for a public health approach. Published online 2021. https://www.who.int/publications/i/item/9789240031593

National Institutes of Health, USA. Recommendations for the Use of Antiretroviral Drugs During Pregnancy and Interventions to Reduce Perinatal HIV Transmission in the United States. Accessed April 19, 2024. https://clinicalinfo.hiv.gov/en

DISCLOSURE

The authors have nothing to disclose.

FUNDING

This work was not supported by a funding source.

REFERENCES

1. UNAIDS. The path that ends AIDS: UNAIDS Global AIDS Update 2023. 2023. Available at: https://www.unaids.org/sites/default/files/media_asset/2023-unaids-global-aids-update_en.pdf. Accessed February 21, 2024.
2. UNFPA. UNFPA estimates. 2022. Available at: https://esaro.unfpa.org/en/topics/adolescent-pregnancy.
3. World Health Organisation recommendations on antenatal care for a positive pregnancy experience - WHO/RHR/16.12. 2016. Available at: http://apps.who.int/iris/bitstream/handle/10665/250800/WHO-RHR-16.12-eng.pdf;jsessionid=659D46528F57D8F89A6F67399101C1C7?sequence=1. Accessed November 25, 2018.
4. Geneva, World Health Organisation. Introducing a framework for implementing triple elimination of mother-to-child transmission of HIV, syphilis and hepatitis B virus: policy brief. 2023. Available at: https://www.who.int/publications/i/item/9789240086784.
5. Geneva, World Health Organisation, IMPAACT network, International AIDS Society. Research for informed choices: accelerating the study of new drugs for HIV in pregnant and breastfeeding women: a call to action. Available at: https://cdn.who.int/media/docs/default-source/hq-hiv-hepatitis-and-stis-library/call-to-action-to-accelerate-study-of-new-arv-for-pregnant-breastfeeding-women.pdf?sfvrsn=bb4febdc_14.
6. Geneva, World Health Organisation, IMPAACT network, International AIDS Society. Research for informed choices: accelerating the study of new drugs for HIV in pregnant and breastfeeding women: a call to action. Available at: https://cdn.who.int/media/docs/default-source/hq-hiv-hepatitis-and-stis-library/call-to-action-to-accelerate-study-of-new-arv-for-pregnant-breastfeeding-women.pdf?sfvrsn=bb4febdc_14.
7. Riley MF. Including pregnant and lactating women in clinical research: moving beyond legal liability. JAMA 2024. https://doi.org/10.1001/jama.2024.6874.
8. Nematadzira TG, Murnane PM, Odiase OJ, et al. Antiretroviral therapy adherence during and postbreastfeeding cessation measured by tenofovir levels in hair. JAIDS J Acquir Immune Defic Syndr 2022;91(3):237–41.
9. Nesheim SR, FitzHarris LF, Mahle Gray K, et al. Epidemiology of perinatal HIV transmission in the United States in the era of its elimination. Pediatr Infect Dis J 2019;38(6):611–6.
10. Geneva, World Health Organisation. Consolidated guidelines on HIV prevention, testing, treatment, service delivery and monitoring: recommendations for a public health approach. 2021. Available at: https://www.who.int/publications/i/item/9789240031593.

11. National Institutes of Health, USA. Recommendations for the use of antiretroviral drugs during pregnancy and interventions to reduce perinatal HIV transmission in the United States. Available at: https://clinicalinfo.hiv.gov/en. Accessed April 19, 2024.
12. Brooks KM, Scott RK, Best BM, et al. Translating clinical pharmacology data in pregnancy to evidence-based guideline recommendations: perspectives from the HIV field. J Clin Pharmacol 2023;63(S1). https://doi.org/10.1002/jcph.2240.
13. Brooks KM, Scarsi KK, Mirochnick M. Antiretrovirals for human immunodeficiency virus treatment and prevention in pregnancy. Obstet Gynecol Clin North Am 2023;50(1):205–18.
14. Eke AC, Gebreyohannes RD, Fernandes MFS, et al. Physiologic changes during pregnancy and impact on small-molecule drugs, biologic (monoclonal antibody) disposition, and response. J Clin Pharmacol 2023;63(S1). https://doi.org/10.1002/jcph.2227.
15. Colbers A, Mirochnick M, Schalkwijk S, et al. Importance of prospective studies in pregnant and breastfeeding women living with human immunodeficiency virus. Clin Infect Dis 2019;69(7):1254–8.
16. Watts DH, Stek A, Best BM, et al. Raltegravir pharmacokinetics during pregnancy. JAIDS J Acquir Immune Defic Syndr 2014;67(4):375–81.
17. Mulligan N, Best BM, Wang J, et al. Dolutegravir pharmacokinetics in pregnant and postpartum women living with HIV. AIDS 2018;32(6):729–37.
18. Waitt C, Orrell C, Walimbwa S, et al. Safety and pharmacokinetics of dolutegravir in pregnant mothers with HIV infection and their neonates: a randomised trial (DolPHIN-1 study). In: Mofenson LM, editor. PLoS Med 2019;16(9):e1002895.
19. Bollen P, Freriksen J, Konopnicki D, et al. The effect of pregnancy on the pharmacokinetics of total and unbound dolutegravir and its main metabolite in women living with human immunodeficiency virus. Clin Infect Dis 2020;26:ciaa006.
20. Zhang H, Hindman JT, Lin L, et al. A study of the pharmacokinetics, safety, and efficacy of bictegravir/emtricitabine/tenofovir alafenamide in virologically suppressed pregnant women with HIV. AIDS Lond Engl 2024;38(1):F1–9.
21. Powis KM, Pinilla M, Bergam L, et al. Pharmacokinetics and virologic outcomes of bictegravir in pregnancy and postpartum. Presented at: conference on Retroviruses and Opportunistic Infections. 2023. Available at: https://www.croiconference.org/wp-content/uploads/sites/2/posters/2023/IMPAACT_PHARMACOKINETICS_AND_VIROLOGIC_15Feb23-133209845782009090.pdf.
22. Stek A, Best B, Luo W, et al. Effect of pregnancy on emtricitabine pharmacokinetics. HIV Med 2012;13(4):226–35.
23. Benaboud S, Tréluyer JM, Urien S, et al. Pregnancy-related effects on lamivudine pharmacokinetics in a population study with 228 women. Antimicrob Agents Chemother 2012;56(2):776–82.
24. Brooks KM, Momper JD, Pinilla M, et al. Pharmacokinetics of tenofovir alafenamide with and without cobicistat in pregnant and postpartum women living with HIV. AIDS 2021;35(3):407–17.
25. Brooks KM, Pinilla M, Stek AM, et al. Pharmacokinetics of tenofovir alafenamide with boosted protease inhibitors in pregnant and postpartum women living with HIV: results from IMPAACT P1026s. JAIDS J Acquir Immune Defic Syndr 2022;90(3):343–50.
26. Bukkems VE, Necsoi C, Hidalgo Tenorio C, et al. Tenofovir alafenamide plasma concentrations are reduced in pregnant women living with human immunodeficiency virus (HIV): data from the PANNA network. Clin Infect Dis 2022;75(4):623–9.

27. Kreitchmann R, Schalkwijk S, Best B, et al. Efavirenz pharmacokinetics during pregnancy and infant washout. Antivir Ther 2019;24(2):95–103.
28. Lartey M, Kenu E, Lassey A, et al. Pharmacokinetics of efavirenz 600 mg once daily during pregnancy and post partum in Ghanaian women living with HIV. Clin Therapeut 2020;42(9):1818–25.
29. Tran AH, Best BM, Stek A, et al. Pharmacokinetics of rilpivirine in HIV-infected pregnant women. JAIDS J Acquir Immune Defic Syndr 2016;72(3):289–96.
30. Osiyemi O, Yasin S, Zorrilla C, et al. Pharmacokinetics, antiviral activity, and safety of rilpivirine in pregnant women with HIV-1 infection: results of a phase 3b, multicenter, open-label study. Infect Dis Ther 2018;7(1):147–59.
31. Mulligan N, Schalkwijk S, Best BM, et al. Etravirine pharmacokinetics in HIV-infected pregnant women. Front Pharmacol 2016;7. https://doi.org/10.3389/fphar.2016.00239.
32. Bukkems VE, Van Hove H, Roelofsen D, et al. Prediction of maternal and fetal doravirine exposure by integrating physiologically based pharmacokinetic modeling and human placenta perfusion experiments. Clin Pharmacokinet 2022;61(8):1129–41.
33. Boyd SD, Sampson MR, Viswanathan P, et al. Cobicistat-containing antiretroviral regimens are not recommended during pregnancy: viewpoint. AIDS 2019;33(6):1089–93.
34. Colbers A, Best B, Schalkwijk S, et al. Maraviroc pharmacokinetics in HIV-1–Infected pregnant women. Clin Infect Dis 2015;61(10):1582–9.
35. Best BM, Mirochnick M, Capparelli EV, et al. Impact of pregnancy on abacavir pharmacokinetics. AIDS 2006;20(4):553–60.
36. Schalkwijk S, Colbers A, Konopnicki D, et al. The pharmacokinetics of abacavir 600 mg once daily in HIV-1-positive pregnant women. AIDS 2016;30(8):1239–44.
37. Best B, Burchett S, Li H, et al. Pharmacokinetics of tenofovir during pregnancy and postpartum: tenofovir pharmacokinetics in pregnancy. HIV Med 2015;16(8):502–11.
38. Conradie F, Zorrilla C, Josipovic D, et al. Safety and exposure of once-daily ritonavir-boosted atazanavir in HIV-infected pregnant women: atazanavir in HIV-infected pregnant women. HIV Med 2011;12(9):570–9.
39. Mirochnick M, Best BM, Stek AM, et al. Atazanavir pharmacokinetics with and without tenofovir during pregnancy. JAIDS J Acquir Immune Defic Syndr 2011;56(5):412–9.
40. Kreitchmann R, Best BM, Wang J, et al. Pharmacokinetics of an increased atazanavir dose with and without tenofovir during the third trimester of pregnancy. JAIDS J Acquir Immune Defic Syndr 2013;63(1):59–66.
41. Rana A, Bao Y, Zheng L, et al. Long-acting injectable CAB/RPV is superior to oral ART in PWH with adherence challenges: ACTG A5359. In: Special session: clinical late-breaking oral abstracts. 2024. Available at: https://www.croiconference.org/abstract/long-acting-injectable-cab-rpv-is-superior-to-oral-art-in-pwh-with-adherence-challenges-actg-a5359/. Accessed April 17, 2024.
42. Eke AC. Adherence predictors in pregnant women living with HIV on tenofovir alafenamide and tenofovir disoproxil fumarate. J Pharm Drug Res 2022;5(1):585–93.
43. Zhou J, Yun J, Ye X, et al. Interventions to improve antiretroviral adherence in HIV-infected pregnant women: a systematic review and meta-analysis. Front Public Health 2022;10:1056915.
44. Abuogi LL, Castillo-Mancilla J, Hampanda K, et al. Tenofovir diphosphate in dried blood spots in pregnant and postpartum women with HIV in Kenya: a novel

approach to measuring peripartum adherence. JAIDS J Acquir Immune Defic Syndr 2022;89(3):310–7.
45. Patel P, Ford SL, Baker M, et al. Pregnancy outcomes and pharmacokinetics in pregnant women living with HIV exposed to long-acting cabotegravir and rilpivirine in clinical trials. HIV Med 2023;24(5):568–79.
46. Eke AC, Mirochnick M, Lockman S. Antiretroviral therapy and adverse pregnancy outcomes in people living with HIV. Hardin CC. N Engl J Med 2023;388(4): 344–56.
47. Eke AC, Lockman S, Mofenson LM. Antiretroviral treatment of HIV/AIDS during pregnancy. JAMA 2023;329(15):1308.
48. Lockman S, Brummel SS, Ziemba L, et al. Efficacy and safety of dolutegravir with emtricitabine and tenofovir alafenamide fumarate or tenofovir disoproxil fumarate, and efavirenz, emtricitabine, and tenofovir disoproxil fumarate HIV antiretroviral therapy regimens started in pregnancy (IMPAACT 2010/VESTED): a multicentre, open-label, randomised, controlled, phase 3 trial. Lancet 2021;397(10281):1276–92.
49. Calmy A, Tovar Sanchez T, Kouanfack C, et al. Dolutegravir-based and low-dose efavirenz-based regimen for the initial treatment of HIV-1 infection (NAMSAL): week 96 results from a two-group, multicentre, randomised, open label, phase 3 non-inferiority trial in Cameroon. Lancet HIV 2020;7(10):e677–87.
50. Venter WDF, Sokhela S, Simmons B, et al. Dolutegravir with emtricitabine and tenofovir alafenamide or tenofovir disoproxil fumarate versus efavirenz, emtricitabine, and tenofovir disoproxil fumarate for initial treatment of HIV-1 infection (ADVANCE): week 96 results from a randomised, phase 3, non-inferiority trial. Lancet HIV 2020;7(10):e666–76.
51. João EC, Morrison RL, Shapiro DE, et al. Raltegravir versus efavirenz in antiretroviral-naive pregnant women living with HIV (NICHD P1081): an open-label, randomised, controlled, phase 4 trial. Lancet HIV 2020;7(5):e322–31.
52. Kintu K, Malaba TR, Nakibuka J, et al. Dolutegravir versus efavirenz in women starting HIV therapy in late pregnancy (DolPHIN-2): an open-label, randomised controlled trial. Lancet HIV 2020;7(5):e332–9.
53. Institute of Medicine (US) and National Research Council (US) Committee to Reexamine IOM Pregnancy Weight GuidelinesKathleen M Rasmussen, Ann L Yaktine, editors. Washington (DC): National Academies Press (US); 2009. The National Academies Collection: Reports funded by National Institutes of Health.-PMID: 20669500 Bookshelf ID: NBK32813 DOI: 10.17226/12584.
54. Eke AC, Gebreyohannes RD, Powell AM. Understanding clinical outcome measures reported in HIV pregnancy studies involving antiretroviral-naive and antiretroviral-experienced women. Lancet Infect Dis 2023;23(4):e151–9.
55. Patel K, Huo Y, Jao J, et al. Dolutegravir in pregnancy as compared with current HIV regimens in the United States. N Engl J Med 2022;387(9):799–809.
56. Zash R, Makhema J, Shapiro RL. Neural-tube defects with dolutegravir treatment from the time of conception. N Engl J Med 2018;379(10):979–81.
57. Zash R, Holmes L, Diseko M, et al. Neural-tube defects and antiretroviral treatment regimens in Botswana. N Engl J Med 2019;381(9):827–40.
58. Heather Watts D. Teratogenicity risk of antiretroviral therapy in pregnancy. Curr HIV AIDS Rep 2007;4(3):135–40.
59. Venkatesh KK, Morrison L, Tuomala RE, et al. Profile of chronic comorbid conditions and obstetrical complications among pregnant women with human immunodeficiency virus and receiving antiretroviral therapy in the United States. Clin Infect Dis 2021;73(6):969–78.

60. Abdul Massih S, Eke AC. Direct antiviral agents (DAAs) and their use in pregnant women with hepatitis C (HCV). Expert Rev Anti Infect Ther 2022;20(11):1413–24.
61. Jones AJ, Mathad JS, Dooley KE, et al. Evidence for implementation: management of TB in HIV and pregnancy. Curr HIV AIDS Rep 2022;19(6):455–70.
62. Cohn J, Owiredu MN, Taylor MM, et al. Eliminating mother-to-child transmission of human immunodeficiency virus, syphilis and hepatitis B in sub-Saharan Africa. Bull World Health Organ 2021;99(4):287–95.
63. Rybak-Krzyszkowska M, Górecka J, Huras H, et al. Cytomegalovirus infection in pregnancy prevention and treatment options: a systematic review and meta-analysis. Viruses 2023;15(11):2142.
64. Condrat CE, Filip L, Gherghe M, et al. Maternal HPV infection: effects on pregnancy outcome. Viruses 2021;13(12):2455.
65. Eke AC, Kerry VB. Ethical challenges to improving access to human papillomavirus vaccines in low- and middle-income countries. NEJM Evid 2022;1(5). https://doi.org/10.1056/EVIDe2200069.
66. Gupta A, Montepiedra G, Aaron L, et al. Isoniazid preventive therapy in HIV-infected pregnant and postpartum women. N Engl J Med 2019;381(14):1333–46.
67. Geneva: World Health Organization. Guide for integration of perinatal mental health in maternal and child health services. 2022. Available at: https://iris.who.int/bitstream/handle/10665/362880/9789240057142-eng.pdf?sequence=1.
68. Fukunaga R, Pierre P, Williams JK, et al. Prioritizing mental health within HIV and tuberculosis services in PEPFAR. Emerg Infect Dis 2024;30(4). https://doi.org/10.3201/eid3004.231726.
69. Zhu QY, Huang DS, Lv JD, et al. Prevalence of perinatal depression among HIV-positive women: a systematic review and meta-analysis. BMC Psychiatr 2019;19(1):330.
70. Mollan KR, Smurzynski M, Eron JJ, et al. Association between efavirenz as initial therapy for HIV-1 infection and increased risk for suicidal ideation or attempted or completed suicide: an analysis of trial data. Ann Intern Med 2014;161(1):1.
71. Allen Reeves A, Fuentes AV, Caballero J, et al. Neurotoxicities in the treatment of HIV between dolutegravir, rilpivirine and dolutegravir/rilpivirine: a meta-analysis. Sex Transm Infect 2021;97(4):261–7.

Research on Maternal Vaccination for HIV Prevention

Krithika P. Karthigeyan, PhD[a], Christian Binuya, BS[a], Kenneth Vuong, BS[a], Sallie R. Permar, MD, PhD[b,*], Ashley N. Nelson, PhD[b,*]

KEYWORDS

- Human immunodeficiency virus-1
- Broadly neutralizing antibodies
- Passive immunization

KEY POINTS

- A major challenge to prevention of vertical human immunodeficiency virus (HIV) transmission involves barriers associated with antiretroviral therapy (ART) access, coverage, and adherence, as well as the lack of interventions to prevent vertical transmission following acute maternal HIV infection.
- Immune-based interventions that synergize with ART will be required to end the pediatric HIV epidemic.
- Active and passive immunization strategies are the 2 promising approaches to boost HIV-1 specific antibodies in pregnancy to be passively transferred to the infant and confer protection in the perinatal and postnatal periods.
- Both active and passive immunization approaches for pregnancy will need to be properly evaluated for their impact on viral fitness to mitigate the generation of viral escape variants more fit for transmission to the infant.
- There remains a deficit in the inclusion of pregnant people living with HIV in current clinical trials evaluating state-of-the-art active or passive immunization strategies, further hindering progress toward achieving an HIV-free generation.

INTRODUCTION

The elimination of pediatric human immunodeficiency virus (HIV) via vertical transmission continues to pose a significant global health challenge. Vertical transmission of

[a] Department of Pediatrics, Weill Cornell Medicine, 413 East 69th Street, BB-869E, New York City, NY 10021, USA; [b] Department of Pediatrics, Weill Cornell Medicine, Drukier Institute for Children's Health, 413 East 69th Street, New York City, NY 10021, USA
* Corresponding authors. Department of Pediatrics, Weill Cornell Medicine, NewYork-Presbyterian Komansky Children's Hospital NewYork-Presbyterian Hospital/ Weill Cornell Medical Center, 525 East 68th Street, Box 225, New York, NY 10065.
E-mail addresses: sap4017@med.cornell.edu (S.R.P.); asn4002@med.cornell.edu (A.N.N.)

Clin Perinatol 51 (2024) 769–782
https://doi.org/10.1016/j.clp.2024.08.007 perinatology.theclinics.com
0095-5108/24/

HIV strains and variants can occur perinatally or postnatally, with perinatal transmission occurring before (placental transmission) or around the time of delivery, while postnatal transmission occurs primarily via breastfeeding. Implementation of prevention of vertical transmission programs has provided access to better care, contributed to increased awareness of HIV status among women living with HIV, and greater than 82% uptake of anti-retroviral therapy (ART) among pregnant people living with HIV.[1,2] Despite these significant efforts, progress toward reduction in vertical transmission rates has remained stagnant over recent years, primarily driven by remaining shortfalls in testing, access to treatment, adherence to daily ART regimens, and retention in care during pregnancy.[3] Moreover, while ART during pregnancy and lactation can significantly reduce the number of infant infections, it does not eliminate the transmission risk. Moreover, this strategy does not prevent vertical HIV transmission following acute infection during pregnancy or lactation. Even with optimal prophylaxis, transmission of HIV-1 occurs at a rate of 1% to 5% at 6 mo of age in infants born to persons living with HIV who breastfeed.[1]

In 2022, approximately 130,000 children under 5 years of age newly acquired HIV.[2] Among these children, approximately 48% were born to individuals that did not receive or had discontinued treatment during pregnancy, and 8% were on treatment but were not able to maintain virologic suppression.[1,2,4] Furthermore, incident HIV infections during pregnancy and breastfeeding contribute to an increasing proportion of new pediatric infections.[2] Therefore, recent research into HIV-1 prevention strategies have focused on both active and passive immunization strategies centered around HIV-1 broadly neutralizing antibodies (bnAbs), which have shown efficacy against prevention of acquisition of susceptible viral strains.[5] This review focuses on the potential for immune-based interventions that can be administered in conjunction with current ART-based strategies to the birthing parent for prevention of vertical transmission, and the potential challenges of each approach.

HUMAN IMMUNODEFICIENCY VIRUS-1 TRANSMISSION: THE UNIQUE CONTEXT OF PREGNANCY

During pregnancy, passive transfer of maternal antibodies to fetuses may play a role in blocking vertical HIV transmission and exert immune selection pressure on viruses, but this mechanism is still poorly understood.[6] The placenta is a physical barrier that provides protection against infections; however, vertical transmission of HIV still occurs through the placenta in about 5% to 10% of pregnant people living with untreated HIV,[7] and transmissions that occur during the postnatal period, specifically via breastfeeding, make up about one-third to half of all vertical transmission events in the world, especially in the absence of interventions.[8] Moreover, as vertical transmission rates are only around 15% to 30% in the absence of ART,[7] understanding those immune factors in pregnancy that confer natural protection against vertical transmission will be important for informing immune-based interventions and evaluating their efficacy.

Many studies have shown that despite having a diverse array of HIV-1 variants circulating in pregnant persons,[7,9–13] only 1 or a few variants get transmitted to the infant, known as the infant transmitted/founder (T/F) variant(s). This genetic bottleneck suggests that the maternal immune system selects for viruses that are transmitted to the infants. A recent study from Marichannegowda and colleagues, looked at a total of 721 HIV envelope (Env) genes by single genome amplification from 12 pairs of mothers and infants, and all paired sequences were clustered together in a phylogenetic tree. These neonates acquired HIV *in utero* and are from 2 cohorts: Women and Infant Transmission Study[14] and Center for HIV/Acquired Immunodeficiency Syndrome (AIDS) Vaccine

Immunology Protocol 9.[15] The genetic diversity of the viral population in neonates who experienced estimated earlier *in utero* HIV acquisition was significantly higher (only 3-fold lower than their mother) than neonates with a shorter period of *in utero* infection (13-fold lower compared to the longer infected neonate).[6] In addition, neonate viral populations formed lineages independent to their mothers, suggesting a distinguished evolutionary pathway of HIV during *in utero* infection when compared to the virus from their cognate mothers.[6] In fact, our group and others have observed that vertically-transmitted variants are significantly more resistant to plasma autologous virus neutralizing antibodies from the birthing parent compared to non-transmitted variants.[10,11,16,17] Further, the viruses transmitted to infants frequently contain bnAb mutations.[16] Thus, vertical transmission of HIV *in utero* and immediately peripartum suggests that placentally-transferred antibodies do not fully prevent HIV acquisition, and that the presence of viral escape variants with resistance to circulating neutralizing antibodies in pregnancy is a determinant feature of vertically transmitted variants.

Another barrier to the development of immune-based interventions to prevent vertical transmission is the lack of established immune correlates of protection. Several studies have suggested that antibodies against conserved, vulnerable regions of the HIV Env may serve as immune correlates of protection against vertical transmission of HIV-1, yet there has been no consensus across studies (reviewed in[18]), which varied by virus clade, transmission mode, and ART status during pregnancy. Similarly, there is a lack of consensus regarding whether non-neutralizing antibodies capable of mediating antibody-dependent cellular cytotoxicity (ADCC) or phagocytosis (ADCP)[19–21] correlate with reduced risk of vertical transmission, despite these responses being correlated with protection in vaccine studies[22,23] and improved outcomes in natural infection.[24,25] A recent study reported higher virus-specific immunoglobulin (IgG) FcR-engagement among non-transmitting mothers, with consistently higher virus-specific FcRn-engagement among non-transmitting dyads compared to transmitting dyads.[20] As a major limitation of many of these studies is the evaluation of small cohorts, it is thus critical that more large-scale comprehensive analyses be performed to establish true immune correlates of protection of vertical transmission of HIV-1 to guide advancements in prevention strategies.

BOOSTING MATERNAL AUTOLOGOUS VIRUS NEUTRALIZATION RESPONSES VIA ACTIVE IMMUNIZATION FOR PREVENTION OF VERTICAL TRANSMISSION OF HIV-1

A HIV-1 vaccine capable of temporarily boosting neutralizing antibody responses against circulating viruses in pregnant people living with HIV could lead to further reductions in vertical transmission risk. While the safety and immunogenicity of an HIV vaccine administered in pregnancy has not been well-established, a few historic HIV vaccine trials have provided some insight into this approach.

The safety and immunogenicity of a maternal HIV Env active vaccination regimen to reduce vertical transmission has previously been evaluated in a phase I clinical trial conducted by the AIDS Vaccine Evaluation Group (AVEG). The clinical trials (protocols 104 and 102) enrolled 26 pregnant women living with HIV in the United States from 1993 to 1995, to evaluate the safety and immunogenicity of an HIV Env gp120 and gp160 subunit vaccine.[26] AVEG 104 participants were randomized 2:1 to receive 300 μg Env subunit MN recombinant gp120 with aluminum phosphate (alum) or placebo control with alum. AVEG 102 participants were randomized 1:1 to receive 640 μg Env subunit recombinant gp160 with alum or placebo control with alum. Overall, the vaccines were well-tolerated with no local or systemic reactions in the mothers and no adverse outcomes in the infants attributable to the vaccine, yet there was no consistent increase in the maternal immune responses elicited by the vaccines. Wright and colleagues reported that 2 women had measurable autologous virus neutralization on entry to the trial and that 2 more women, 1 vaccinee and 1 placebo recipient, developed detectable neutralizing antibodies during the course of the trial. While the small sample size limited their ability to identify factors that might influence transmission, this study demonstrated that an HIV Env vaccine can be safely administered to pregnant women with HIV. In a recent follow-up study, we have found that while the vaccine increased MN gp120-specific binding responses, it failed to enhance maternal autologous virus neutralization responses.[27] Therefore, more advanced approaches are needed to induce potent B cell stimulation and drive development of robust autologous virus neutralization during pregnancy.

To further assess the ability of a heterologous HIV Env gp120 immunization strategy to boost autologous neutralizing antibody responses, our group performed additional preclinical studies in nonhuman primates. In this study, female rhesus macaques (RMs) were infected with SHIV.C.CH505 (n = 12) and started on a daily ART regimen at 12 w post-infection. Starting 2 w after ART initiation, RMs received 3 immunizations in monthly intervals with HIV b.63521/1086.C gp120 or placebo (n = 6/group) vaccine with STR8S-C, a squalene-based emulsion adjuvant containing the toll-like receptor agonists R848 and CpG (CpG oligodeoxynucleotide).[28] Compared to the placebo-immunized animals, Env-vaccinated, SHIV-infected RMs exhibited enhanced IgG binding, avidity, and ADCC responses against the vaccine immunogens and the autologous SHIV.C.CH505 Env. Moreover, we observed the preferential expansion of Env-specific memory B cells that recognized the SHIV.C.CH505 Env, the antigen of primary exposure, following heterologous vaccination. This study provided proof of concept that heterologous HIV Env vaccination in the setting of lentiviral infection and ART suppression can augment functional antibody responses against the Env antigen of primary exposure (ie, the circulating virus variant).

While there remains a hiatus in the evaluation of active immunization strategies for prevention of vertical transmission due to gaps in enrollment of pregnant people in vaccine trials,[29] there has been a substantial increase in the number of HIV vaccine trials focused on adult populations over the last decade.[5] Recognizing that pregnancies can potentially occur during these trials despite recommendations around contraception, Stranix-Chibanda and colleagues performed a retrospective, cross-protocol analysis to identify and compare pregnancy outcomes reported in 53 phase I and phase IIa HIV-1 vaccine clinical trials conducted by the HIV Vaccine Trials Network (HVTN).[30] A total of 193 pregnancies were reported across the 53 trials, with 82% (n = 159 of 193) of pregnancies occurring after all vaccinations had been completed. Amongst the 193 pregnancies following enrollment in HVTN studies through December 31, 2018, there were 22 maternal or fetal adverse events (AEs) reported that were classified anywhere from moderate to severe, but all deemed unrelated to the study product. Of the 22 AEs, 3 were congenital anomalies, which included 1 case of hepatic mesenchymal hamartoma, 1 case of Poland's syndrome, and 1 unspecified anomaly. Overall, 11% (n = 17 of 154) of women who received at least one study product experienced a moderate to severe AE among themselves or in their offspring compared to 12% (n = 5 of 39) of women who received placebo. A secondary evaluation of 111 pregnancies that had documented outcomes and occurred within 1 y of the last product administration, revealed no significant differences in reported rates of adverse pregnancy outcomes between vaccinees and placebo recipients when vaccine vectors, adjuvant used, or geographic region were examined.[30] This study provides a preliminary assessment of the safety of HIV vaccines in pregnancy and can inform the next phase of clinical trials.

While flu and Tdap vaccines are recommended by the Centers for Disease Prevention and Control during pregnancy, many vaccines such as the human papillomavirus vaccine, the measles, mumps, and rubella trivalent vaccine are not.[31] Aside from safety concerns around administering an HIV vaccine during pregnancy, it should also be recognized that induction of HIV Env-specific antibody responses in pregnant people with long-standing or newly-acquired HIV by active vaccination comes with the potential risk of promoting viral escape variants in maternal plasma that will be more fit for transmission to the infant.[16,32,33] Thus, it will be important to evaluate the impact of immunization on viral fitness and evolution, as well as optimize the timing of vaccination during pregnancy to achieve maximal transplacental transfer of vaccine-elicited antibodies.

PASSIVE IMMUNIZATION WITH BROADLY NEUTRALIZING ANTIBODIES FOR PREVENTION OF VERTICAL HUMAN IMMUNODEFICIENCY VIRUS-1 TRANSMISSION

Over the past decade, passive immunization via administration of monoclonal antibodies has proven to be an effective approach for targeting infectious pathogens,[34] including Severe Acute Respiratory Syndrome-Coronavirus-2[35] and Respiratory Syncytial Virus,[36] in the absence of protective humoral responses acquired either naturally or through active immunization. In HIV, passive immunization with bnAbs is an attractive approach for prevention of virus acquisition and thus, merit exploration for prevention of vertical transmission. HIV-1-specific bnAbs target distinct epitopes on the HIV-1 Env trimer and have demonstrated the ability to robustly reduce viremia in people living with HIV not on ART and to prevent virus acquisition in adults at risk for HIV infection.[37] Moreover, many bnAbs can mediate Fc-dependent functions such as ADCC and ADCP,[38,39] enhancing their protectiveness. An added benefit of bnAb administration for passive protection is fewer adverse effects compared to ART drugs.[40]

Several clinical trials have been conducted to optimize passive immunization strategies and evaluate the efficacy of bnAbs against HIV-1 acquisition.[41] Many of the early trials evaluated HIV bnAbs as monotherapy, using a single highly potent and broad bnAb with specificity against 1 distinct epitope on the HIV Env. All of these studies resulted in eventual treatment failure due to the rapid selection of neutralization-resistant viral variants,[41–43] suggesting that administration of a combination of bnAbs targeting a variety of epitopes would improve coverage breadth in comparison to a single bnAb therapy. In macaque models, it has been shown that passive immunization using human monoclonal bnAbs with diverse Env epitope specificity that potently neutralize the challenge virus can reduce vertical transmission of escape variants.[44] Currently, there are a number of clinical trials that have recently evaluated combination bnAb therapy in adults and/or children living with HIV[41,45] (**Table 1**), yet none have incorporated pregnant people. It will be important for future studies to evaluate passive immunization strategies in this vulnerable group in conjunction with ART as this approach offers several potential benefits including, reduction of the viral reservoir in pregnancy, prevention of *in utero* and peripartum transmission, and transplacental transfer of antibodies to the infant for protection against postnatal exposure. Moreover, passive bnAb immunization during pregnancy could protect pregnant people living in areas of high HIV prevalence from acute infection during pregnancy and/or lactation, a high-risk setting for vertical virus transmission. It will also be imperative to address potential adverse effects, such as bnAb administration in pregnancy driving viral escape variants that can then be transmitted to the infant.

Table 1
Summary of most recent clinical trials assessing combination broadly neutralizing antibodies therapy

Clinical Trial	bnAb Combination	Study Summary	Trial Status
NCT03707977	VRC01LS and 10–1074	A 2-phase trial, evaluating the efficacy and significance of 2 bnAbs combination, VRC01LS and 10–1074, in suppressing HIV in a children cohort that was getting ART treatment	Completed; 12/2021
NCT02824536	3BNC117 + 10–1074	A phase 1 trial, evaluated the PK and safety of administering a dual bnAb combination in HIV uninfected adults in support to find a prophylaxis against HIV	Completed; 01/2018
NCT05245292	3BNC117-LS, 10–1074-LS, and N803	A phase 1 trial, evaluating the safety of a combination of 2 bnAb infusion in ART-treated adults living with HIV during ATI	Recruiting; 12/2025 (estimated)
NCT03721510	PGT121, VRC07–523LS, and PGDM1400	A phase 1/2a trial, evaluating the safety and PK of using these antibodies for HIV prevention and therapy in HIV-uninfected and HIV-infected adults	Completed; 05/2022
NCT04212091	PGT121.414.LS and VRC07–523LS	A phase 1 trail, evaluating the safety and PK, conducted in 2 parts: (A) PGT121.414.LS was administered alone and (B) administered in combination with VRC07–523LS in HIV-uninfected adults	Completed; 01/2023
NCT05890963	VRC07–523LS	An open-labeled phase 1b trial, evaluating the safety and the antiviral effect of a bnAb in combination with bispecific antibody in people living with HIV while on ART	Recruiting; 02/2025 (estimated)

Table 2
Summary of studies identifying broadly neutralizing antibodies escape in response to passive immunization

Year	bnAb Combination	Summary of the Study
2005,[44]	2G12; 2F5; 4E10	• Administration of this combination bnAbs delayed viral rebound. • Increase in viral load occurred at a time when 2F5 and 4E10 had already been weaned out. • Viruses that rebounded early, as well as viruses that emerged after prolonged suppression of viremia, both had escaped inhibition of 2G12, suggesting 2G12's role in controlling viremia. • No escape to the 2F5 and 4E10 monoclonal antibodies. • Only 2G12 had achieved plasma concentration required for *in vivo* activity. • Hypothesis 1: 2G12 was the weakest of the 3 antibodies compared to 2F5 and 4E10, indicated by rapid appearance of 2G12 escape mutants • Hypothesis 2: Only 2G12 was active in vivo; hence, only 2G12 escape occurs.
2021,[48]	PG9; VRC01; DH512; DH429	• VRC01 and DH512 neutralized all viruses tested during the study, and large number of the viruses was resistant to PG9 and DH429. • Genetic motifs associated with resistance against PG9, VRC01, and DH512. • Some motifs are also associated with sensitivity to the same bnAbs that had signature sites conferring resistance. • bnAb-mediated immune pressure may be a major force driving selections of escape mutations.
2022,[49]	VRC01 alone	• Despite high serum concentration, VRC01 alone did not prevent HIV acquisition more effectively than placebo.
2022,[50]	VRC07–523LS; PGT121	• VRC07–523LS was more efficacious at a higher dose for intervals of up to 24 wk whereas PGT121 was more effective at lower dose with shorter intervals. • High-dose groups had higher titers at peak; however, neutralization response decreased to almost similar level as the lower-dose groups at the same time ~24 wk post immunization. • Neutralizing antibody titers increased again after dose 2, but declined to undetectable level after week 24 post dose 2.

DEVELOPMENT OF BROADLY NEUTRALIZING ANTIBODIES ESCAPE VARIANTS: A MAJOR CHALLENGE IN PREVENTION AND CURE STRATEGIES FOR HUMAN IMMUNODEFICIENCY VIRUS-1

Although passive immunization of bnAbs during pregnancy has great potential for reducing the risk of vertical transmission of HIV, it also comes with the added risk of driving escape variants that can be selectively transmitted to the infant. There are several instances under which viral escape can occur. Firstly, innate resistance where the participant's circulating virus pool contains resistant variants prior to bnAbs infusion and, secondly, *de novo* escape mutations, which only arise after administration of specific bnAbs.[46] In the setting of pregnancy, it is important to understand the role of bnAbs in the birthing parent on vertical transmission to design effective passive immunization strategies that can synergize with ART to further reduce transmission risk.[33]

As previously discussed, the field of passive immunization using HIV-1 bnAbs has recognized the need for combination therapy and it is possible that this approach in pregnancy can also minimize the risk of escape variants being transmitted to the infant. However, several studies have revealed the development of bnAb resistant variants arising even in the context of combination therapy (**Table 2**). A study from Trkola and colleagues, evaluated the efficacy of passive immunization with 3 bnAbs—2G12, 2F5, and 4E10—in suppressing viral rebound. In this study, 2 individuals with chronic infection and 4 individuals with acute infection showed evidence of prolonged delay in viral rebound after ART interruption. While this confirmed that a bnAb combination therapy can prevent viremia, 12 other participants in this study, with 2G12-sensitive circulating virus variants at baseline, eventually developed escape mutants to this

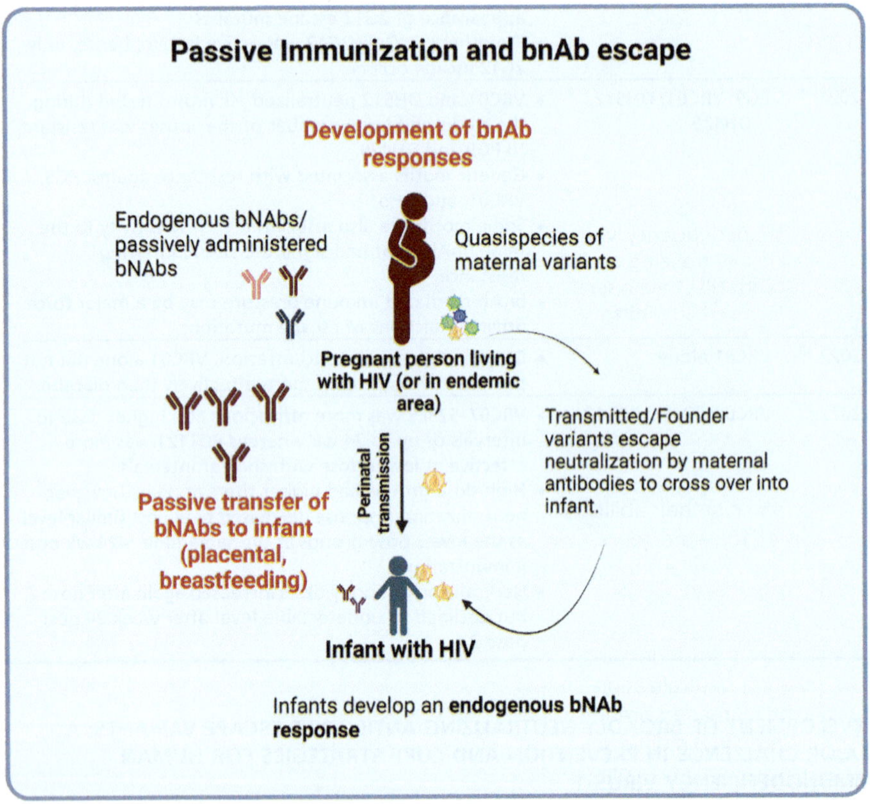

Fig. 1. Passive immunization via broadly neutralizing antibodies (bnAb) administration can potentially drive viral escape. Passive administration of bnAbs to pregnant people living with human immunodeficiency virus (HIV), or residing in HIV endemic regions, as well as endogenous bnAbs (in pregnant persons living with HIV) can contribute to escape of viral variants driving development of transmitted/founder (T/F) variants that are resistant to neutralization by bnAbs. These variants are selected for transmission to the infant along with antibodies (placental transfer or via breastfeeding), which can then lead to the development of an endogenous bnAb response in infants with HIV. (*Created with* BioRender.com.)

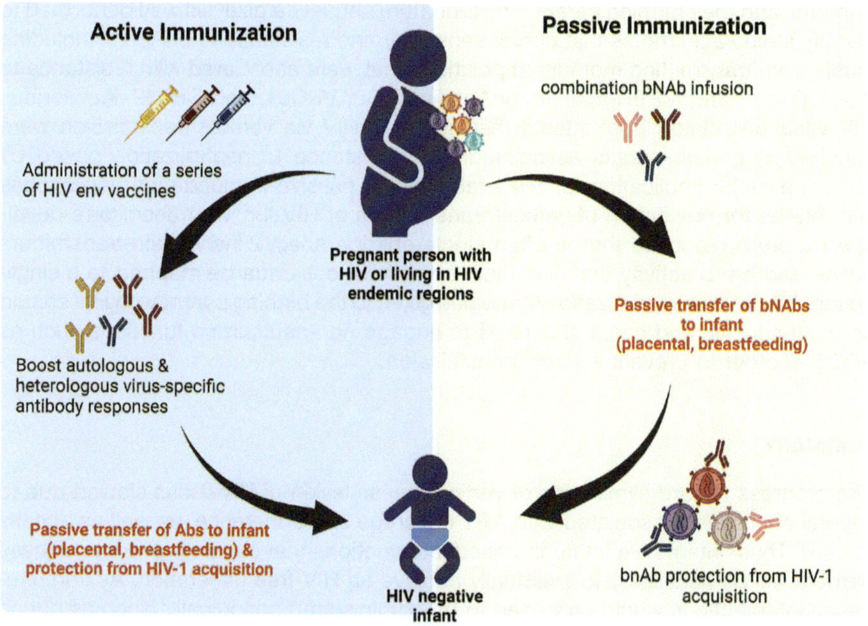

Fig. 2. Active and passive immunization strategies for prevention of vertical transmission of human immunodeficiency virus (HIV-1). Active immunization strategies involve boosting HIV-1 specific neutralizing antibody responses against circulating variants in pregnant persons living with HIV-1 via a series of immunizations during gestation. Passive immunization strategies involved administration of a combination of HIV broadly neutralizing antibodies, associated with protection from HIV-1 acquisition. In both cases, antibody responses will be boosted in pregnant people living with HIV, or those pregnant persons living in endemic regions, to levels for maximal transfer through placenta or breastfeeding to confer protection to the infant. (*Created with* BioRender.com.)

antibody and lost their ability to control viremia. The remaining monoclonal antibodies (2F5 and 4E10) were too weak to maintain and control viremia, thus viral rebound occurred.[47] A similar study also looked into the potential of a dual combination of bnAbs—3BNC117 and 10-1074—in eradicating HIV viremia also saw prolonged virologic suppression on treatment interruption as long as bNAb-resistant viruses were not present at study initiation.[45] As seen in these studies, bnAb combinations can have differing neutralization effects; hence, future studies may require incorporating bnAbs with increased breadth and potency to reach virologic control.[48] It should also be considered that a different combination of bnAbs may prove efficacious for preventing vertical transmission of HIV-1, as at least 1 study has reported differing sensitivity of heterosexually transmitted viral variants to bnAbs compared to vertically transmitted variants.[49] This finding further highlights the importance of including pregnant people living with HIV in future clinical trials.

Although combination bnAb therapy for passive immunization has yet to be evaluated for efficacy in reducing vertical transmission, several studies suggest that plasma bnAb responses or generation of potent heterologous virus neutralization responses in the birthing parent can drive bnAb escape variants that are transmitted to the infant (**Fig. 1**).[32,50] To determine whether acquired variants by the infant were mutants that escaped maternal plasma bnAb activity, our group analyzed HIV-1 *env* sequences in infants and their birthing parent.[32,33] Signature sequence analysis was performed to identify amino acid motifs that confer sensitivity and resistance to bnAbs,[32] including motifs from transmitting mothers at positions that were associated with resistance to V2-, CD4bs-, and MPER-specific bnAbs like PG9, VRC01, and DH512. Autologous HIV variants isolated from infants that acquired HIV via vertical transmission were enriched in genetic motifs associated with resistance to neutralization posed by bnAbs, a major implication for the evaluation of passive immunization approaches with bnAbs for prevention of vertical transmission of HIV-1.[33] As transmitters developed a bnAb response that is often single-epitope specific, while non-transmitters possessed bnAb activity that was multi-specific or could not be mapped to a single epitope,[33] passive immunization strategies given to the birthing parent with HIV should be multi-specific and might also need to engage non-neutralizing functions such as ADCC in order to prevent *in utero* transmission.

SUMMARY

The progress toward elimination of vertical transmission of HIV-1 has slowed due to several challenges associated with ART coverage and adherence, as well as access to care. Thus, alternative immune-based interventions that can help overcome these barriers will be necessary to eventually achieve an HIV-free generation. As immune-based interventions would only need to be administered periodically, such as during the duration of a pregnancy, they can help overcome adherence issues observed with daily multi-drug ART regimens. As highlighted in this article, both active and passive immunization approaches should be further explored to boost the HIV-1-specific neutralizing antibody responses in pregnancy for transplacental transfer to confer protection to the infant during the intrapartum and postnatal period (**Fig. 2**). However, given that a key determinant of vertical transmission events is the HIV-1 neutralizing antibody response in the birthing parent, which can alter viral fitness and promote escape variants that are more likely to be transmitted, these approaches warrant some caution. Most importantly, a lack of incorporation of pregnant people living with HIV in the current clinical trials will continue to contribute to this major gap in knowledge in the field, leaving this group vulnerable to transmission risks, particularly those in resource-limited settings.

Best Practices

What is the current practice for preventing vertical transmission of HIV-1?

- HIV-1 testing prior to and during pregnancy.
- Pregnant and lactating people should be informed on ways to avoid HIV-1 infection with HIV-1 and offered pre-exposure prophylaxis (PrEP)
- Persons living with HIV should be on an ART therapy regimen during pregnancy and childbirth.
- HIV-exposed infants should be placed on prophylactic therapy based on gestational age, and HIV-infected infants should be placed on a risk-based ART prophylaxis regimen.

What changes in current practice are likely to improve outcomes?

- Increased access to HIV-1 testing and PrEP for pregnant and lactating people, particularly in endemic areas.
- Immune-based interventions to prevent HIV-1 infection of pregnant and lactating people and vertical transmission could improve outcomes, though further studies/trials are needed before this can become clinical point-of-care.

Pearls/Pitfalls at the point-of-care:

- Patients may decline testing.
- Delayed care for those who test positive for HIV-1 due to requirements for patient-initiated follow-up care, as well as social stigma.
- Often symptoms of acute HIV-1 infection may go unrecognized as these are usually mild, nonspecific, and self-limiting, and thus never brought to clinical attention.

Major Recommendations:

- All pregnant and lactating persons living with HIV-1 should be on, or immediately started on, the recommended ART regimen.
- Further studies to determine the efficacy of immune-based interventions on prevention of vertical HIV-1 transmission and their impact on viral escape/fitness.
- Further studies to understand of the role of non-neutralizing antibodies in preventing vertical transmission.

Bibliographic Source(s): This is important: list current sources/references to support info above

1. https://hivinfo.nih.gov/understanding-hiv/fact-sheets/preventing-perinatal-transmission-hiv
2. https://clinicalinfo.hiv.gov/en/guidelines/perinatal/management-infants-arv-hiv-exposure-infection
3. Swinkels HM, Justiz Vaillant AA, Nguyen AD, et al. HIV and AIDS. [Updated 2024 May 6]. In: StatPearls [Internet]. Treasure Island (FL): StatPearls Publishing; 2024 Jan-. Available from: https://www.ncbi.nlm.nih.gov/books/NBK534860/

DISCLOSURE

S.R. Permar serves as a consultant to Moderna, Merck, Pfizer, Dynavax, and GSK vaccine programs for CMV, and leads sponsored research programs with Moderna, United States, Dynavax, and Pfizer, United States on CMV vaccines. All other authors have nothing to disclose.

REFERENCES

1. Shetty AK, Maldonado Y. Antiretroviral drugs to prevent mother-to-child transmission of HIV during breastfeeding. Curr HIV Res 2013;11(2):102–25.
2. UNAIDS (2024). Global HIV Statistics Fact Sheet 2024. Available at: https://www.unaids.org/sites/default/files/media_asset/UNAIDS_FactSheet_en.pdf. (Accessed September 4, 2024).
3. Ruel T, Penazzato M, Zech JM, et al. Novel approaches to postnatal prophylaxis to eliminate vertical transmission of HIV. Glob Health Sci Pract 2023;11(2).
4. Eke AC, Lockman S, Mofenson LM. Antiretroviral treatment of HIV/AIDS during pregnancy. JAMA 2023;329(15):1308–9.
5. Kim J, Vasan S, Kim JH, et al. Current approaches to HIV vaccine development: a narrative review. J Int AIDS Soc 2021;24(Suppl 7):e25793.
6. Marichannegowda MH, Mengual M, Kumar A, et al. Different evolutionary pathways of HIV-1 between fetus and mother perinatal transmission pairs indicate unique immune selection in fetuses. Cell Rep Med 2021;2(7):100315.
7. Wolinsky SM, Wike CM, Korber BT, et al. Selective transmission of human immunodeficiency virus type-1 variants from mothers to infants. Science 1992; 255(5048):1134–7.

8. Rainwater SM, Wu X, Nduati R, et al. Cloning and characterization of functional subtype A HIV-1 envelope variants transmitted through breastfeeding. Curr HIV Res 2007;5(2):189–97.
9. Ahmad N, Baroudy BM, Baker RC, et al. Genetic analysis of human immunodeficiency virus type 1 envelope V3 region isolates from mothers and infants after perinatal transmission. J Virol 1995;69(2):1001–12.
10. Dickover RE, Garratty EM, Plaeger S, et al. Perinatal transmission of major, minor, and multiple maternal human immunodeficiency virus type 1 variants in utero and intrapartum. J Virol 2001;75(5):2194–203.
11. Scarlatti G, Leitner T, Hodara V, et al. Neutralizing antibodies and viral characteristics in mother-to-child transmission of HIV-1. AIDS 1993;7:S45–8.
12. Verhofstede C, Demecheleer E, Cabooter ND, et al. Diversity of the human immunodeficiency virus type 1 (HIV-1) *env* sequence after vertical transmission in mother-child pairs infected with HIV-1 subtype A. J Virol 2003;77(5):3050–7.
13. Kwiek JJ, Russell ES, Dang KK, et al. The molecular epidemiology of HIV-1 envelope diversity during HIV-1 subtype C vertical transmission in Malawian mother–infant pairs. AIDS 2008;22(7):863–71.
14. Permar SR, Fong Y, Vandergrift N, et al. Maternal HIV-1 envelope-specific antibody responses and reduced risk of perinatal transmission. J Clin Invest 2015; 125(7):2702–6.
15. Moody MA, Pedroza-Pacheco I, Vandergrift NA, et al. Immune perturbations in HIV-1–infected individuals who make broadly neutralizing antibodies. Science immunology 2016;1(1):aag0851.
16. Kumar A, Smith CE, Giorgi EE, et al. Infant transmitted/founder HIV-1 viruses from peripartum transmission are neutralization resistant to paired maternal plasma. PLoS Pathog 2018;14(4):e1006944.
17. Baan E, de Ronde A, Stax M, et al. HIV-1 autologous antibody neutralization associates with mother to child transmission. PLoS One 2013;8(7):e69274.
18. Mangold JF, Goswami R, Nelson AN, et al. Maternal intervention to prevent mother-to-child transmission of HIV: moving beyond antiretroviral therapy. Pediatr Infect Dis J 2021;40(5S):S5–10.
19. Pollara J, McGuire E, Fouda GG, et al. Association of HIV-1 envelope-specific breast milk IgA responses with reduced risk of postnatal mother-to-child transmission of HIV-1. J Virol 2015;89(19):9952–61.
20. Barrows BM, Krebs SJ, Jian N, et al. Fc receptor engagement of HIV-1 Env-specific antibodies in mothers and infants predicts reduced vertical transmission. Front Immunol 2022;13:1051501.
21. Mabuka J, Nduati R, Odem-Davis K, et al. HIV-specific antibodies capable of ADCC are common in breastmilk and are associated with reduced risk of transmission in women with high viral loads. PLoS Pathog 2012;8(6):e1002739.
22. Haynes BF, Gilbert PB, McElrath MJ, et al. Immune-correlates analysis of an HIV-1 vaccine efficacy trial. N Engl J Med 2012;366(14):1275–86.
23. Perez LG, Martinez DR, Decamp AC, et al. V1V2-specific complement activating serum IgG as a correlate of reduced HIV-1 infection risk in RV144. PLoS One 2017;12(7):e0180720.
24. Milligan C, Richardson BA, John-Stewart G, et al. Passively acquired antibody-dependent cellular cytotoxicity (ADCC) activity in HIV-infected infants is associated with reduced mortality. Cell Host Microbe 2015;17(4):500–6.
25. Ackerman ME, Mikhailova A, Brown EP, et al. Polyfunctional HIV-specific antibody responses are associated with spontaneous HIV control. PLoS Pathog 2016; 12(1):e1005315.

26. Wright PF, Lambert JS, Gorse GJ, et al. Immunization with envelope MN rgp120 vaccine in human immunodeficiency virus-infected pregnant women. J Infect Dis 1999;180(4):1080–8.
27. Hompe ED, Jacobson DL, Eudailey JA, et al. Maternal humoral immune responses do not predict postnatal HIV-1 transmission risk in antiretroviral-treated mothers from the IMPAACT PROMISE Study. mSphere 2019;4(5). https://doi.org/10.1128/mSphere.00716-19.
28. Nelson AN, Dennis M, Mangold JF, et al. Leveraging antigenic seniority for maternal vaccination to prevent mother-to-child transmission of HIV-1. NPJ Vaccines 2022;7(1):87.
29. Salloum M, Paviotti A, Bastiaens H, et al. The inclusion of pregnant women in vaccine clinical trials: an overview of late-stage clinical trials' records between 2018 and 2023. Vaccine 2023;41(48):7076–83.
30. Stranix-Chibanda L, Yu C, Isaacs MB, et al. A retrospective analysis of incident pregnancy in phase 1 and 2a HIV-1 vaccine study participants does not support concern for adverse pregnancy or birth outcomes. BMC Infect Dis 2021;21(1):802.
31. Centers for disease C. Vaccine safety for moms-to-Be. 2021. Available at: https://www.cdc.gov/vaccines/pregnancy/vacc-safety.html. Accessed June 7, 2024.
32. Kumar A, Giorgi EE, Tu JJ, et al. Mutations that confer resistance to broadly-neutralizing antibodies define HIV-1 variants of transmitting mothers from that of non-transmitting mothers. PLoS Pathog 2021;17(4):e1009478.
33. Tu JJ, Kumar A, Giorgi EE, et al. Vertical HIV-1 transmission in the setting of maternal broad and potent antibody responses. J Virol 2022;96(11):e0023122.
34. Recent interventions to improve retention in HIV care and adherence to antiretroviral treatment among adolescents and youth: a systematic review. AIDS Patient Care STDS 2019;33(6):237–52.
35. Focosi D, McConnell S, Casadevall A, et al. Monoclonal antibody therapies against SARS-CoV-2. Lancet Infect Dis 2022;22(11):e311–26.
36. Jones JM. Use of nirsevimab for the prevention of respiratory syncytial virus disease among infants and young children: recommendations of the Advisory Committee on Immunization Practices—United States, 2023. MMWR Morbidity and mortality weekly report 2023;72.
37. Reeves DB, Mayer BT, deCamp AC, et al. High monoclonal neutralization titers reduced breakthrough HIV-1 viral loads in the Antibody Mediated Prevention trials. Nat Commun 2023;14(1):8299.
38. Asokan M, Dias J, Liu C, et al. Fc-mediated effector function contributes to the in vivo antiviral effect of an HIV neutralizing antibody. Proc Natl Acad Sci USA 2020;117(31):18754–63.
39. Wang P, Gajjar MR, Yu J, et al. Quantifying the contribution of Fc-mediated effector functions to the antiviral activity of anti-HIV-1 IgG1 antibodies in vivo. Proc Natl Acad Sci U S A 2020;117(30):18002–9.
40. Stephenson KE, Wagh K, Korber B, et al. Vaccines and broadly neutralizing antibodies for HIV-1 prevention. Annu Rev Immunol 2020;38:673–703.
41. Frattari GS, Caskey M, Sogaard OS. Broadly neutralizing antibodies for HIV treatment and cure approaches. Curr Opin HIV AIDS 2023;18(4):157–63.
42. Cohen YZ, Lorenzi JC, Krassnig L, et al. Relationship between latent and rebound viruses in a clinical trial of anti–HIV-1 antibody 3BNC117. J Exp Med 2018;215(9):2311–24.
43. Riddler SA, Zheng L, Durand CM, et al. Randomized clinical trial to assess the impact of the broadly neutralizing HIV-1 monoclonal antibody VRC01 on HIV-1

persistence in individuals on effective ART. Open Forum Infect Dis 2018;5(10): ofy242.
44. Himes JE, Goswami R, Mangan RJ, et al. Polyclonal HIV envelope-specific breast milk antibodies limit founder SHIV acquisition and cell-associated virus loads in infant rhesus monkeys. Mucosal Immunol 2018;11(6):1716–26.
45. Sneller MC, Blazkova J, Justement JS, et al. Combination anti-HIV antibodies provide sustained virological suppression. Nature 2022;606(7913):375–81.
46. Williamson C, Lynch RM, Moore PL. Anticipating HIV viral escape - resistance to active and passive immunization. Curr Opin HIV AIDS 2023;18(6):342–8.
47. Trkola A, Kuster H, Rusert P, et al. Delay of HIV-1 rebound after cessation of antiretroviral therapy through passive transfer of human neutralizing antibodies. Nat Med 2005;11(6):615–22.
48. Sneller MC, Blazkova J, Justement JS, et al. Combination anti-HIV antibodies provide sustained virological suppression. Nature 2022;606(7913):375–81.
49. Mabuka J, Goo L, Omenda MM, et al. HIV-1 maternal and infant variants show similar sensitivity to broadly neutralizing antibodies, but sensitivity varies by subtype. AIDS 2013;27(10):1535–44.
50. Martinez DR, Tu JJ, Kumar A, et al. Maternal broadly neutralizing antibodies can select for neutralization-resistant, infant-transmitted/founder HIV variants. mBio 2020;11(2).

Human Immunodeficiency Virus and Breastfeeding

Clinical Considerations and Mechanisms of Transmission in the Modern Era of Combined Antiretroviral Therapy

Jenna S. Powers, MD[a], Medrine Kihanga, BS[b],
Lisa Marie Cranmer, MD, MPH[c,d,*]

KEYWORDS

• HIV • Breastfeeding • Antiretroviral therapy (ART) • Risk reduction

KEY POINTS

- Postnatal human immunodeficiency virus (HIV) transmission through breastfeeding is a rare event when risk reduction strategies are in place.
- Cell-associated HIV in breast milk may be a source of transmission in the setting of sustained undetectable maternal viral load.
- The "gut-breast" axis plays an important role in potential mechanisms of increased transmission in the setting of mixed breast feeding and is a critical area for future studies.

INTRODUCTION

The optimization and widespread use of combined antiretroviral therapy (cART) have significantly transformed the landscape of human immunodeficiency virus (HIV) care during pregnancy and through the postpartum period. Without cART, the risk of HIV transmission through breastfeeding is estimated to be around 15%, depending on several factors including maternal HIV viral load, breastfeeding duration, and feeding practices.[1,2] Consequently, historic guidelines have recommended a zero-risk strategy in high-income settings where infant formula is widely accessible, advising replacement feeding with formula or banked, pasteurized donor human milk for women living with HIV (WLHIV). However, with sustained cART-induced HIV viral

[a] Emory School of Medicine, Emory University, Atlanta, GA 30322, USA; [b] Earlham College, Richmond, IN 47374, USA; [c] Department of Pediatrics, Emory University, 2015 Uppergate Drive, Suite 534, Atlanta, GA 30322, USA; [d] Department of Epidemiology, Emory University, 1518 Clifton Road, Atlanta, GA 30322, USA
* Corresponding author. 2015 Uppergate Drive, Suite 534, Atlanta, GA 30322.
E-mail address: lisa.marie.cranmer@emory.edu

Clin Perinatol 51 (2024) 783–799
https://doi.org/10.1016/j.clp.2024.08.001 perinatology.theclinics.com
0095-5108/24/

suppression, transmission of HIV through breastfeeding has become exceedingly rare, dropping to less than 1%.[3–5] Reflecting advancements in cART, the American Academy of Pediatrics (AAP) and the United States Department of Health and Human Services (DHHS) Panel on Treatment of HIV During Pregnancy and Prevention of Perinatal Transmission have made pivotal changes in clinical guidance to support breastfeeding for WLHIV with sustained undetectable viral loads throughout pregnancy and postpartum.[6,7] Similarly, the British HIV Association, the European AIDS Clinical Society, and other high-income countries have developed formal guidance to support breastfeeding as an option for WLHIV.[8–11]

This review examines the current state of knowledge on HIV transmission through breast milk in the cART era. The authors explore the risk factors and transmission mechanisms relevant to WLHIV with sustained viral suppression, identify research gaps with direct implications for clinical practice, and highlight risk reduction strategies employed globally.

STATEMENT OF INCLUSION

The authors endorse a broad perspective on gender and acknowledge the challenges posed by gender bias in health care. We also recognize the historic underrepresentation of women in HIV research. Consequently, we will use the term "women" to refer to individuals assigned female sex at birth, which may include people of other gender identities (transgender male individuals and nonbinary individuals). The term "breastfeeding" denotes the act of feeding a child with milk produced from human mammary glands. We acknowledge that some transgender and nonbinary individuals may prefer the term "chest feeding" and that medical providers should consider an individual's preference of terminology when providing patient care. Our goal is to respect and honor people of diverse gender identities within the scope of this review.

EPIDEMIOLOGY OF HUMAN IMMUNODEFICIENCY VIRUS TRANSMISSION THROUGH BREASTFEEDING IN THE COMBINED ANTIRETROVIRAL THERAPY ERA

Without maternal cART, breast milk transmission (BMT) risk is estimated to be around 15% (95% confidence interval [CI] 7, 22%).[12] Clinical risk factors associated with BMT identified in studies from the pre-cART era include elevated maternal plasma and breast milk HIV viral load, low maternal CD4+ T-cell count, and early introduction of formula or solid foods ("mixed feeding"; **Fig. 1**).[13–16] Risk is higher during early lactation (~6% in the first 4–6 weeks), with ongoing risk of transmission risk estimated at 0.9% per month for the duration of breastfeeding.[1,13] Maternal cART initiated during or before pregnancy is associated with lower rates of BMT, but estimates vary by geographic region and timing of maternal cART initiation. A meta-analysis of 6 studies in low-income settings found low rates of BMT among mothers on cART during the first 6 months of breastfeeding (1.1% [95% CI 0.3, 1.9%]); not all mothers had documented sustained viral supression.[5] Maternal cART discontinuation, detectable plasma or breast milk HIV RNA, and lack of sustained plasma viral suppression have been associated with BMT in the context of maternal access to cART.[5,17] A secondary analysis of the Breastfeeding, Antiretrovirals, and Nutrition study in Malawi found that detectable HIV viral load in plasma (>40 copies/mL) was associated with 40-fold increased risk of infant transmission (hazard ratio [HR] 40 [95% CI 15, 107]); detection of HIV in maternal breast milk (>56 copies/mL) was associated with approximately 8-fold higher risk of infant transmission (HR 7.8 [95% CI 3.1, 19.2]). No transmission events occurred in this study when maternal plasma viral load remained below 100 copies/mL.[17] In published studies including over 3000 mother–infant pairs with

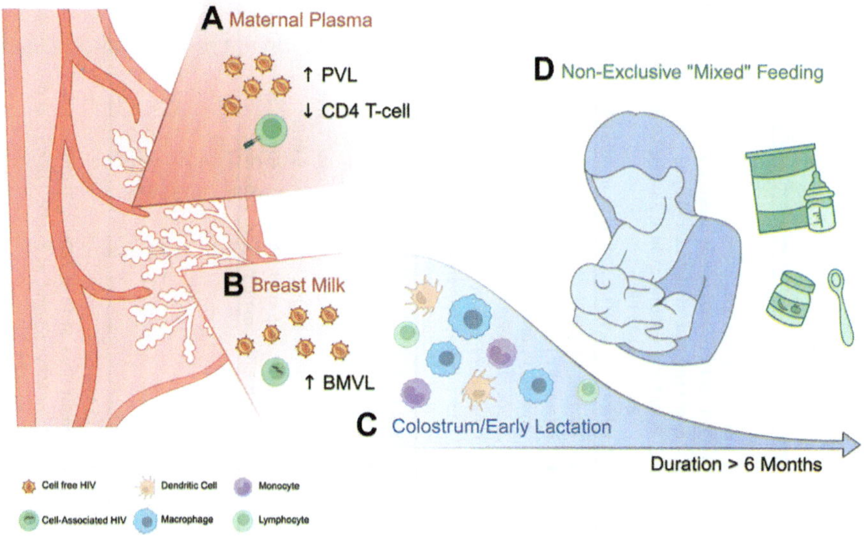

Fig. 1. Risk factors for infant HIV transmission through breastfeeding. (A) Elevated maternal plasma viral load (PVL) and diminished CD4 T-cell counts increase risk of BMT. (B) Breast milk viral load (BMVL) including cell-free and cell-associated HIV is associated with increased risk of BMT.[13–16] (C) Longitudinal analyses have demonstrated higher BMVLs in the first few weeks of breast feeding, possibly related to the increased cellularity of colostrum and early lactation.[53,84] However, cumulative exposure is also an important risk factor.[5,16,68] (D) Mixed breastfeeding (MBF) has been consistently shown to increase transmission risk in the pre-cART era.[58–61] (Created with BioRender.com.)

detailed data on BMT timing and serial maternal viral load monitoring in the era of cART, a total of 19 BMT cases occurred under the following conditions: maternal plasma viral load greater than 50 copies/mL (n = 10), report of poor maternal ART adherence (n = 2), or maternal cART initiation less than 3 months prior to delivery (n = 7) (**Table 1**).[3,18–22] Of note, for 3 BMT transmission cases, mothers had sustained viral suppression (>3 months) prior to the detection of HIV infection of their infants, but maternal cART was started late during the third trimester of pregnancy and mothers had detectable plasma or breast milk viral loads in the early postpartum period. For example, an infant from the DolPHIN-2 trial had confirmed HIV infection at 18 months of age after serial negative HIV PCR tests from delivery through the age of 12 months. While the mother of this infant had documented viral suppression less than 50 copies/mL for 6 months before the infant's HIV was diagnosed, the mother did not achieve viral suppression until 12 weeks postpartum.[22,23] No infant transmission events have been reported among mothers who initiated cART preconception and demonstrated sustained viral suppression throughout pregnancy and breastfeeding[21,24–32] (see **Table 1**).

MECHANISMS OF BREAST MILK TRANSMISSION

For BMT to occur, HIV virions must first bypass the mammary epithelium, remain infectious within the breast milk, traverse infant mucosal barriers, and establish infection in the infant oropharynx or gastrointestinal (GI) tract.[33] This route involves a complex

Table 1
Breast milk transmission

Maternal cART Initiation	Study	Population *(N, Location)*	Timing and Type of cART *[Duration Median (IQR)]*	Breastfeeding Practices *(Duration Median [IQR])*	Infant BMT *(Overall rate, transmission details)*
Postpartum	PROMISE Flynn et al,[3] 2018	N = 1220 Sub-Saharan Africa India	7–14 d PP (N = 527) 2nd/3rd Trimester (N = 648) • 26 w GA (IQR 21, 31) LPV/r + (AZT/3 TC) or (TDF/FTC)	EBF/MBF not specified	7/1219 (0.6%) • 1 infant HIV+ at 3 m; MPVL <40 c/mL Prior MPVL >200 c/mL at delivery, PVL>50 c/mL 6 w PP • 1 infant HIV+ at 9m; MPVL <40 c/mL; Prior MPVL <40c/mL at 14 w, 26 w PP, MPVL >200 c/mL at delivery, 6 w PP • 5 infants HIV+, MPVL >200 c/mL (median 13,479 c/mL)
Pregnancy	Mma Bna Shapiro et al,[19] 2010	N = 527 Botswana	2nd/3rd Trimester • 26–34 w GA LPV/r or ABC + (AZT/3 TC)	EBF (93%)/MBF	2/517(0.4%); 10 LTFU • 1 infant HIV+ at 3 m, MPVL and BM VL <50 c/mL Prior MPVL at delivery 257 c/mL, MPVL and BMVL <50 c/mL at 1 m PP • 1 infant HIV+ at 3 m, MPVL and BMVL <50 c/mL Prior MPVL at delivery <50, PVL and BMVL at 1 m PP <50 c/mL. Mother reported cART adherence challenges
	Safe Milk for African Children (SMAC) Giuliano et al,[20] 2013	N = 288 Malawi	2nd/3rd Trimester • 26w GA (IQR 24, 30) • 83 d (IQR 62, 87) AP among BMT NVP+ (AZT/3 TC) or (d4T/3 TC)	EBF 26w (IQR 25, 26)	6/278 (2.1%) • 1 infant HIV+ at 3 m, MPVL <40 c/mL, BMVL 90 c/mL Prior MPVL and BMVL <40 c/mL at 1 m PP • 1 infant HIV+ at 12 m, MPVL <40 c/mL, BMVL unknown Prior MPVL<40 c/mL at 1 m, 3 m, 6 m PP; BMVL 293 c/mL at 1 m PP, BMVL <40 c/mL at 3 m, 6 m PP • 4 infants HIV+, maternal PVL >200 c/mL
	Tshilo Dikotla Study Volpe et al,[85] 2022	N = 247 Bostwana	2nd/3rd Trimester • 16–36 w GA DTG or EFV + (TDF/FTC)	EBF/MBF All: 24.7 w (range .1, 86) EBF: 18 w (range 0, 41)	0/247 (0.0%)
	DOLPHIN-2 Malaba et al,[22] 2022	N = 268 South Africa, Uganda	3rd Trimester • 55 d (IQR 33, 77) AP EFV or DTG + (TDF/FTC) or (TDF/3TC)	EBF/MBF	1/242 (0.4%) • 1 infant HIV+ at 18 m, MPVL <50 c/mL Prior MPVL 69 c/mL at 6 w PP, 126 c/mL at delivery and 24 w PP

Preconception	KIULARCO Luoga et al,[18] 2018	N = 228 Tanzania	3rd Trimester/preconception • 23 m (IQR 4, 52) AP EFV+ (TDF/FTC) or (TDF/3 TC)	EBF/MBF 52 w (IQR 41, 54)	2/186 (1%); 19 LTFU; 18 Died • 1 infant HIV+, MPVL 144,111 copies/mL at 5 wk PP • 1 infant HIV+, mother discontinued cART
	Crisinel et al,[24] 2021	N = 20 Switzerland	Preconception (18), 1st trimester (2)	EBF/MBF 6.3 m (IQR 2.5, 11.1)	0/20 (0%)
	Nashid et al,[25] 2020	N = 3 Canada	Preconception	EBF/MBF	0/3 (0%)
	ISOSS[28] 2022	N = 150 England	Preconception/Pregnancy	EBF/MBF 56 d (IQR 23 d, 140 d)	0/106 (0%)
	Yusuf et al,[27] 2021	N = 10 US	Preconception	EBF 4.4 m (1.0, 8.5)	0/10 (0%)
	Koay et al,[31] 2022	N = 7 US	Preconception/Pregnancy	EBF/MBF 2 w–6 m	0/7 (0%)
	Prestileo et al,[29] 2022	N = 13 Italy	Preconception (9), 1st trimester (4) LPV/r or RAL + (TDF/FTC)	EBF/MBF not specified 5.4 m	0/13 (0%)
	Weiss et al,[30] 2022	N = 30 Germany	Preconception INSTI, NNRTI, or PI-based cART	EBF/MBF 2 w–12 m	0/22 (0%); 8 LTFU
	Levison et al,[26] 2023	N = 72[a] US and Canada	Preconception (62)/Pregnancy INSTI, NNRTI, or PI-based cART	EBF/MBF 24 w (range 1 d, 72 w)	0/68 (0%); 4 LTFU
	Abuogi et al,[32] 2023	N = 13 US	Preconception (11)/Pregnancy • 39 w (37, 40) AP	EBF/MBF 62 d (16, 188)	0/10 (0%)
	Boyce et al,[21] 2024	N = 7 US	Preconception/pregnancy	EBF/MBF 2 m–20 m	1/7 (14%) • 1 Infant HIV+ at 17 m, MPVL 5.9 million c/mL, LTFU after 4 w

Abbreviations: 3 TC, lamivudine; AP, antepartum; AZT, zidovudine; BMT, breast milk transmission; BMVL, breast milk viral load; cART, combination antiretroviral therapy; d, days; DTG, dolutegravir; EBF, exclusive breastfeeding; EFV, efavirenz; FTC, emtricitabine; GA, gestational age; LPV/r, lopinavir/ritonavir; m, months; MBF, mixed breastfeeding; MPVL, maternal plasma viral load; NFV, nelfinavir; NNRTI, non-nucleoside reverse transcriptase inhibitor; NSTI, integrase strand transfer inhibitor; NVP, nevirapine; PI, protease inhibitor; PP, postpartum; RAL, raltegravir; TDF, tenofovir disoproxil fumarate; w, weeks; y, years.

[a] N, 51 unique cases not reported by Yusuf, Koay or Abuogii.

interplay of HIV viral dynamics with maternal and infant immunologic and microbiologic factors that shape transmission risk (**Fig. 2**).

Human Immunodeficiency Virus Viral Dynamics in Breast Milk

Breast milk of WLHIV contains both cell-free and cell-associated viruses. Cell-free HIV RNA is detected in over half of WLHIV in the absence of cART and is strongly positively associated with concurrent plasma RNA levels.[34] Documented temporal correlation of intermittent HIV RNA in plasma and breast milk suggests that cell-free virus in breast milk arises from plasma transport, though local replication and/or virion production may also occur.[34,35] HIV infects several types of cells in breast milk, including CD4+ T-cells, macrophages, and mammary epithelial cells.[33] The cellular composition of breast milk is dynamic overtime; overall cellularity is higher in colostrum and early breast milk, but frequencies of T lymphocytes and macrophages can fluctuate in response to pathogen exposure and hormonal changes.[33] The CD4+ T-cell reservoir is thought to be primarily responsible for cell-associated BMT, but HIV-infected macrophages and epithelial cells may facilitate cell-to-cell T lymphocyte infection and contribute to HIV viral persistence in breast milk.[33] Cell-associated HIV DNA in breast milk independently predicts transmission after adjusting for plasma and breast milk cell-free viral load from pre-cART studies.[36] Sequence analysis of viral envelope fragments in maternal breast milk and plasma of infants who acquired HIV postnatally suggested that transmission from cell-associated HIV DNA in breast milk occurs throughout early and late breastfeeding periods, whereas cell-free HIV RNA was associated only with infant transmissions that occurred after 9 months of breastfeeding.[36]

Treatment with cART suppresses cell-free RNA in both plasma and breast milk, but cell-associated DNA can persist in latent memory CD4+ T-cells or macrophages after cART initiation and is a potential source for BMT.[33–35,37] Studies characterizing cell-associated HIV reservoirs in breast milk among women with long-term viral suppression are lacking; proviral DNA levels in breast milk after cART initiation have been followed for less than 6 months.[33–35,37] In addition, latent CD4+ T-cell reservoirs in breast milk may have a lower activation threshold for latency reversal and more robust production of replication-competent HIV virions. In vitro activation resulted in a higher number of HIV Gag-secreting cells in breast milk compared to peripheral blood (500 vs 45), even when the quantity of HIV DNA was comparable between compartments.[38]

Mastitis, or breast inflammation, is known to influence breast milk HIV viral dynamics. Mastitis is characterized by compromised epithelial barriers, enhanced recruitment and translocation of neutrophils, macrophages, lymphocytes, and elevated levels of cell-free HIV RNA in breast milk in pre-cART studies.[15,35,39,40] Subclinical mastitis, as measured by the ratio of sodium to potassium (Na:K) and/or neutrophil count, was associated with higher levels of cell-free HIV RNA but not cell-associated HIV DNA among mothers not taking cART.[41] Clinical circumstances leading to mastitis, such as infrequent breast emptying or rapid weaning, should be avoided among WLHIV as a precaution, although it is unknown if mastitis induces virus production from breast milk cellular reservoirs and/or an influx of virus-containing cells into the milk in the setting of cART.[42–44]

The Influence of Breast Milk Immunity on Human Immunodeficiency Virus Transmission

Studies from the pre-cART era demonstrate that innate and adaptive immune responses in the breast milk compartment influence HIV replication and the risk for BMT. Innate immune factors in human milk such as mucins, lactoferrin, and bile salt stimulating lipase inhibit cell-free HIV replication but are less protective against cell-

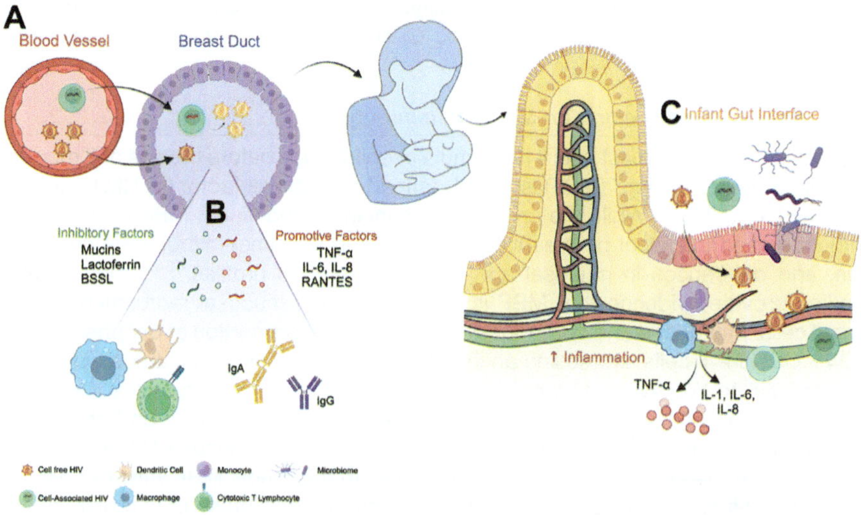

Fig. 2. Maternal and infant immune factors that impact postnatal HIV transmission through breast milk. (A) The mammary epithelium prevents HIV entry, maintaining at least a 100 fold lower HIV RNA level compared to plasma.[48] (B) Breast milk contains inhibitory factors, including innate components (lactoferrins, homeostatic cytokines, and mucins) that may protect against cell-free HIV replication.[45–47] Pro-inflammatory cytokine profiles (TNF, IL-6, IL-8 and RANTES) are associated with increased risk for BMT.[49,50] HIV-specific cytotoxic T lymphocytes (CTL), IgA, and IgG antibodies affect BMT. (C) Disruption of the infant gut interface enables HIV to traverse the epithelial layer, leading to microbiota disturbance and allowing the virus to establish infection in CD4+ CCR5+ T cells.[54] (Created with BioRender.com.)

associated virus.[45–49] Pro-inflammatory cytokines, such as TNF, IL-6, IL-8, and RANTES, in breast milk are associated with elevated breast milk viral loads and increased transmission risk.[49,50] Breast milk HIV-specific cellular IFN-γ responses lowered transmission risk by 70% (adjusted odds ratio [aOR] 0.29 [95% CI 0.092, 0.91]) in a Kenyan cohort.[51] In addition, passively transferred maternal IgA and immunoglobulin G (IgG) in breast milk may exert virologic control through direct neutralization and other Fc-mediated functions. Pollara and colleagues[52] found that HIV-1 envelope-specific breast milk IgA levels were associated with reduced risk of BMT, but no such association was found for HIV-specific IgG in breast milk.

The Infant Gastrointestinal Tract Immune Interface

The link between breast milk and the infant GI tract (also called the "gut-breast axis") is essential for both GI tract and systemic infant immune development. The infant GI tract is relatively permeable or "leaky," allowing low-dose systemic exposure to dietary antigens or pathogens while sustaining a tolerant immune environment characterized by increased regulatory T-cells (Tregs), Th17, and Th2 cells.[53] However, these conditions may inadvertently be conducive to HIV transmission. The infant gut is populated with high levels of CD4+ CCR5+ T-cells that are the targets for initial HIV infection (see **Fig. 2**B).[54] Cell-free HIV may also bypass the permeable GI tract epithelium by transcytosis or breaks in the epithelial barrier.[55,56] Epithelial barrier integrity is heavily influenced by the gut microbiome, and breastfeeding plays a vital role in its development by promoting structural integrity, functionality, and maintenance of mucosal barrier properties. Conditions that dysregulate infant GI microbiome, increase epithelial permeability, or also increase mucosal immune cell trafficking, such as infant oral thrush and GI illness, have the potential to increase risk of HIV transmission.[57]

The Effect of Mixed Feeding on Mucosal Immunity

Coadministration of breast milk with formula or solid foods before the age of 6 months, or "mixed breastfeeding" (MBF) is a well-defined clinical risk factor for BMT from the pre-cART era.[58–60,61] While the precise mechanism is undefined, MBF is associated with increased intestinal permeability, alterations in intestinal microbiome composition, and differences in mucosal and systemic immune profiles.[62–65] Two notable studies provide evidence that MBF is associated with mucosal recruitment of HIV target cells. McFarland and colleagues[66] found a higher proportion of peripheral blood CD4+ CCR5+ T-cells expressing an intestinal homing profile (β7hi) among Ugandan infants born to WLHIV who were MBF compared to exclusive breastfeeding (EBF). Wood and colleagues[67] observed higher expression of chemokines and chemokine receptors implicated in recruiting HIV target cells in the oral mucosa of South African infants who experienced MBF compared to EBF. In this study, MBF was also associated with greater diversity of bacterial species in the infant's intestinal microbiome and higher levels of peripheral CD4+ T-cell activation. Additional studies are needed to understand how the type of mixed feeding (nonhuman milk vs solid food) influences the intestinal microbiome, mucosal, and systemic immune maturation and BMT risk. A pooled analysis of West and South African mother–infant pairs in the pre-cART era found similar rates of postnatal HIV transmission among infants whose mothers practiced MBF with nonhuman milk compared to EBF infants, while introduction of solid foods before 2 months of life was associated with a 3 fold higher risk of BMT.[68] It is unknown whether mixed feeding is associated with BMT among infants born to mothers on sustained cART. Njom Nlend and colleagues[69] demonstrated higher BMT for MBF versus EBF infants (3 out of 14 [21%] vs 25 out of 658 [3.8%]) in a cohort of mother–infant pairs from Cameroon, of whom 52% of mothers were taking cART, but the risk of MBF on BMT was not stratified by maternal cART use. In a recent systematic review and meta-analysis of breast milk HIV transmission in the cART era, no studies provided data on mixed feeding.[5] Investigating the mechanism of increased BMT risk in mixed feeding will inform future studies needed to define the actual risk with long-term ART suppression. Similarly, understanding relative BMT risk related to infant gut mucosal inflammation induced by liquid formula and solid food introduction in the context of maternal cART will be important to strengthen evidence-driven and patient-centered counseling.

CLINICAL MANAGEMENT OF BREASTFEEDING MOTHERS WITH HUMAN IMMUNODEFICIENCY VIRUS AND THEIR INFANTS TO REDUCE BREAST MILK TRANSMISSION

The clinical care of WLHIV who choose to breastfeed and their infants involves multidisciplinary care by obstetricians, pediatricians, lactation specialists, and infectious disease specialists. Interventions to reduce BMT extend from preconception through pregnancy, infant delivery, and postpartum follow-up.

Maternal Antiretroviral Therapy

Initiation of maternal cART as early as possible, ideally preconception, and maintenance of viral suppression through pregnancy and breastfeeding are critical to avoid BMT. The postpartum period, often called "the fourth trimester," introduces unique individual and structural barriers for WLHIV to maintain cART adherence, including sleep deprivation while caring for a newborn, hormonal changes associated with mood disturbance, and increased financial burden. Studies have consistently demonstrated increased rates of viral rebound, poorer adherence to ART, and poor retention in care during the postpartum period.[70–72] Frequent maternal virologic monitoring (every 1–2 months) while breastfeeding is recommended, alongside endorsement of behavioral health strategies to optimize adherence, including use of mobile phone alarm reminders, pill boxes or prepackaged medications, and identification of an adherence support partner.[73,74] In the future, long-acting antiretroviral agents could be of particular benefit to ensure optimal drug levels while breastfeeding, and pharmacokinetic studies are underway.[75,76]

Infant Antiretroviral Prophylaxis

Infant antiretroviral prophylaxis serves as an added layer of protection against BMT, but the selection of optimal agents and duration of prophylaxis for breastfeeding infants vary considerably among published guidelines. The Promoting Maternal and Infant Survival Everywhere (PROMISE) trial compared infant prophylaxis with nevirapine to maternal cART and found no difference in transmission rates at 6 months or 12 months.[3] Some experts recommend single-drug prophylaxis (zidovudine or nevirapine) through 4 to 6 weeks after breastfeeding cessation, while others endorse prophylaxis for only 2 to 4 weeks, similar to non-breastfeeding populations.[30,32] A more conservative approach includes 3 drug prophylaxis (nevirapine or raltegravir with zidovudine and lamivudine) for 4 to 6 weeks, followed by nevirapine or zidovudine through 4 to 6 weeks after breastfeeding cessation.[27] More studies are needed to provide insight into the duration of infant prophylaxis and whether or not triple ART infant prophylaxis could be beneficial in the early stages of breastfeeding when there may be a higher theoretic risk for HIV transmission informed by pre-cART studies. Infants taking prolonged antiretroviral prophylaxis should have periodic screening for antiretroviral drug toxicities including neutropenia or hepatic dysfunction at baseline and after 2 to 4 weeks, with additional follow-up testing for abnormal results or clinical symptoms. Virologic monitoring of infants who are breastfeeding should include HIV DNA or RNA PCR at 14 to 21 days of life, 1 to 2 months of life, 4 to 6 months of life, and every 2 months thereafter if breastfeeding continues. Infants should receive additional HIV DNA or RNA PCR 6 weeks, 3 months, and 6 months after breastfeeding cessation.[7]

In the future, use of broadly neutralizing antibodies (bNAbs) targeting the HIV envelope for infant prophylaxis could lessen the burden of ART toxicity and decrease frequency of administration. Phase 1 clinical trials in infants exposed to HIV have shown a positive safety profile.[77,78] The Tatelo study, a 1 out of 2 clinical trial in Botswana, demonstrated sustained viral suppression for 24 weeks among 11 out of 25 infants with HIV who received bNAb-only treatment, pointing to the potential for bNAbs as infant prophylaxis.[79] Use of long-acting injectable antiretroviral agents is being evaluated for pre-exposure prophylaxis in adults; age-de-escalation pharmacokinetic studies could also inform infant use in the setting of breastfeeding.

Establishing Exclusive Breastfeeding and Addressing Clinical Complications

Less than 25% of the general US population practices EBF for the first 6 months, and proactive involvement of a lactation specialist is beneficial to support WLHIV to establish and maintain EBF.[80] Prenatal consultation to provide education and ensure access to lactation pump supplies in advance of delivery, in-hospital assistance with optimal positioning and infant latch and outpatient follow-up to address challenges with milk supply enhance the potential for successful EBF.

Close collaboration between a lactation specialist and a pediatrician is essential for management of breastfeeding complications. Short-term supplementation with pasteurized human donor milk, flash-heated breast milk, or infant formula may be needed in particular circumstances, such as delayed milk production, mastitis, severe infant thrush or GI illness, and detectable maternal viremia.[7] In the case of mastitis, or cracked/bleeding nipples, a mother can feed from the non-affected breast while pumping and disposing breast milk from the affected breast until resolution. Management of maternal viremia should involve temporary cessation of breastfeeding while obtaining a repeat HIV viral load. If maternal viremia persists, breastfeeding cessation should be strongly considered and some experts recommend initiation of 3 drug infant prophylaxis for 4 to 6 weeks.[32] If maternal viremia resolves on repeat testing and any adherence challenges have been addressed, breastfeeding may continue. Guidance on the duration of breastfeeding varies; some experts advise mothers to wean after 6 months, while others defer to maternal preference. Parents should be counseled to introduce a bottle before the of age 1 month to prepare for eventual weaning. Slow weaning over 2 to 4 weeks is recommended, replacing one feed with formula every 2 to 3 days.[32]

Approach to Shared Decision-making and Infant Feeding Counseling

Shared decision-making between WLHIV and medical providers regarding infant feeding choices is endorsed by updated clinical guidelines, and health care providers should initiate early conversations about feeding options for WLHIV who are pregnant or considering pregnancy. Prior to changes in AAP and DHHS guidance, many WLHIV opted to breastfeed without communicating their choice to their health care provider due to fear of stigma and lack of perceived support.[5] Feeding choices among WLHIV are influenced by many individual, cultural, and health care system factors.[81] Providers should explore an individual's motivations for breastfeeding and discuss all feeding options with patients in a nonjudgmental manner. Replacement feeding with certified donor human milk or formula is the only option to ensure 0% risk of HIV transmission after delivery; however, even in high-income settings, social inequities that disproportionally affect WLHIV may limit access to replacement feeding options. The well-established benefits of breastfeeding for maternal and child health should also be acknowledged. Breastfeeding is associated with lower risk of metabolic syndrome, obstetric complications, and cancer among mothers.[82] Breastfeeding lowers rates of infant sudden infant death syndrome, necrotizing enterocolitis, and sepsis and has longer term benefits, including reduced incidence of obesity, asthma, diabetes, and autoimmunity during childhood.[82,83] As health care providers discuss feeding options with WLHIV, a variety of clinical and social factors should be considered for an individualized risk assessment, including history of cART adherence, duration of viral suppression, mental health and substance use history, and the social, emotional, and financial support systems available to the patient during the breastfeeding period. Preemptive discussions should include the planned clinical schedule for maternal and infant viral load monitoring, potential side effects of infant antiretroviral prophylaxis, potential complications that may warrant temporary or permanent breastfeeding cessation, and parental coping strategies if the infant were to acquire HIV.

KNOWLEDGE GAPS AND RESEARCH PRIORITIES

Addressing knowledge gaps and setting research priorities is essential to support collaborative efforts between patients and providers, ensuring optimal outcomes in the context of breastfeeding and HIV transmission during the modern cART era. Basic science studies employing advanced technology for reservoir cell detection in breast milk of long-term ART-suppressed individuals would be beneficial to assess persistence of cell-associated HIV from longitudinal clinical samples. Epidemiology studies on the risk of HIV transmission from MBF among mothers on cART should distinguish between formula supplementation and solid food introduction and include precise exposure time measures. Development and evaluation of point-of-care laboratory tests to evaluate qualitative and/or quantitative cell-free RNA in breast milk could guide clinical management decisions. Additionally, clinical risk-assessment tools to aid in decision-making for both providers and WLHIV would be beneficial.

SUMMARY

Postnatal HIV transmission through breastfeeding is a rare event when risk reduction strategies are in place, including maternal cART, infant prophylaxis, and close maternal and infant virologic monitoring. Early conversations about feeding options between patients and health care providers are important to review current evidence on transmission risk in the cART era and consider an individual's preferences, clinical history, and social support. Future research to evaluate HIV viral dynamics in breast milk among women with sustained viral suppression will be important to inform evidence-driven clinical guidance.

FUNDING

This work was supported by an NIAID, United States Career Development Award (K23AI143479 to LMC) and the Program for Retaining, Supporting, and EleVating Early-career Researchers at Emory from the Emory School of Medicine, a gift from the Doris Duke Charitable Foundation and through the Georgia Clinical and Translational Science Award (UL1-TR002378; to LMC).

Best Practices

What is the current practice for WLHIV who desire to breastfeed?

- Health care providers should provide education to WLHIV regarding infant feeding options, communicating that (1) replacement feeding with formula or certified donor human milk is the only way to ensure 0% risk of HIV transmission after birth; and (2) breastfeeding is associated with less than 1% risk of HIV transmission to the infant if maternal viral suppression is maintained throughout pregnancy and breastfeeding.
- If a WLHIV with sustained viral suppression during pregnancy chooses to breastfeed, health care providers should support this decision, and clinical care of the mother and infant should include the following:
  - Prenatal and postnatal lactation support to establish and maintain EBF.
  - Continuation of maternal cART with virologic monitoring every 1 to 2 months through the breastfeeding period.
  - Provision of infant antiretroviral prophylaxis according to guidance from a pediatric HIV specialist, with serial infant virologic monitoring (at 14–21 days, 1–2 months and 4–6 months of life, followed by every 2 months thereafter if breastfeeding continues, and 4–6 weeks, 3 months, and 6 months after breastfeeding cessation).
  - Gradual weaning over 2 to 4 weeks.

Pearls/pitfalls at the point-of-care:

- Early education and open communication about feeding choices are crucial for shared decision-making between health care providers and WLHIV.

- Prenatal referral to a lactation specialist and pediatric HIV provider is optimal to ensure that WLHIV who choose to breastfeed are prepared for EBF and outpatient follow-up for infant antiviral prophylaxis and virologic monitoring.
- Risk reduction interventions involve coordination among multidisciplinary health care providers, including obstetricians, pediatricians, lactation consultants, and adult and pediatric HIV specialists.
- Management of complications that arise during breastfeeding including maternal mastitis, infant thrush or GI illness, maternal viremia, or maternal cART adherence challenges can include temporary supplementation with certified human donor milk, flash-heated breast milk, or formula, followed by continuation of breastfeeding if the complication resolves. In the United States, guidance for nuanced clinical decisions is available through the National Perinatal HIV Hotline (1–888–448–8765).

Bibliographic Source(s):

Abuogi L, Noble L, Smith C; COMMITTEE ON PEDIATRIC AND ADOLESCENT HIV; SECTION ON BREASTFEEDING. Infant Feeding for Persons Living with and at Risk for HIV in the United States: Clinical Report. Pediatrics. 2024 Jun 1;153(6):e2024066843. https://doi.org/10.1542/peds.2024-066843. PMID: 38766700.

Panel on Treatment of HIV during Pregnancy and Prevention of Perinatal Transmission. Recommendations for the use of antiretroviral drugs during pregnancy and interventions to reduce perinatal HIV transmission in the United States. Published online January 31, 2024. Accessed June 3, 2024. https://clinicalinfo.hiv.gov/en/guidelines/perinatal

ACKNOWLEDGMENTS

J.S. Powers, M. Kihanga and L.M.C. wrote the initial draft of the manuscript. J.S. Powers designed figures. L.M. Cranmer revised the final manuscript.

DISCLOSURE

All authors declare no financial conflicts of interest.

REFERENCES

1. Nduati R, John G, Mbori-Ngacha D, et al. Effect of breastfeeding and formula feeding on transmission of HIV-1: a randomized clinical trial. JAMA 2000; 283(9):1167–74.
2. De Cock KM, Fowler MG, Mercier E, et al. Prevention of mother-to-child HIV transmission in resource-poor countries: translating research into policy and practice. JAMA 2000;283(9):1175–82.
3. Flynn PM, Taha TE, Cababasay M, et al. Prevention of HIV-1 transmission through breastfeeding: efficacy and safety of maternal antiretroviral therapy versus infant nevirapine prophylaxis for duration of breastfeeding in HIV-1-Infected women with high CD4 cell count (IMPAACT PROMISE): a randomized, open-label, clinical trial. J Acquir Immune Defic Syndr 2018;77(4):383–92.
4. Davis NL, Corbett A, Kaullen J, et al. Antiretroviral drug concentrations in breastmilk, maternal HIV viral load, and HIV transmission to the infant: results from the BAN study. J Acquir Immune Defic Syndr 2019;80(4):467–73.
5. Bispo S, Chikhungu L, Rollins N, et al. Postnatal HIV transmission in breastfed infants of HIV-infected women on ART: a systematic review and meta-analysis. J Int AIDS Soc 2017;20(1):21251.

6. Update to clinical guidelines for infant feeding supports shared decision making: clarifying breastfeeding guidance for people with HIV | national institutes of health. Available at: https://oar.nih.gov/news-and-updates/oar-updates/update-clinical-guidelines-infant-feeding-supports-shared-decision-making. Accessed December 28, 2023.
7. Abuogi L, Noble L, Smith C, Committee on pediatric and adolescent HIV, section on breastfeeding. Infant feeding for Persons living with and at risk for HIV in the United States: clinical report. Pediatrics 2024;53(6):e2024066843.
8. Reeves I, Cromarty B, Deayton J, et al. British HIV Association guidelines for the management of HIV-2 2021. HIV Med 2021;22(Suppl 4):1–29.
9. Ambrosioni J, Levi L, Alagaratnam J, et al. Major revision version 12.0 of the European AIDS Clinical Society guidelines 2023. HIV Med 2023;24(11):1126–36.
10. Khan S, Tsang KK, Brophy J, et al. Canadian Pediatric & Perinatal HIV/AIDS Research Group consensus recommendations for infant feeding in the HIV context. J Assoc Med Microbiol Infect Dis Can 2023;8(1):7–17.
11. Keane A, Lyons F, Aebi-Popp K, et al. Guidelines and practice of breastfeeding in women living with HIV-Results from the European INSURE survey. HIV Med 2024; 25(3):391–7.
12. Dunn DT, Newell ML, Ades AE, et al. Risk of human immunodeficiency virus type 1 transmission through breastfeeding. Lancet 1992;340(8819):585–8.
13. Coutsoudis A, Dabis F, Fawzi W, et al. Late postnatal transmission of HIV-1 in breast-fed children: an individual patient data meta-analysis. J Infect Dis 2004; 189(12):2154–66.
14. Teasdale CA, Marais BJ, Abrams EJ. HIV: prevention of mother-to-child transmission. BMJ Clin Evid 2011;2011:0909.
15. Rutagwera DG, Molès JP, Kankasa C, et al. Prevalence and determinants of HIV shedding in breast milk during continued breastfeeding among Zambian mothers not on antiretroviral treatment (ART): a cross-sectional study. Medicine (Baltim) 2019;98(44):e17383.
16. Rousseau CM, Nduati RW, Richardson BA, et al. Longitudinal analysis of human immunodeficiency virus type 1 RNA in breast milk and of its relationship to infant infection and maternal disease. J Infect Dis 2003;187(5):741–7.
17. Davis NL, Miller WC, Hudgens MG, et al. Maternal and breastmilk viral load: impacts of adherence on peripartum HIV infections averted-the breastfeeding, antiretrovirals, and nutrition study. J Acquir Immune Defic Syndr 2016;73(5):572–80.
18. Luoga E, Vanobberghen F, Bircher R, et al. Brief report: No HIV transmission from virally suppressed mothers during breastfeeding in rural Tanzania. J Acquir Immune Defic Syndr 2018;79(1):e17–20.
19. Shapiro RL, Hughes MD, Ogwu A, et al. Antiretroviral regimens in pregnancy and breast-feeding in Botswana. N Engl J Med 2010;362(24):2282–94.
20. Giuliano M, Andreotti M, Liotta G, et al. Maternal antiretroviral therapy for the prevention of mother-to-child transmission of HIV in Malawi: maternal and infant outcomes two years after delivery. PLoS One 2013;8(7):e68950.
21. Boyce TG, Havens PL, Henderson SL, et al. From guidelines to practice: a programmatic model for implementation of the updated infant feeding recommendations for people living with HIV. J Pediatric Infect Dis Soc 2024;13(7):381–5.
22. Malaba TR, Nakatudde I, Kintu K, et al. 72 weeks post-partum follow-up of dolutegravir versus efavirenz initiated in late pregnancy (DolPHIN-2): an open-label, randomised controlled study. Lancet HIV 2022;9(8):e534–43.

23. Malaba TR, Nakatudde I, Kintu K, et al. DolPHIN-2 final results: dolutegravir vs efavirenz in late pregnancy to 72W postpartum. Presented at: March 6, 2021; Conference on Retroviruses and Opportunistic Infections (CROI) (Virtual).
24. Crisinel PA, Kusejko K, Kahlert CR, et al. Successful implementation of new Swiss recommendations on breastfeeding of infants born to women living with HIV. Eur J Obstet Gynecol Reprod Biol 2023;283:86–9.
25. Nashid N, Khan S, Loutfy M, et al. Breastfeeding by women living with human immunodeficiency virus in a resource-rich setting: a case series of maternal and infant management and outcomes. J Pediatric Infect Dis Soc 2020;9(2):228–31.
26. Levison J, McKinney J, Duque A, et al. Breastfeeding among people with human immunodeficiency virus in north America: a multisite study. Clin Infect Dis 2023; 77(10):1416–22.
27. Yusuf HE, Knott-Grasso MA, Anderson J, et al. Experience and outcomes of breastfed infants of women living with HIV in the United States: findings from a single-center breastfeeding support initiative. J Pediatric Infect Dis Soc 2021; 11(1):24–7.
28. ISOSS HIV report 2022. GOV.UK. Available at: https://www.gov.uk/government/publications/infectious-diseases-in-pregnancy-screening-isoss-hiv-report-2022/isoss-hiv-report-2022. Accessed March 28, 2024.
29. Prestileo T, Adriana S, Lorenza DM, et al. From undetectable equals untransmittable (U=U) to breastfeeding: is the jump short? Infect Dis Rep 2022;14(2): 220–7.
30. Weiss F, von Both U, Rack-Hoch A, et al. Brief report: HIV-positive and breastfeeding in high-income settings: 5-year experience from a perinatal center in Germany. J Acquir Immune Defic Syndr 2022;91(4):364–7.
31. Koay WLA, Rakhmanina NY. Supporting mothers living with HIV in the United States who choose to breastfeed. J Pediatric Infect Dis Soc 2022;11(5):239.
32. Abuogi L, Smith C, Kinzie K, et al. Development and implementation of an interdisciplinary model for the management of breastfeeding in women with HIV in the United States: experience from the children's hospital Colorado immunodeficiency Program. J Acquir Immune Defic Syndr 2023;93(5):395–402.
33. Van de Perre P, Rubbo PA, Viljoen J, et al. HIV-1 reservoirs in breast milk and challenges to elimination of breast-feeding transmission of HIV-1. Sci Transl Med 2012;4(143):143sr3.
34. Slyker JA, Chung MH, Lehman DA, et al. Incidence and correlates of HIV-1 RNA detection in the breast milk of women receiving HAART for the prevention of HIV-1 transmission. PLoS One 2012;7(1):e29777.
35. Gantt S, Carlsson J, Heath L, et al. Genetic analyses of HIV-1 env sequences demonstrate limited compartmentalization in breast milk and suggest viral replication within the breast that increases with mastitis. J Virol 2010;84(20):10812.
36. Koulinska IN, Villamor E, Chaplin B, et al. Transmission of cell-free and cell-associated HIV-1 through breast-feeding. J Acquir Immune Defic Syndr 2006; 41(1):93–9.
37. Shapiro RL, Ndung'u T, Lockman S, et al. Highly active antiretroviral therapy started during pregnancy or postpartum suppresses HIV-1 RNA, but not DNA, in breast milk. J Infect Dis 2005;192(5):713–9.
38. Becquart P, Petitjean G, Tabaa YA, et al. Detection of a large T-cell reservoir able to replicate HIV-1 actively in breast milk. AIDS 2006;20(10):1453–5.
39. Semba RD, Kumwenda N, Hoover DR, et al. Human immunodeficiency virus load in breast milk, mastitis, and mother-to-child transmission of human immunodeficiency virus type 1. J Infect Dis 1999;180(1):93–8.

40. Lunney KM, Iliff P, Mutasa K, et al. Associations between breast milk viral load, mastitis, exclusive breast-feeding, and postnatal transmission of HIV. Clin Infect Dis 2010;50(5):762–9.
41. Gantt S, Shetty AK, Seidel KD, et al. Laboratory indicators of mastitis are not associated with elevated HIV-1 DNA loads or predictive of HIV-1 RNA loads in breast milk. J Infect Dis 2007;196(4):570–6.
42. Kuhn L, Aldrovandi GM, Sinkala M, et al. Effects of early, abrupt weaning on HIV-free survival of children in Zambia. N Engl J Med 2008;359(2):130–41.
43. Kuhn L, Kim HY, Walter J, et al. HIV-1 concentrations in human breast milk before and after weaning. Sci Transl Med 2013;5(181):181ra51.
44. Thea DM, Aldrovandi G, Kankasa C, et al. Post-weaning breast milk HIV-1 viral load, blood prolactin levels and breast milk volume. AIDS 2006;20(11):1539–47.
45. Mall AS, Habte H, Mthembu Y, et al. Mucus and Mucins: do they have a role in the inhibition of the human immunodeficiency virus? Virol J 2017;14:192.
46. Ballard O, Morrow AL. Human milk composition: nutrients and bioactive factors. Pediatr Clin North Am 2013;60(1):49–74.
47. Saeland E, de Jong MAWP, Nabatov AA, et al. MUC1 in human milk blocks transmission of human immunodeficiency virus from dendritic cells to T cells. Mol Immunol 2009;46(11–12):2309–16.
48. Lyimo MA, Howell AL, Balandya E, et al. Innate factors in human breast milk inhibit cell-free HIV-1 but not cell-associated HIV-1 infection of CD4+ cells. J Acquir Immune Defic Syndr 2009;51(2):117–24.
49. Lyimo MA, Mosi MN, Housman ML, et al. Breast milk from Tanzanian women has divergent effects on cell-free and cell-associated HIV-1 infection in vitro. PLoS One 2012;7(8):e43815.
50. Farquhar C, Mbori-Ngacha DA, Redman MW, et al. CC and CXC chemokines in breastmilk are associated with mother-to-child HIV-1 transmission. Curr HIV Res 2005;3(4):361–9.
51. Lohman BL, Slyker J, Mbori-Ngacha D, et al. Prevalence and magnitude of human immunodeficiency virus (HIV) type 1-specific lymphocyte responses in breast milk from HIV-1-Seropositive women. J Infect Dis 2003;188:1666–74.
52. Pollara J, McGuire E, Fouda GG, et al. Association of HIV-1 envelope-specific breast milk IgA responses with reduced risk of postnatal mother-to-child transmission of HIV-1. J Virol 2015;89(19):9952–61.
53. Tobin NH, Aldrovandi GM. Immunology of pediatric HIV infection. Immunol Rev 2013;254(1):143–69.
54. Bunders MJ, van der Loos CM, Klarenbeek PL, et al. Memory CD4(+)CCR5(+) T cells are abundantly present in the gut of newborn infants to facilitate mother-to-child transmission of HIV-1. Blood 2012;120(22):4383–90.
55. Bomsel M. Transcytosis of infectious human immunodeficiency virus across a tight human epithelial cell line barrier. Nat Med 1997;3(1):42–7.
56. Alfsen A, Yu H, Magérus-Chatinet A, et al. HIV-1-infected blood mononuclear cells form an integrin- and agrin-dependent viral synapse to induce efficient HIV-1 transcytosis across epithelial cell monolayer. Mol Biol Cell 2005;16(9): 4267–79.
57. Embree JE, Njenga S, Datta P, et al. Risk factors for postnatal mother-child transmission of HIV-1. AIDS 2000;14(16):2535–41.
58. Coutsoudis A, Pillay K, Spooner E, et al. Influence of infant-feeding patterns on early mother-to-child transmission of HIV-1 in Durban, South Africa: a prospective cohort study. South African Vitamin A Study Group. Lancet 1999;354(9177): 471–6.

59. Coovadia HM, Rollins NC, Bland RM, et al. Mother-to-child transmission of HIV-1 infection during exclusive breastfeeding in the first 6 months of life: an intervention cohort study. Lancet 2007;369(9567):1107–16.
60. Iliff PJ, Piwoz EG, Tavengwa NV, et al. Early exclusive breastfeeding reduces the risk of postnatal HIV-1 transmission and increases HIV-free survival. AIDS 2005; 19(7):699–708.
61. Kuhn L, Sinkala M, Kankasa C, et al. High uptake of exclusive breastfeeding and reduced early post-natal HIV transmission. PLoS One 2007;2(12):e1363.
62. Bezirtzoglou E, Tsiotsias A, Welling GW. Microbiota profile in feces of breast- and formula-fed newborns by using fluorescence in situ hybridization (FISH). Anaerobe 2011;17(6):478–82.
63. Penders J, Thijs C, Vink C, et al. Factors influencing the composition of the intestinal microbiota in early infancy. Pediatrics 2006;118(2):511–21.
64. Le Huërou-Luron I, Blat S, Boudry G. Breast- v. formula-feeding: impacts on the digestive tract and immediate and long-term health effects. Nutr Res Rev 2010; 23(1):23–36.
65. Siigur U, Ormisson A, Tamm A. Faecal short-chain fatty acids in breast-fed and bottle-fed infants. Acta Paediatr 1993;82(6–7):536–8.
66. McFarland EJ, Powell TM, Onyango-Makumbi C, et al. Ontogeny of CD4+ T lymphocytes with phenotypic susceptibility to HIV-1 during exclusive and nonexclusive breastfeeding in HIV-1-Exposed Ugandan infants. J Infect Dis 2017;215(3): 368–77.
67. Wood LF, Brown BP, Lennard K, et al. Feeding-related gut microbial composition associates with peripheral T-cell activation and mucosal gene expression in African infants. Clin Infect Dis 2018;67(8):1237–46.
68. Becquet R, Bland R, Leroy V, et al. Duration, pattern of breastfeeding and postnatal transmission of HIV: pooled analysis of individual data from West and South African cohorts. PLoS One 2009;4(10):e7397.
69. Njom Nlend AE, Motaze ACN, Sandie A, et al. HIV-1 transmission and survival according to feeding options in infants born to HIV-infected women in Yaoundé, Cameroon. BMC Pediatr 2018;18:69.
70. Nachega JB, Uthman OA, Anderson J, et al. Adherence to antiretroviral therapy during and after pregnancy in low-income, middle-income, and high-income countries: a systematic review and meta-analysis. AIDS 2012;26(16):2039–52.
71. Gertsch A, Michel O, Locatelli I, et al. Adherence to antiretroviral treatment decreases during postpartum compared to pregnancy: a longitudinal electronic monitoring study. AIDS Patient Care STDS 2013;27(4):208–10.
72. Siddiqui R, Bell T, Sangi-Haghpeykar H, et al. Predictive factors for loss to postpartum follow-up among low income HIV-infected women in Texas. AIDS Patient Care STDS 2014;28(5):248–53.
73. Axelsson JM, Hallager S, Barfod TS. Antiretroviral therapy adherence strategies used by patients of a large HIV clinic in Lesotho. J Health Popul Nutr 2015;33:10.
74. Davies G, Koenig LJ, Stratford D, et al. Overview and implementation of an intervention to prevent adherence failure among HIV-infected adults initiating antiretroviral therapy: lessons learned from Project HEART. AIDS Care 2006;18(8): 895–903.
75. IMPAACT 2040 | IMPAACT. Available at: https://www.impaactnetwork.org/studies/impaact2040. Accessed June 3, 2024.
76. Patel P, Ford SL, Baker M, et al. Pregnancy outcomes and pharmacokinetics in pregnant women living with HIV exposed to long-acting cabotegravir and rilpivirine in clinical trials. HIV Med 2023;24(5):568–79.

77. Cunningham CK, McFarland EJ, Morrison RL, et al. Safety, tolerability, and pharmacokinetics of the broadly neutralizing human immunodeficiency virus (HIV)-1 monoclonal antibody VRC01 in HIV-exposed newborn infants. J Infect Dis 2020;222(4):628–36.
78. McFarland EJ, Cunningham CK, Muresan P, et al. Safety, tolerability, and pharmacokinetics of a long-acting broadly neutralizing human immunodeficiency virus type 1 (HIV-1) monoclonal antibody VRC01LS in HIV-1-Exposed newborn infants. J Infect Dis 2021;224(11):1916–24.
79. Shapiro RL, Ajibola G, Maswabi K, et al. Broadly neutralizing antibody treatment maintained HIV suppression in children with favorable reservoir characteristics in Botswana. Sci Transl Med 2023;15(703):eadh0004.
80. Centers for Disease Control and Prevention. Breastfeeding report card, United States. Atlanta: Centers for Disease Control and Prevention; 2022.
81. Tuthill EL, Tomori C, Van Natta M, et al. "In the United States, we say, 'No breastfeeding,' but that is no longer realistic": provider perspectives towards infant feeding among women living with HIV in the United States. J Int AIDS Soc 2019;22(1):e25224.
82. Gross MS, Taylor HA, Tomori C, et al. Breastfeeding with HIV: an evidence-based case for new policy. J Law Med Ethics 2019;47(1):152–60.
83. Henrick BM, Rodriguez L, Lakshmikanth T, et al. Bifidobacteria-mediated immune system imprinting early in life. Cell 2021;184(15):3884–98.e11.
84. Miotti PG, Taha TE, Kumwenda NI, et al. HIV transmission through breastfeeding: a study in Malawi. JAMA 1999;282(8):744–9.
85. Volpe LJ, Powis KM, Legbedze J, et al. A counseling and monitoring approach for supporting breastfeeding women living with HIV in Botswana. J Acquir Immune Defic Syndr 2022;89(2):e16.

When Black and White Turns Gray

Navigating the Ethical Challenges of Implementing Shared Infant Feeding Decisions for Persons Living with Human Immunodeficiency Virus in the United States

Kira J. Nightingale, MS, MBA[a,*],
Elizabeth D. Lowenthal, MD, MSCE[a,b,1],
Marielle S. Gross, MD, MBE[c,2]

KEYWORDS

• HIV • Breastfeeding • Ethics • Clinical guidelines • Health policy • Autonomy • Equity • Harm reduction

KEY POINTS

- The revised US guidelines supporting breastfeeding for perinatally human immunodeficiency virus (HIV)-exposed infants represent a significant departure from longstanding practices, improving autonomy, justice, and beneficence, while introducing new, more complex ethical challenges.
- Patient autonomy depends on comprehensive, unbiased counseling that is culturally competent and consistent with the patient's level of health literacy.
- Justice remains a significant concern, as marginalized racial, ethnic, and socioeconomic groups for whom breastfeeding present greatest potential health benefits experience disproportionate barriers to providing breast milk for their infants, including psychological and legal risks from HIV criminalization.

Continued

[a] Department of Biostatistics, Epidemiology, and Informatics, University of Pennsylvania School of Medicine, Philadelphia, PA, USA; [b] Department of Pediatrics, University of Pennsylvania School of Medicine, Children's Hospital of Philadelphia, Philadelphia, PA, USA; [c] Johns Hopkins Berman Institute of Bioethics, Baltimore, MD, USA
[1] Present address: 734 Schuylkill Avenue, Room 11241, Philadelphia, PA 19146.
[2] Present address: 1809 Ashland Avenue, Baltimore, MD 21205.
* Corresponding author. 423 Guardian Drive, Office 110, Philadelphia, PA 19104.
E-mail address: Kira.Nightingale@pennmedicine.upenn.edu

Clin Perinatol 51 (2024) 801–816
https://doi.org/10.1016/j.clp.2024.08.002 perinatology.theclinics.com

Continued

- Ascertaining patients' best interests is not straightforward and may be complicated by diverse experiences, perspectives, and priorities of multiple clinicians, patients, and considerations relevant to each unique case.
- Successful implementation of new guidelines requires patient engagement, clinical collaboration, and coordinated social services, with an approach grounded in humility, respect, flexibility, and allyship in navigating nuanced ethical considerations.

INTRODUCTION

In January 2023, the US Department of Health and Human Services (DHHS) revised the infant feeding guidelines for perinatally human immunodeficiency virus (HIV)-exposed infants, for the first time stating that persons living with HIV (PLHIV) should receive "evidence-based, patient-centered counseling to support shared decision-making about infant feeding."[1] The American Academy of Pediatrics (AAP) followed suit in 2024, advising that pediatricians should follow a "family-centered, nonjudgmental, harm reduction approach" when working with PLHIV who desire to breastfeed.[2] Previous US guidelines strongly recommended avoidance of breastfeeding in PLHIV to avoid the possibility of HIV transmission through breast milk (**Table 1**).[3] Importantly, this change was not due to recent updates in the medical literature or changes in our understanding of the clinical equipoise, but rather as a response to mounting pressure from patients, and advocates that collaborative decision-making for infant feeding was essential for parental autonomy, maximizing benefit over harm, and ensuring reproductive justice in light of existing US health disparities.[4–7]

The 2023 guidelines provide specific recommendations for patient counseling, maternal use of antiretroviral therapy (ART) during pregnancy and breastfeeding, and HIV transmission risk-mitigation practices. These changes bring US guidelines closer in line with the World Health Organization standards, which have long advocated for exclusive breastfeeding through 6 months in PLHIV on ART with suppressed HIV viral loads.[8] The risk of infant HIV transmission can be made very low (<1%) with the use of maternal suppressive ART and/or infant HIV prophylaxis and is countered by breastfeeding benefits including lower rates of morbidity and mortality for both dyad members.[8–13]

Historically, in high-income countries (HICs), any risk of HIV transmission to an infant was seen as unacceptable, regardless of potential benefits conferred by breastfeeding. Although the overall risk of infectious diseases that can be prevented through breastfeeding, such as diarrhea and pneumonia, is much lower in the United States than lower income countries, there are numerous benefits of breastfeeding in HICs.14[,15] Breastfeeding has been associated with several important short-term and long-term outcomes including a decreased risk of sepsis, gastroenteritis, and sudden infant death syndrome, improved school performance, decreased likelihood of childhood obesity or asthma, and improved immunity.[16–18] There are also benefits conferred to the mother[a], such as decreased risk of cardiovascular diseases, type II diabetes, breast and ovarian cancer, obstetric complications in subsequent pregnancy, anxiety and depression, and improved infant bonding.[19–23] In light of these

[a] Although this article uses women-focused language, these ethical arguments also apply to any birthing person who may breastfeed or chestfeed.

Table 1
History of infant feeding guidelines in the United States for perinatally human immunodeficiency virus-exposed infants, beginning with the initial statement from the Centers for Disease Control and Prevention (CDC) in 1985

1985: CDC Morbidity and Mortality Weekly Report (MMWR)[63]	"HTLV-III/LAV-infected women should be advised against breastfeeding to avoid postnatal transmission to a child who may not yet be infected."
2015: DHHS Recommendations for Use of Antiretroviral Drugs in Pregnant HIV-1-Infected Women for Maternal Health and Interventions to Reduce Perinatal HIV Transmission in the United States	"In discussing the avoidance of breastfeeding as the strong, standard recommendation for HIV-infected women in the United States, the Panel notes that women may face social, familial, and personal pressures to breastfeed despite this recommendation and that it is important to begin addressing possible barriers to formula feeding during the antenatal period."
2023: DHHS Recommendations for the Use of Antiretroviral Drugs during Pregnancy and Interventions to Reduce Perinatal HIV Transmission in the United States	"People with HIV should receive evidence-based, patient-centered counseling to support shared decision-making about infant feeding. Counseling about infant feeding should begin prior to conception or as early as possible in pregnancy; information about and plans for infant feeding should be reviewed throughout pregnancy and again after delivery."

health considerations, in addition to the improved HIV outcomes, categorically prohibiting breastfeeding among PLHIV is no longer justified. The authors review the complex ethical considerations applicable to implementation of the new guidelines as they relate to autonomy, justice, and beneficence. Also included are clinical vignettes that illustrate key ethical considerations and tensions (clinical vignettes are composite cases and do not represent any individual patient **Boxes 1–3**).

ETHICAL CONSIDERATIONS

Autonomy

As with other health decisions, PLHIV have the right to exercise autonomy in infant feeding decisions. Autonomy is a core tenet of medical ethics and encompasses an individual's ability to form beliefs, opinions, and preferences and act upon these thoughts and values.[24] The concept of autonomy is linked to shared decision-making, which includes (1) provision of clear, accurate, and unbiased medical evidence about reasonable alternatives and the risks and benefits of each; (2) clinician expertise in communicating and tailoring evidence to individual patients; and (3) patients' values, goals, informed preferences, and concerns, including treatment burdens.[25] In considering infant feeding, we must note that there are 2 patients, the infant and the mother. In general, parents have the responsibility and authority to make medical and care decisions for their children, guided by the best interests of the child. However, health providers sometimes believe that a paternalistic approach toward "prohibiting" breastfeeding makes sense when considering the risk of HIV transmission.[26] This poses a risk to patient autonomy, as decisions cannot be considered freely made if the counseling provided to patients is biased or coercive.

Patients are also unable to make autonomous decisions without an understanding of the relative risks and benefits of a given choice. This can be made more challenging due to 2 key factors: the patient's level of individual health literacy and the extent of clinical uncertainty that exists around the topic. Both issues are salient when considering infant feeding decisions within the context of maternal HIV. The DHHS's Healthy People 2030 initiative defines individual health literacy as "the degree to which individuals have the ability to find, understand, and use information and services to inform health-related decisions and actions for themselves and others."[27] Persons living with and susceptible to HIV in the United States are overrepresented by individuals of lower socioeconomic status or racial and ethnic minorities, and these populations are also among those with the lowest health literacy.[28,29] Lower health literacy itself is associated with lower likelihood of ART use, higher HIV viral load, lower CD4 count, and poorer understanding of HIV risk factors and associated comorbidities.[30,31] Health literacy directly impacts individual autonomy, as being free to make a choice requires understanding the options. Counseling by even the most well-intentioned provider can be undermined by low health literacy, as accurately assessing health literacy and communicating information at the appropriate level can be time-consuming, a luxury that many providers, especially those at high-volume clinics, may not have.

The provision of clear, accurate, and unbiased medical evidence in the context of maternal HIV and breastfeeding is additionally complicated by the many unknowns regarding how to optimally minimize HIV transmission risk. For instance, it is unknown how often the mother's viral load should be monitored to ensure continued suppression, whether mixed feeding (ie, provision of both breast milk and formula/solids) increases transmission risk to the infant when maternal ART is used, and what approach to infant prophylaxis is best for minimizing both transmission risk and medication toxicities.[1] The communication of uncertainty in medical practice has long posed challenges to providers, although recent papers have suggested various frameworks and strategies to ensure that clinical uncertainty is communicated effectively.[32,33] The uncertainty surrounding best practices complicates the process of weighing risks, benefits, and burdens. It is vital that clinicians acknowledge and address clinical uncertainty, as studies have shown that effective communication of uncertainty improves patient trust and satisfaction.[34–36] Successful communication of uncertainty also creates an opportunity for providers to assess patient preferences and values and to collaboratively develop and articulate a clear plan for how to move forward, and when the plan should be reassessed. This process can help provider and patient feel confident about and align on their understanding of the plan and its underlying rationale.

Some providers and institutions use checklists or informed consent forms both to guide communication about clinical uncertainty and to document that the parent understands and is willing to accept the risk of HIV transmission.[2,37] An ethical challenge with these tools is whether their use is driven by a desire to improve patient understanding or simply as a legal instrument to protect the institution. When implemented well, a checklist can be an effective teaching and comprehension-assessment tool, built on the premise that there are key concepts a parent should understand prior to making a feeding decision. Providers must be cautious, however, that any such tools present unbiased information in a way that is easily understood and do not stray into the territory of simply asking patients to sign an assumption of risk.

While institutions with existing breastfeeding policies may be revising their policies in light of the guideline change, many institutions are considering policy documents for the first time, and it is important that they are aware of the ethical issues at hand. One report from before the guideline change describes an institution's practices, which include completion of a waiver acknowledging breastfeeding risk, agreeing to monthly follow-up and blood work for both mother and infant, and a triple ART regimen for the infant beginning at birth.[37] These practices, while intended to maximize benefits and reduce potential harm, may be experienced as punitive and are not fully supported by evidence. They also frequently disproportionately address risks without attending to benefits of breastfeeding, for the purpose of guarding against any institutional liability. Informed consent documents and waivers of this nature pose a risk to patient autonomy by oftentimes failing to give equal attention to the benefits of breastfeeding, impacting the patient's ability to make a truly informed choice.

As previously mentioned, a patient's ability to exercise autonomy hinges on his/her ability to fully understand the issues at hand. To ensure that patients benefit from unbiased and comprehensive counseling that represents a diversity of perspectives and relevant evidence, patients should be provided with access to materials from third-party resources and referral to community-based support networks, for example, The Well Project.[38] In the case where a provider's views differ from that of a parent, it is up to the provider to determine whether it is due to inadequate parental understanding or simply differing priorities. While the former indicates the need for additional education and counseling, the latter represents a scenario in which the provider should respect parental autonomy (see **Box 1** for a related clinical vignette). In these circumstances, providers should be forthcoming with their patients about the specific details of their concerns, while at the same time expressing explicit intent to support the patient through the process, regardless of their chosen feeding method. Likewise, as institutions craft or revise protocols for implementation of the new guidelines, educational materials should be reviewed to ensure balanced presentation of benefits and risks, and unnecessary waivers or written informed consent forms should be eliminated in favor of shared decision-making with appropriate clinical documentation to align breastfeeding counseling with comparable practices in other medical domains.

Finally, when considering autonomy in the context of pediatric care, we must ask the question, "autonomy for whom?" While autonomy of the would-be breastfeeding parent is clearly at stake, the autonomy of co-parents, other family members, caregivers, multiple intersecting clinical specialists, as well as infants themselves is ethically relevant for feeding decisions. The AAP advocates for patient-centered and family-centered care, stating that "patients and families are integral partners with the health care team" and that "families' perspectives and information are important

Box 1
Clinical vignette: autonomy

A woman living with perinatally acquired HIV and a history of sustained viral suppression is currently pregnant and desires to breastfeed her baby. She and the baby's father understand that the risk of HIV transmission to the infant is low, but not zero. The mother's lived experience has resulted in the strongly held belief that the importance of improved mother–infant bonding through breastfeeding vastly outweighs the less than 1% risk of infant HIV acquisition. Her pediatrician, however, will not support breastfeeding based on his belief that any risk of HIV transmission to his patient (the infant) is unacceptable. In this case, while the pediatrician is attempting to protect the interests of the infant (beneficence), he is discounting what the parents believe is in their baby's best interest. The mother's lived experience with HIV and desire to breastfeed are driving her to seek autonomy to make a feeding decision for herself and her infant that will be supported by a skilled professional.

in clinical decision-making."[39] Meanwhile, infants are not autonomous agents, as their parent/guardian and/or clinicians must make decisions for them, while the capacities and attendant rights emerge and grow with a child as they approach adulthood. Thus, an infant's interests in autonomy are framed around optimizing that individual's future ability to be self-directing. Ethical challenges emerge when respecting present-day parental autonomy may be at odds with maximizing an infant's future autonomy.

For example, both Obstetricians and Pediatricians in the United States may perform neonatal circumcision out of respect for parental autonomy, though they are necessarily eliminating the infant's future ability to decide this matter for himself. As with the case of breastfeeding, we accept that parents, and the mother in particular, are within their rights to provide informed consent on behalf of their infant. In both examples, there are significant health and cultural factors at play, and both options are considered within a reasonable standard of care, though there are different potential risks and benefits to each.[40–42] Importantly, both circumcision and HIV-exposed breastfeeding have low-frequency risks of potentially serious complications, and yet both are consistent with a sufficiently open future for the child. In the case of circumcision, clinicians not only respect the parent's decision to circumcise their newborn, but they will perform the procedure to facilitate realizing the parent's decision prior to discharge from the hospital, thereby minimizing the newborn's risks from the procedure. By contrast, we do not afford parents the freedom to neglect or abuse their children, as such actions unambiguously threaten their health and well-being, unduly foreclosing the potential of an adequately open future and therefore prompting clinical and/or state interventions.[43]

In the case of infant feeding, when there is a co-parent such as a father, the ideal situation would be that both the mother and co-parent share similar understanding, beliefs, and preferences and make the infant feeding decision together. However, this is not always the case and can be complicated in the context of maternal HIV, when the co-parent as well as other family or community members may be unaware of the mother's HIV status.[44] In some circumstances, disclosure can pose risks to the mother and child.[45] Co-parents cannot participate in truly informed decision-making if they are not aware of the HIV-related risk their infant faces from breastfeeding. However, we would argue that in this situation, clinicians should assume the primacy of maternal autonomy, including her relevant health privacy and safety interests, barring any explicit concerns for neonatal neglect or abuse.

To effectively ensure protection of patient autonomy, clinicians should become familiar with current evidence surrounding infant and maternal benefits of breastfeeding, risks of HIV transmission through breast milk, best practices for risk mitigation, and the sociologic, structural, and economic considerations most likely to influence infant feeding decisions for PLHIV in the United States. This information should be used to support collaborative decision-making, supporting parental autonomy through unbiased accounting of what is currently known and unknown. Providers should also carefully consider whether the use of tools such as checklists is intended as teaching instruments, or if they serve only as waivers that solely emphasize risks and aim to protect the institution from liability. Patient autonomy can only be fully realized when counseling is unbiased, complete, and presented in an accessible manner.

Justice

The principle of distributive justice in a health care setting mandates that every individual be treated equitably, with the same access to resources and services.[46] This is, unfortunately, rarely the case in the United States. Because the adverse health outcomes that can be mitigated by breastfeeding disproportionately impact minority and lower socioeconomic status individuals, and this population has significant overlap with the individuals most impacted by HIV, where a categorical prohibition on breastfeeding appeared to exacerbate existing health disparities. The prior prohibition also worked in opposition to the concept of reproductive justice, in which the ability to parent a child in a safe and healthy environment is a core value.[47] The new guidelines therefore have advanced health equity and reproductive justice by supporting PLHIV to choose breastfeeding, and therefore to receive maternal and neonatal health benefits, but it also opens the door to new justice concerns.

As stated in the revised guidelines, minimizing HIV transmission risk requires heightened surveillance throughout breastfeeding, including regular monitoring of maternal viral load and prompt diagnosis and treatment of issues such as cracked nipples and mastitis. However, the optimal frequency for checking the viral load of PHLIV who breastfeed in HICs is unknown, and thus, recommendations are vague, suggesting that testing once every 1 or 2 months is an appropriate option, mirroring frequency of laboratory evaluation utilized in clinical trials.[1] This heightened frequency of laboratory draws and clinical evaluations adds financial and time burdens for new parents, and requires that the birthing parent has a work schedule, social support, and child care that allow for frequent absences as well as reliable transportation. The burdens of adhering to these recommendations may make breastfeeding impractical or infeasible for many US women, particularly for those individuals with lower socioeconomic means who are also disproportionately impacted by HIV. Likewise, rurality, the need to maintain confidentiality of an HIV diagnosis, and other structural barriers may render such surveillance paradigms inaccessible to many PLHIV. In contrast, follow-up and monitoring regimens for PLHIV who formula feed are less onerous, indirectly pushing lower income families into making infant feeding decisions based on financial or logistical considerations rather than health reasons or personal values.

The financial consideration of infant feeding choice encompasses not only the clinical costs, but those of the feeding method itself. For many families, formula feeding is the most cost-effective option, with US families spending approximately $800 to $2500 per year on infant formula and related accessories (eg, bottles, bottle sterilization supplies); costs may be even lower for low-income families who qualify for the US Department of Agriculture's (USDA) Special Supplemental Nutrition Program for Women, Infants, and Children (WIC) and receive formula at no cost.[48–50] Breastfeeding, in contrast, has been estimated to cost families between $8640 and 11,611 during the infant's first year, which includes the opportunity costs of lost income from maternity leave and missed working hours.[51] The most medically equivalent alternative to breastfeeding is human donor milk, but it also the most cost prohibitive, with an ounce of donor milk costing anywhere from $3.50 to 5 in the United States, equating to over $20,000 in the first 6 months of life alone.[52,53] These cost barriers to non-formula options are a threat to distributive justice, given that individuals of lower socioeconomic status are less likely to be able to receive the benefits of breastfeeding simply because providing human milk, either their own or from a donor, to their infant is prohibitively expensive.

Finally, HIV criminalization creates the potential for disparity in the implementation of national breastfeeding guidelines, as a number of states maintain broad statutes proscribing the knowing transmission of bodily fluids that may contain HIV to another individual. Thus, exposure of an infant to potentially infectious breast milk or blood during feeding may raise legal concerns for patients and providers alike, even if breastfeeding is undertaken or supported in accordance with current medical guidelines.[54,55] Additionally, HIV-related laws are disproportionately enforced based on race and sex, with Black individuals and women significantly more likely to be arrested, convicted, and face longer sentences for HIV-related crimes.[56] This confluence of differing state laws, enforcement disparities, and the epidemiology of US PLHIV reinforces a long-standing threat to justice in the United States. Many have argued against the criminalization of HIV, and indeed some states have made significant revisions to HIV-related law in recent years. However, it is important to recognize that as of the writing of this study, breastfeeding may be legally risky for PLHIV in some US states, especially for Black women and for patients with substance-use disorder history.[57–59] These laws raise further concerns for the routine use of CPS referrals in this setting, as patients may inadvertently be exposed to unjust state interventions that may reflect objectives that diverge from the dyad's rights, interests, and well-being.

There is a long history of structural injustice and disparities within the US health care and legal system. Structural injustice refers to the idea that "social arrangements, including certain institutions and social practices, have highly consequential, differential, and sometimes unjust effects on individuals because they are members of identifiable social groups."[60] It is important that in implementing the new infant feeding guidelines, clinicians are intentional about minimizing these inequities and guarding against potentially reinforcing existing structural injustice. Providers should ensure that they are supporting PLHIV who desire to breastfeed by taking into account their unique life context, including financial barriers to various feeding methods, and challenges that may be posed by some of the more stringent monitoring requirements. Remote monitoring, such as leveraging telemedicine solutions, should be enacted to minimize the burden of participation in surveillance during breastfeeding. Likewise, in-person visits for the mother may be coordinated with pediatric surveillance and routine check-ups to cluster care. Development of local protocols must consider the burdens as well as prospective benefits of surveillance, and patient input should be sought by authorities and incorporated into the local testing paradigms. Long-acting injectable antiretrovirals should be studied for this use case, as the potential to guarantee more consistent viral suppression over several months with a single injection may make providers and patients more confident and more frequent testing unwarranted.

Finally, while providers may be unable to directly address potential legal concerns, they should be cognizant of their existence and appreciate the imperative of maintaining confidentiality of HIV diagnoses and the punitive role that tools such as CPS referrals and breastfeeding waivers may have within the current legal framework (see **Box 2** for a related clinical vignette).

Beneficence and Non-maleficence

The revision to the infant feeding guidelines recognized the existing clinical equipoise and serves to improve patient autonomy and justice. However, the very real risk of infant HIV transmission should not be underemphasized. Risk mitigation strategies and their burdens must be comprehensively understood. At the same time, the potential to cause harm by refusing to support PLHIV who are interested in breastfeeding must be acknowledged. Even before the recent guideline change, it was recognized that refusing to support breastfeeding could be more harmful than beneficial. Mothers who desire to breastfeed but cannot find a supportive clinician may breastfeed anyway, without appropriate risk mitigation practices in place.[7] A patient who feels unsupported by her clinician is less likely to honestly discuss her medical concerns and choices during an encounter,[61] resulting in an increased risk of harm that can be directly attributed to the clinician's unwillingness to support a valid medical choice.

Box 2
Clinical vignette: justice

A woman living with HIV and her husband had a previous child who had difficulty tolerating infant formulas and was hospitalized with failure to thrive. They were counseled about risks and benefits of breastfeeding in the context of maternal HIV and both want the mother to breastfeed their new infant. Both parents have a history of substance use and mental health disorders that are well controlled under established long-term care. The mother has an undetectable HIV viral load and her care team and the infant's pediatrician agreed with the parents on a plan to support breastfeeding. This plan allows the family unit, which lives with multiple stigmatized conditions, to experience the benefits of breastfeeding (justice). However, the team at the birthing hospital was less familiar with breastfeeding in the context of maternal HIV. With heightened concerns due to the parental substance use and mental health histories as well as the prior child with a history of failure to thrive, the medical team at the birthing hospital involved CPS with the goal of ensuring close supervision post-discharge. Involvement of CPS put stress on the mother's mental health that made it more difficult for her to initiate exclusive breastfeeding. While the medical team had the infant's best interests at heart, from the parents' perspective the CPS referral placed them under undue additional stress with their new baby, and compromising their ability to successfully initiate and sustain exclusive breastfeeding. Power asymmetry between the patients and institutional actors in this case illustrates a pervasive pattern of structural injustice in which intersectional vulnerabilities are compounded and multiple core elements of the family's well-being are negatively impacted as a result.

Within medical ethics, beneficence is the concept that clinicians do "good," providing care that is in the best interests of the patient. This poses challenges when differences of opinion exist regarding what is "in the best interest of the patient." It is easy to see how beneficence could come into conflict with patient autonomy, for example, if a clinician disagrees with a mother's desire to breastfeed. A holistic view of both the risks and benefits of breastfeeding, rather than a focus only on the HIV transmission risk, is vital to ensuring that beneficence is truly achieved. Clinician experiences cannot be overlooked when considering what beneficence means to the infant feeding decision-making process. Clinicians who were practicing in the 1980s and 1990s, when an infant HIV diagnosis was considered a lethal sentence, may take the stance that it is always in the best interest of the pediatric patient to maintain an HIV transmission risk of zero. In contrast, clinicians who have experienced HIV as a manageable chronic illness and who daily see the impacts of structural health inequalities on child wellness might be more comfortable with prioritizing the benefits of breastfeeding. Complicating matters further is the fact that providers may have differing views on who exactly their patient is—the mother, the infant, or the family as a whole. A clinician who views the mother as his/her patient might be more willing to engage in collaborative decision-making with the mother as primary partner, whereas a clinician who views his/her primary responsibility as infant-focused and who has had prior infants with poor HIV outcomes may view the only beneficent approach as breastfeeding avoidance. Provider experiences can help inform care but also have the potential to get in the way of evidence-based practice and to discount parental values that are not concordant with those of the provider.

A paternalistic stance may be taken for the sake of beneficence, particularly when dealing with a person whose freedom of choice is limited, such as the case of an infant. Under the revised guidelines, there are circumstances when the advised approach bends toward paternalism. For example, it is considered not advisable for a woman living with HIV to breastfeed when she has 2 or more consecutive detectable HIV viral loads. This recommendation is made with the knowledge that maternal viremia increases transmission risk to the infant but fails to acknowledge that infant prophylaxis can still be protective in this scenario. Therefore, balancing beneficence and autonomy, parents might want to discuss the option of initiating or increasing infant prophylaxis or pumping and pasteurizing the mother's milk while addressing the causes of maternal viremia and maintaining the benefits of maternal milk. It is important that practitioners take the time to weigh risks and benefits at an individual patient level in order to best balance beneficence, non-maleficence, and patient autonomy (see **Box 3** for related clinical vignettes).

Acknowledging that engagement of child protective services (CPS) may play a punitive rather than supportive role for already disadvantaged families, the revised guidelines take a strong stance against engaging CPS or similar agencies in response to the infant feeding choices of an individual with HIV. True cases of suspected child abuse and neglect should not be ignored. However, clinical equipoise surrounding the issue of supported breastfeeding in the context of maternal HIV now dictates that the feeding decision itself is not a reason to involve CPS. Communication and coordination of care has the potential to play an important role in avoiding unwarranted CPS involvement, by ensuring that all of the involved care providers are aware of the mother's feeding intentions, even when providers may be located at different institutions with different policies and norms. Gray areas may still arise in relationship to decisions that extend beyond the feeding choice itself. For example, breastfeeding without consistent monitoring of maternal treatment and viral loads can create the concern that there may be immediate, modifiable risks to the infant. In ideal circumstances, CPS could help put support services in place to mitigate this risk. However, the very real risk of a CPS referral resulting in penalizing actions toward well-intentioned parents that threaten the child's well-being necessitates strong caution. It is also important that in situations where a CPS referral is deemed necessary, clinicians communicate with the local agents who will be handling the case and ensure that an evidence-based management plan is in place and appropriate clinical contacts are available if questions arise.

To effectively balance beneficence and non-maleficence with other ethical principles, we advocate for a holistic approach to infant feeding counseling and advising,

Box 3
Clinical vignettes: beneficence and non-maleficence

Scenario 1: A mother with long-term HIV viral suppression is breastfeeding and is diagnosed with coronavirus disease. Despite continued excellent ART adherence, she has 2 sequential detectable HIV viral loads (both <100 copies/mL). A provider may feel that beneficence/non-maleficence dictates strict adherence to current guidelines that advise cessation of breastfeeding in the context of 2 sequential detectable viral loads. The mother wants to continue breastfeeding while mitigating transmission risks. This scenario would benefit from an individualized assessment of the mother's personal history, risks, and preferences, which may result in a solution such as provision or increase of infant prophylaxis until the mother's viral load returns to an undetectable level.

Scenario 2: A mother with a detectable viral load during the third trimester has been advised against breastfeeding by her provider. She understands the risk of transmission to her infant and given that prefers to formula feed. However, she receives financial support from her mother-in-law who is strongly opposed to formula feeding and threatens to withdraw support if the new mother does not breastfeed. As with scenario 1, a comprehensive assessment of the patient's individual situation could result in risk mitigation strategies, such as pumping and pasteurization, that minimize HIV transmission risk while still ensuring that the mother's other concerns and needs are met.

including consideration of the risks and benefits to all parties involved. Communication and coordination of care across the mother–child dyad's provider team is also essential to ensure that benefits are achieved while preventing unintended harm. Providers should remain up to date on best practices for infant feeding in this population and encourage other members of the patient support team to do so as well to ensure that transient increases in risk, such as low detectable viral loads or mastitis, are managed in a way that is evidence based and in line with patient desires and goals.

SUMMARY

The revision to the DHHS infant feeding guidelines represents a unique case in which significant updates were made to long-standing guidelines as a result of ethical concerns and pressure from patients and advocates rather than because of new changes in our understanding of the science. A change of this nature, while not unprecedented, is unusual. An analogous change recently occurred for blood donation, when in 2023, the Food and Drug Administration revised national policy prohibiting men who have sex with men from donating blood, instead implementing a universal screening process to assess HIV risk regardless of sexual orientation.[62] In the case of blood donation, there was strong cultural pressure to revise donation requirements. While there is in fact an increased HIV risk for men who have sex with men, a categorical prohibition on blood donation only served to eliminate the potential benefits of increasing the pool of blood donors while perpetuating stigma and discounting modern evidence-based blood screening. Similarly, the universal recommendation against breastfeeding in PLHIV attempted to eliminate any risk of transmission of HIV to the infant while ignoring the numerous potential benefits of breastfeeding. While the recent guideline changes are ethically justified, the fact that ethical challenges remain in the implementation of the guidelines must not be overlooked. In this article, we summarize some of the key ethical issues that care providers should consider in the care of PLHIV who are considering breastfeeding. The topics raised should be viewed as a starting point for a robust relational and pragmatic approach to ethical decision-making.

As a brief call to action, we would like to stress the importance of ensuring that institutional policies are consistent with current national guidelines, and that the spectrum of clinicians and community workers who interact with PLHIV are acquainted with the guideline and resources available to support their implementation. We also encourage journal editors to consider addendums to published articles discussing breastfeeding in PLHIV in the United States that have become outdated since the issuance of the revised guidelines, particularly those that are highly cited. This will help to ensure that health care workers have access to updated information to guide their ethical support of PLHIV and their infants. Finally, we hope that the issuance of these revised guidelines will inspire an increase in breastfeeding research within high-income settings so that the clinical unknowns will be addressed.

In closing, we would like to acknowledge that these updated guidelines represent a major change that departs from a well-established practice norm, and care providers may experience personal discomfort as they implement new guidelines that substantially differ from their previous practices. Even the most well-intentioned providers are likely to face challenges in the implementation of the new guidelines. It is vital that providers recognize that breastfeeding in the context of maternal HIV requires dynamic engagement, and that risk mitigation measures can and should change as patients' situations evolve. Successful implementation of the revised infant feeding guidelines will require communication and buy-in from providers across specialties, authentic engagement with patients, and thoughtful attention to the ethical challenges.

Best Practices

What is the current practice for ethical consideration of infant feeding for individuals living with HIV in the United States?

Best practice/guideline/care path objective(s):

- The DHHS issued revised infant feeding guidelines in January 2023 for perinatally HIV-exposed infants, which for the first time encourage collaborative decision-making. The guidelines support evidence-based, patient-centered counseling and state that PLHIV who choose to breastfeed and meet appropriate risk-mitigation criteria should be supported in that decision, as should parents who choose to formula feed. Care providers should be up to date on current infant feeding guidelines and leverage support from resources such as the National Perinatal HIV/AIDS hotline (1–888–448–8765) and colleagues with a high patient volume in this population. Conversations surrounding infant feeding should be patient and family-focused, collaborative and include a discussion of both the current knowledge on the topic and gaps in the data.

Pearls/pitfalls at the point-of-care:

- The ethical considerations relating to infant feeding decisions are complex and patient dependent.
- Situations are likely to arise in which multiple ethical principles appear to be in conflict, and thoughtful consideration must be given to determine which principle(s) should take primacy.
- All care providers who play a role in supporting the infant and mother should be given the same information on the infant feeding plan and help support its implementation.

Major recommendation:

- Care providers should engage in thoughtful, patient-centered counseling of PLHIV who are making infant feeding decisions, recognizing that a holistic approach to feeding decisions is necessary and that there is no one-size-fits-all solution.

Bibliographic source(s):

- Panel on Treatment of HIV during Pregnancy and Prevention of Perinatal Transmission. Recommendations for the Use of Antiretroviral Drugs during Pregnancy and Interventions to Reduce Perinatal HIV Transmission in the United States. 2023. Department of Health and Human Services. https://clinicalinfo.hiv.gov/en/guidelines/perinatal

DISCLOSURE

The authors have nothing to disclose.

REFERENCES

1. Panel on Treatment of HIV During Pregnancy and Prevention of Perinatal Transmission. Recommendations for the use of antiretroviral Drugs during pregnancy and interventions to reduce perinatal HIV transmission in the United States. Rockville, MD: Department of Health and Human Services; 2023. Available at: https://clinicalinfo.hiv.gov/en/guidelines/perinatal.
2. Abuogi L, Smith C, Kinzie K, et al. Development and implementation of an interdisciplinary model for the management of breastfeeding in women with HIV in the United States: experience from the children's hospital Colorado immunodeficiency Program. J Acquir Immune Defic Syndr 2023;93(5):395–402.

3. Panel on treatment of HIV during pregnancy and prevention of perinatal transmission. Recommendations for use of antiretroviral Drugs during pregnancy and interventions to reduce perinatal HIV transmission in the United States. 2022. Available at: https://clinicalinfo.hiv.gov/sites/default/files/guidelines/documents/Perinatal_GL.pdf. Accessed March 17, 2022.
4. Gross MS, Taylor HA, Tomori C, et al. Breastfeeding with HIV: an evidence-based case for new policy. J Law Med Ethics 2019;47(1):152–60.
5. Gostin LO, Kavanagh MM. The ethics of breastfeeding by women living with HIV/AIDS: a concrete proposal for reforming department of health and human services recommendations. J Law Med Ethics 2019;47(1):161–4.
6. Johnson G, Levison J, Malek J. Should providers discuss breastfeeding with women living with HIV in high-income countries? an ethical analysis. Clin Infect Dis 2016;63(10):1368–72.
7. EL Tuthill, Tomori C, Van Natta M, et al. "In the United States, we say,'No breastfeeding,'but that is no longer realistic": provider perspectives towards infant feeding among women living with HIV in the United States. J Int AIDS Soc 2019;22(1):e25224.
8. World Health Organization. Infant and Young Child Feeding. 2021. Available at: https://www.who.int/news-room/fact-sheets/detail/infant-and-young-child-feeding (Accessed 5 September 2024).
9. Flynn PM, Taha TE, Cababasay M, et al. Association of maternal viral load and CD4 count with perinatal HIV-1 transmission risk during breastfeeding in the PROMISE postpartum component. J Acquir Immune Defic Syndr 2021;88(2):206–13.
10. Flynn PM, Taha TE, Cababasay M, et al. Prevention of HIV-1 transmission through breastfeeding: efficacy and safety of maternal antiretroviral therapy versus infant nevirapine prophylaxis for duration of breastfeeding in HIV-1-infected women with high CD4 cell count (IMPAACT PROMISE): a randomized, open-label, clinical trial. J Acquir Immune Defic Syndr 2018;77(4):383–92.
11. Sankar MJ, Sinha B, Chowdhury R, et al. Optimal breastfeeding practices and infant and child mortality: a systematic review and meta-analysis. Acta Paediatr 2015;104(467):3–13.
12. Lamberti LM, Fischer Walker CL, Noiman A, et al. Breastfeeding and the risk for diarrhea morbidity and mortality. BMC Publ Health 2011;11(Suppl 3):S15.
13. Lamberti LM, Zakarija-Grković I, Fischer Walker CL, et al. Breastfeeding for reducing the risk of pneumonia morbidity and mortality in children under two: a systematic literature review and meta-analysis. BMC Publ Health 2013;13(Suppl 3):S18.
14. The Institute for Health Metrics and Evaluation. Data from: Global Burden of Disease. 2019. Seattle, WA. Available at: https://vizhub.healthdata.org/lbd/diarrhoea (Accessed 5 September 2024).
15. World Health Organization. Pneumonia in children, Available at: https://www.who.int/news-room/fact-sheets/detail/pneumonia, 2022. (Accessed 5 September 2024).
16. Victora CG, Bahl R, Barros AJD, et al. Breastfeeding in the 21st century: epidemiology, mechanisms, and lifelong effect. Lancet 2016;387(10017):475–90.
17. Horta BL, Bahl R, Martinés JC, et al. Evidence on the long-term effects of breastfeeding : systematic review and meta-analyses. Geneva: World Health Organization; 2007.
18. Ip S, Chung M, Raman G, et al. Breastfeeding and maternal and infant health outcomes in developed countries. Evid Rep Technol Assess 2007;(153):1–186.

19. Sattari M, Serwint JR, Levine DM. Maternal implications of breastfeeding: a review for the internist. Am J Med 2019;132(8):912–20.
20. Godfrey J, Lawrence R. Toward optimal health: the maternal benefits of breastfeeding. J Wom Health 2010;19(9):1597–602.
21. Sibolboro Mezzacappa E, Endicott J. Parity mediates the association between infant feeding method and maternal depressive symptoms in the postpartum. Arch Wom Ment Health 2007;10(6):259–66.
22. Chowdhury R, Sinha B, Sankar MJ, et al. Breastfeeding and maternal health outcomes: a systematic review and meta-analysis. Acta Paediatr 2015;104(S467): 96–113.
23. Peñacoba C, Catala P. Associations between breastfeeding and mother-infant relationships: a systematic review. Breastfeed Med 2019;14(9):616–29.
24. Gillon R. Autonomy and the principle of respect for autonomy. Br Med J 1985; 290(6484):1806–8.
25. National Quality Forum. Shared decision making: a standard of care for all patients, Available at: https://www.qualityforum.org/Publications/2017/10/NQP_Shared_Decision_Making_Action_Brief.aspx, 2017. (Accessed 5 September 2024).
26. Lai A, Young ES, Kohrman H, et al. Tilting the scale: current provider perspectives and practices on breastfeeding with HIV in the United States. AIDS Patient Care STDS 2023;37(2):84–94.
27. Office of disease prevention and health promotion. Healthy People 2030, Available at: https://health.gov/healthypeople/about. (Accessed 5 September 2024).
28. HIV.gov. Impact on racial and ethnic minorities. Available at: https://www.hiv.gov/hiv-basics/overview/data-and-trends/impact-on-racial-and-ethnic-minorities/. Accessed January 16, 2024.
29. Lopez C, Kim B and Sacks K. Health literacy in the United States: enhancing asswssments and reducing disparities, Available at: https://milkeninstitute.org/sites/default/files/2022-05/Health_Literacy_United_States_Final_Report.pdf, 2022. (Accessed 5 September 2024).
30. Baumann KE, Phillips AL, Arya M. Overlap of HIV and low health literacy in the southern USA. Lancet HIV 2015;2(7):e269–70.
31. Reynolds R, Smoller S, Allen A, et al. Health literacy and health outcomes in persons living with HIV disease: a systematic review. AIDS Behav 2019;23(11): 3024–43.
32. Medendorp NM, Stiggelbout AM, Aalfs CM, et al. A scoping review of practice recommendations for clinicians' communication of uncertainty. Health Expect 2021;24(4):1025–43.
33. Simonovic N, Taber JM, Scherr CL, et al. Uncertainty in healthcare and health decision making: five methodological and conceptual research recommendations from an interdisciplinary team. J Behav Med 2023;46(4):541–55.
34. Bontempo AC. Patient attitudes toward clinicians' communication of diagnostic uncertainty and its impact on patient trust. SSM - Qualitative Research in Health 2023;3:100214.
35. Meyer AND, Giardina TD, Khawaja L, et al. Patient and clinician experiences of uncertainty in the diagnostic process: current understanding and future directions. Patient Educ Counsel 2021;104(11):2606–15.
36. Gordon GH, Joos SK, Byrne J. Physician expressions of uncertainty during patient encounters. Patient Educ Counsel 2000;40(1):59–65.
37. Yusuf HE, Knott-Grasso MA, Anderson J, et al. Experience and outcomes of breastfed infants of women living with HIV in the United States: findings from a

single-center breastfeeding support initiative. J Pediatric Infect Dis Soc 2021; 11(1):24–7.
38. The well Project. Infant feeding and HIV. Available at: https://www.thewellproject.org/resource-highlight-topics/infant-feeding-and-hiv. Accessed June 2, 2024.
39. Committee on Hospital Care and the Institute for Patient- and Family-Centered Care. Patient- and family-centered care and the pediatrician's role. Pediatrics 2012;129(2):394–404.
40. Task Force on Circumcision. Male circumcision. Pediatrics 2012;130(3):e756–85.
41. Circumcision DA Crawford. A consideration of some of the controversy. J Child Health Care 2002;6(4):259–70.
42. Prabhakaran S, Ljuhar D, Coleman R, et al. Circumcision in the paediatric patient: a review of indications, technique and complications. J Paediatr Child Health 2018;54(12):1299–307.
43. Davis DS. Genetic dilemmas and the child's right to an open future. Hastings Cent Rep 1997;27(2):7–15.
44. Greene S, Ion A, Elston D, et al. "Why aren't you breastfeeding?": how mothers living with HIV talk about infant feeding in a "breast is best" world. Health Care Women Int 2015;36(8):883–901.
45. Tam M, Amzel A, Phelps BR. Disclosure of HIV serostatus among pregnant and postpartum women in sub-Saharan Africa: a systematic review. AIDS Care 2015; 27(4):436–50.
46. Olejarczyk JP, Young M. Patient rights and ethics. Treasure Island (FL): StatPearls Publishing; 2022.
47. Loretta R, Erika D, Whitney P, et al. Radical reproductive justice : foundation, theory, practice, critique. New York, NY: The Feminist Press at CUNY; 2017.
48. Rollins NC, Bhandari N, Hajeebhoy N, et al. Why invest, and what it will take to improve breastfeeding practices? Lancet 2016/01/30/2016;387(10017):491–504.
49. Kirkham E. Costs of breastfeeding vs. formula: which actually costs more? plutus foundation. Available at: https://plutusfoundation.org/2020/costs-breastfeeding-formula/. Accessed July 23, 2020.
50. US Department of Agriculture. WIC Food packages - maximum monthly allowances. Available at: https://www.fns.usda.gov/wic/food-packages-maximum-monthly-allowances. Accessed November 7, 2023.
51. Mahoney SE, Taylor SN, Forman HP. No such thing as a free lunch: the direct marginal costs of breastfeeding. J Perinatol 2023;43(5):678–82.
52. Bai Y, Kuscin J. The current state of donor human milk use and practice. J Midwifery Wom Health 2021;66(4):478–85.
53. Jain S. How often and how much should your baby eat? American Academy of Pediatrics Committee on Nutrition. Available at: https://www.healthychildren.org/English/ages-stages/baby/feeding-nutrition/Pages/how-often-and-how-much-should-your-baby-eat.aspx. Accessed January 11, 2024.
54. The Center for HIV Law and Policy. HIV criminalization in the United States: a sourcebook on state and federal HIV criminal law and practice, Available at: https://www.hivlawandpolicy.org/sites/default/files/HIVCriminalizationintheUSASourcebookonStateFedHIVCriminalLawandPractice022722.pdf, 2022. (Accessed 30 January 2024).
55. Symington A, Chingore-Munazvo N, Moroz S. When law and science part ways: the criminalization of breastfeeding by women living with HIV. Ther Adv Infect Dis 2022;9. 20499361221122481.

56. UCLA school of law williams institute. HIV criminalization in the United States. Available at: https://williamsinstitute.law.ucla.edu/visualization/hiv-criminalization/. Accessed January 30, 2024.
57. Hoppe T, McClelland A, Pass K. Beyond criminalization: reconsidering HIV criminalization in an era of reform. Curr Opin HIV AIDS 2022;17(2):100–5.
58. Centers for Disease Control and Prevention, HIV criminalization and ending the HIV epidemic in the U.S, Available at: https://www.cdc.gov/hiv/policies/law/criminalization-ehe.html. (Accessed 30 January 2024).
59. Burris S, Cameron E. The case against criminalization of HIV transmission. JAMA 2008;300(5):578–81.
60. Powers M, Faden R. What structural injustice is. Structural injustice: power, advantage, and human rights. New York, NY: Oxford University Press; 2019.
61. Levy AG, Scherer AM, Zikmund-Fisher BJ, et al. Prevalence of and factors associated with patient nondisclosure of medically relevant information to clinicians. JAMA Netw Open 2018;1(7):e185293.
62. FDA finalizes move to recommend individual risk assessment to determine eligibility for blood donations. 2023. Available at: https://www.fda.gov/news-events/press-announcements/fda-finalizes-move-recommend-individual-risk-assessment-determine-eligibility-blood-donations. Accessed January 18, 2024.
63. Centers for Disease Control and Prevention, MMWR: current trends recommendations for assisting in the prevention of perinatal transmission of human t-lymphotropic virus type III/lymphadenopathy-associated virus and acquired immunodeficiency syndrome, 43(48)(721-726, 731-726). Available at: https://www.cdc.gov/mmwr/preview/mmwrhtml/00033122.htm (Accessed 6 December 2023).

Treatment of HIV Infection in Children Across the Age Spectrum: Achievements and New Prospects

Moherndran Archary, MBChB, DCH(SA), FCPaeds(SA), Paeds ID (SA), PhD(UKZN)[a,b,*], Kagiso Mochankana, MBBS, FCPaeds(SA), MMeD(UB)[b,1], Adrie Bekker, MBChB, DCH(SA), MMed (SU), FCPaeds(SA), Cert Neo(SA), PhD(SU)[c]

KEYWORDS

- Human immunodeficiency virus • Antiretroviral therapy • Neonates • Children
- Adolescents • New strategies

KEY POINTS

- Successful treatment of children with human immunodeficiency virus (HIV) requires a holistic approach, addressing the medical, psychosocial, and economic needs of children and their families.
- Early initiation of highly effective antiretroviral treatment (ART) and maintaining viral suppression prevents HIV-related morbidity and mortality.
- Improved access to antiretroviral (ARV)formulations for neonates allows initiation of treatment soon after birth, limiting HIV reservoir size and enhancing the potential for future HIV cure.
- Newer long-acting ART offer hope of improving adherence and acceptability to lifelong ART.

INTRODUCTION

Approximately 3.2 million children and adolescents globally living with human immunodeficiency virus (HIV) require lifelong antiretroviral (ARV) treatment (ART) to prevent HIV-related morbidity and mortality.[1,2] Progress toward achieving the UNAIDS goals of 95:95:95 in children has lagged behind progress in adults, with only 63% of children

[a] Department of Paediatrics and Child Health, Nelson R Mandela School of Medicine, 4th Floor, Main Building, 719 Umbilo Road, Durban, 4001, South Africa; [b] Department of Paediatrics, Victoria Mxenge Hospital (Previously King Edward VIII Hospital), Sydney Road, Durban, 4001, South Africa; [c] Department of Paediatrics and Child Health, Department of Medicine, 3rd Floor Clinical Building, Francie van Zijl Drive, Tygerberg, 7505, Cape Town, South Africa
[1] Present address: Private Bag X7, Congela, 4013.
* Corresponding author. Private Bag X7, Congela 4013, South Africa.
E-mail address: archary@ukzn.ac.za

Clin Perinatol 51 (2024) 817–832
https://doi.org/10.1016/j.clp.2024.08.003 perinatology.theclinics.com

with an HIV diagnosis, 57% on ART and 46% virologically suppressed.[1] Achieving these goals will require addressing the unique challenges facing children and adolescents with HIV together with their caregivers. These multifaceted challenges underscore the need for a comprehensive and holistic approach to pediatric HIV care, addressing the medical, ethical, and socioeconomic challenges to optimize the efficacy of available treatment strategies.[2–4]

Combination ART (cART) is not only highly effective in suppressing HIV replication but also prevents opportunistic infections and improves the well-being of children with HIV, especially if started early.[3,4] Additionally, prevention of vertical transmission of HIV, family planning, and pre-exposure prophylaxis (PrEP) to reduce adult HIV infections have been crucial strategies in reducing new pediatric HIV infections and changing the landscape of pediatric HIV in sub-Saharan Africa.[5–7]

Progress in licensing child-friendly ARV formulations and simplified regimens has resulted in substantial improvement in the morbidity and mortality outcomes among children living with HIV.[8,9] These advancements underscore the transformative impact of evolving treatment modalities on pediatric HIV outcomes.[9]

CURRENT STATE OF ANTIRETROVIRAL TREATMENT TREATMENT (1)

When to Start?

The optimal timing for initiating ART in children should carefully balance virologic control, disease progression, and long-term toxicity.[10] Immediate or expeditious initiation of ART is generally recommended for all people living with HIV, with specific exceptions for individuals diagnosed with conditions such as cryptococcal meningitis, disseminated Mycobacterium avium complex disease, or Mycobacterium tuberculosis (TB).[10–13]

The START and CHER study evaluated the advantages associated with early initiation of ART for individuals newly diagnosed with HIV.[12,14] Children who are co-infected with TB and HIV are at a higher risk of mortality if ART initiation is delayed.[15] Based on this evidence, many countries have adopted the "test and start" approach, ensuring prompt ART initiation, particularly for children below 15 years.[16] Current guidelines universally advocate for the early commencement of ART in children living with HIV, irrespective of disease stage, coexisting conditions, or immunologic status.[17]

In summary, the evidence from these studies collectively supports early initiation of HIV treatment in children to improve virologic control, reduce disease progression, reduce HIV reservoirs, and resulting in better long-term outcomes.

What Regimen to Start with?

The recommendations for selecting ARV regimens are generally extrapolated from adult populations due to the paucity of randomized, Phase 3 clinical trials directly comparing ART regimens in pediatric patients.[18] Recommended pediatric regimens should demonstrate high rates of viral suppression and immunologic enhancement, acceptable drug toxicity profile, availability of child-friendly formulations and dosing recommendations for children, and limited drug interactions.[6] Typically, an ARV regimen comprises 2 Nucleoside Reverse Transcriptase Inhibitors (NRTIs) combined with an active drug from one of the following classes: Integrase Strand Transfer Inhibitor, Non-Nucleoside Reverse Transcriptase Inhibitor, or boosted Protease Inhibitor. The selection of a specific regimen in high-income countries is individualised based on factors including the characteristics of the proposed regimen, the patient's age, weight, underlying conditions, sexual maturity rating, and the results of drug-resistance testing.[19,20] Guidelines from the World Health Organization (WHO) and many low-middle-income countries emphasize a public health approach with standardized sequencing of regimens based on community prevalence of HIV drug resistance.

Optimal Antiretroviral Regimens and Key Considerations for Initial Regimen Selection

Several pediatric clinical trials have played a pivotal role in guiding the selection of ARV therapies. The IMPAACT P1060 trial demonstrated the superiority of a lopinavir/ritonavir (LPV/r)-based regimen over a nevirapine (NVP)-based regimen in children aged 2 to 35 mo, particularly in those with previous NVP exposure, prompting a shift in guideline recommendations.[21] In contrast, earlier trials had shown comparable virologic efficacy.[22,23]

More recently, the ODYSSEY trial has demonstrated the superior efficacy of dolutegravir (DTG) with 2 nucleoside analogues compared to standard-of-care in children initiating first- or second-line ART, prompting a shift in guidelines.[24] Approval of generic DTG formulations and cost reduction agreements further supported the rapid adoption of DTG globally.[25]

The currently recommended ARV combination for initiating ART in children of different ages and weights is INSTI-based, and is outlined as follows:[20]

- DTG is the preferred medication for infants, children, and adolescents at least 4 w old and weighing greater than or equal to 3 kg. DTG, as a single drug formulation, is available in dispersible tablets for infants weighing at least 3 kg and film-coated tablets for children weighing at least 20 kg. A fixed-dose combination (FDC) containing abacavir (ABC)/DTG/lamivudine(3 TC) is available in dispersible tablets (Triumeq PD) for children weighing at least 10 kg but less than 25 kg and as a single film-coated tablet (Triumeq) for those weighing at least 25 kg.
- Bictegravir (BIC) is not available as a standalone tablet but is part of an FDC tablet containing BIC/emtricitabine (FTC)/tenofovir alafenamide (TAF). This FDC tablet is an alternative treatment for children aged 2 y or older, weighing at least 14 kg. Dosing is weight-dependent, and the tablet comes in 2 strengths.
- Raltegravir (RAL) can be used for infants weighing at least 2 kg from birth. Several formulations are available, including granules, chewable tablets, and tablets.

The preferred NRTI combination consists of FTC plus TAF for children and adolescents weighing 14 kg or more. Several fixed drug combinations are available, including FTC/TAF, BIC/FTC/TAF, Elvitegravir/cobicistat/FTC/TAF (EVG/c/FTC/TAF).[20]

ABC is the most widely recommended NRTI backbone in infants.[24] A multivariate analysis of 5332 ABC-exposed patients revealed a generally lower risk in black populations compared to other ethnic groups, making the HLA-B 5701 allele test-optional in most African countries before ABC initiation.[26]

The preferred initial ART for children based on age, weight, and specific considerations are summarized in **Tables 1** and **2**.[19,20]

Antiretroviral Treatment Monitoring

Routine monitoring of children recently diagnosed with HIV or in chronic care should be comprehensive and holistic. Evaluating viral suppression and immune recovery by measuring plasma viral loads and CD4 counts is the cornerstone of laboratory monitoring response to ART. A holistic evaluation encompasses scrutiny of growth and development, aiming to identify potential HIV-associated abnormalities. A comprehensive history to identify challenges with continuing treatment and new symptoms, together with a detailed physical examination to uncover key physical manifestations

Table 1
Recommended antiretroviral treatment combinations based on age groups[19,20]

	Birth to <14 Days of Age	Aged ≥14 d and ≥2 kg to <4 wk	Aged ≥4 wk and ≥3 kg to <2 y	Aged ≥2 y and ≥14 kg	Aged ≥6 y and ≥25 kg
INSTI-Based Regimens	Two NRTIs *plus* RAL				
				Two NRTIs *plus* BIC	
			Two NRTIs *plus* DTG		
NNRTI-Based Regimens	Two NRTIs *plus* NVP				
PI-Based Regimens		Two NRTIs *plus* LPV/r			

of HIV disease, are important. Additionally, targeted laboratory tests for anemia, leukopenia, thrombocytopenia, hypoalbuminemia, nephropathy (via urinalysis), hyperglycaemia, hepatic transaminitis, and renal insufficiency (creatinine) should be performed if indicated.[19]

Post-initiation of ART, continuous support for adherence and diligent evaluation for clinical adverse events is recommended. The frequency and timing of clinical assessment and laboratory testing must be cost-effective and limit the disruption to schooling and family life.[19,26]

Treatment Failure

Treatment failures can be broadly classified as virologic, immunologic, or clinical. Virologic failure happens when there is an insufficient initial response to therapy or a resurgence of viral activity after achieving suppression. It is an early sign of poor adherence

Table 2
Preferred Dual-nucleoside reverse transcriptase inhibitors backbone options for use in combination with other drugs[19,20]

Age	Dual-NRTI Backbone Options
Neonates Aged Birth to 1 mo	AZT *plus* (3 TC or FTC) ABC *plus* (3 TC or FTC)
Infants and Children Aged >1 mo to <2 y	ABC *plus* (3 TC or FTC)
Children and Adolescents Aged ≥ 2 y with SMRs of 1–3	ABC *plus* (3 TC or FTC) FTC/TAF in children and adolescents weighing ≥14 kg and receiving a regimen that contains an INSTI or an NNRTI FTC/TAF in children and adolescents weighing ≥35 kg and receiving a regimen that includes a boosted PI
Adolescents Aged ≥12 y with SMRs of 4 or 5	*As per the adult's recommendation* TDF or TAF with 3 TC or FTC

Abbreviations: 3 TC, lamivudine; ABC, abacavir; BIC, bictegravir; DTG, dolutegravir; EFV, efavirenz; EVG, elvitegravir; EVG/c, elvitegravir/cobicistat; FDC, fixed-dose combination; FTC, emtricitabine; INSTI, integrase strand transfer inhibitor; LPV/r, lopinavir/ritonavir; NVP, nevirapine; PI, protease inhibitor; RAL, raltegravir; TAF, tenofovir alafenamide; TDF, tenofovir disoproxil fumarate; AZT, zidovudine.

with the potential of developing drug resistance. The definition of virologic suppression is maintaining a plasma viral load below a specified threshold after 6 mo of treatment. Most recommendations use a 50 copies/mL threshold to guide ARV management decisions, while the WHO recommends a 1000 copies/mL threshold.[19,20]

Due to their unique characteristics, infants may take longer to achieve virologic suppression, especially when starting ART with high viral loads. It is essential to closely monitor their progress even if viral load reduction is evident but has yet to reach the target levels. Ongoing viral non-suppression can be selected for HIV drug resistance and further complicate treatment options.[27]

There is still some uncertainty about how to interpret HIV RNA levels ranging between the lower limit of detection and less than 200 copies/mL in patients on ART. Short-term detectable but low plasma viral load levels, known as "blips," are commonly observed and are generally not signs of imminent virologic failure.[28]

Immunologic and clinical failure refers to a situation where there is an inadequate recovery of the CD4 count and clinical evidence of disease progression despite ongoing treatment.[9] It is essential to differentiate between clinical deterioration caused by immune reconstitution inflammatory syndrome and actual treatment failure.[9]

The management of virologic failure requires a thorough assessment of therapy adherence, dosing accuracy, medication intolerance, and potential drug interactions. When all else fails, ARV drug resistance testing may be necessary. This testing can be either phenotypic, genotypic, or both if resources allow. Genotypic assays that detect mutations are more affordable and rapid. Standard databases such as the Stanford Database can be used to interpret genotypic results. If a patient is found to have developed resistance to ARV drugs, it is recommended to switch to a new treatment plan that includes at least 2 fully effective agents. The selection of the new regimen should be based on the patient's medical history, results of drug-resistance tests, and other factors such as age and potential drug interactions.[19,20]

Successful management of pediatric HIV requires collaboration with pediatric HIV specialists, close monitoring of treatment adherence, and continuous evaluation of treatment response. Individualized decisions must be made to optimize outcomes in the event of treatment failure, considering the unique circumstances of each patient.[22]

TREATMENT OF THE NEONATE WITH HUMAN IMMUNODEFICIENCY VIRUS (2)

Commencing ART in neonates (<28 days of age) presents unique challenges to ensure the successful and timely implementation of neonatal ART. Multiple factors should be addressed to attain swift neonatal ART uptake, including involvement of a multidisciplinary team, ensuring early infant HIV diagnosis, development of age-appropriate ARV formulations suitable for use in this population, and optimization of ARV dosing guidance for both term and preterm (<37 weeks gestational age) infants. The WHO recommends immediate initiation of ART for all infants living with HIV, including neonates, irrespective of their clinical or immunologic stage, due to the benefits of improved mortality and morbidity.[12,29] Additional benefits of early ART also include smaller viral reservoirs and improved neurologic outcomes.

Access to Early Infant Human Immunodeficiency Virus Diagnosis

Despite the clear advantages of starting ART shortly after birth, the practical implementation of this strategy can be challenging. The availability of HIV nucleic acid testing (NAT) with a rapid turnaround time should be prioritized in low-resource, high-burden HIV settings to enable early infant HIV diagnosis. HIV NAT is required to diagnose HIV among infants and children younger than 18 mo of age[29] as maternal HIV antibody is transmitted across the placenta and can persist for many months post-delivery. Point-of-care HIV NAT, used at or around birth, has been shown to improve the proportion of infants diagnosed with HIV.[30,31]

Antiretroviral Drug Options and Formulations in Neonates

The need for age-appropriate ARV formulations is another key component within the neonatal HIV treatment care cascade. Of the 23 individual ARV drug agents currently approved by the United States Food and Drug Administration and many more FDCs for adults, less than eight ARV drugs have data for use in term neonates.[32] This situation is worse for preterm infants where only zidovudine (ZDV), 3 TC and NVP have HIV treatment dosing guidance available for preterm infants.

Off-label use of older and less potent ARV drugs is common in neonates where few pediatric ARV regulatory approvals extend to less than 3 mo of age. LPV/r oral solution is only approved from a postmenstrual age of 42 w and a postnatal age of 14 d unless the benefit outweighs the risk of life-threatening events, which was observed mainly in preterm infants within the first week of life. These events were possibly due to the excipients of the LPV/r oral solution containing 42.4% alcohol and 15.3% propylene glycol.[33] A small pharmacokinetics (PK) study using a different LPV/r formulation (granules) showed no serious drug-related safety signal due to different excipients, but more safety data are needed.[34] Similarly, ABC is not approved for use in neonates; however, a neonatal dose is listed in international pediatric HIV guidelines[19,20] following a population PK modeling and simulation study.[35] RAL is a first-generation integrase inhibitor approved in infants weighing greater than 2 kg based on findings from the IMPAACT P1066 and the IMPAACT P1110 studies. However, RAL has a low resistance barrier and is not readily available in low and middle income countrie (LMICs)s. Similarly, maraviroc is also approved for use in combination with other ARV drugs for the treatment of CCR5-tropic HIV-1 infection in infants born term and weighing greater than or equal to 2 kg, but access is limited.[36]

Oral ARV liquid formulations are primarily used in term and preterm infants, lending themselves to precise dosing during a time of rapid weight gain and dynamic developmental changes. However, difficulty procuring individual liquids with frequent stock-outs, poor palatability, and short shelf life has discouraged widespread availability.[37]

Solid ARV formulations, such as RAL granule formulation, can be safely and effectively administered in neonates.[38] As fewer neonates are perinatally infected with HIV, it has become increasingly difficult to procure or develop ARV formulations that will only be used in the neonatal period, which are seldom used and only for a short period after birth. Therefore, the repurposing of existing pediatric formulations, including scored ABC/3 TC dispersible tablets (120/60 mg), LPV/r granules (40/10 mg), and DTG dispersible tablets (10 mg) for use in neonates is an ongoing area of research.[34,39]

Dose Adjustments and Pharmacologic Considerations for Neonates

The first months of life are characterized by rapid weight gain and dynamic developmental, metabolic changes that affect an infant's medication responses. Multiple dose adjustments are often required during this period to enable safe and effective treatment. For example, a typical term neonate will double their weight at 6 mo and triple it by 1 y of age, requiring a higher drug dose over time. Apart from body weight, neonatal dosing considerations are also affected by the immaturity of organs at birth and the rate of organ maturation over time, especially in preterm infants. ZDV, commonly used for the prevention of vertical HIV transmission and primarily eliminated by the liver, is an example of a drug with slow elimination at birth, which rapidly increases over time. Preterm infants require a lower starting dose of ZDV at birth due to reduced clearance, followed by a gradual dose escalation compared to term infants, who require a higher mg/kg starting dose at birth, followed by a more rapid dose increase over time. This reduced clearance of ZDV after birth was demonstrated in a PK study performed in preterm infants, which led to the adoption of more nuanced ZDV dosing recommendations for preterm infants: 2 mg/kg twice daily at birth, increased to 3 mg/kg twice daily by 4 w postnatal age for preterm infants less than 30 w gestational age; and 4 mg/kg twice daily at birth, increased to 12 mg/kg twice daily by 4 w postnatal age, for preterm infants greater than or equal to 35 w gestational age.[40] In young infants, the clearance of ZDV increases rapidly, and by 3 mo of age, the overall ZDV PK is similar to adults.[41]

Novel study designs such as mathematical PK models and extrapolation of adult PK efficacy targets can assist with describing age-dependent physiologic changes and play an important role in predicting initial dosing for neonates.[35,36,38] Moreover, the extrapolation of ARV drugs to neonates and children is supported by similar responses to intervention and the same exposure-response observed in children compared to adults.[32] Using existing efficacy PK targets allow for smaller sample sizes and facilitate and accelerates the execution of neonatal PK studies, contributing toward evidence-based guidelines. However, continuous safety surveillance of ARV drugs is crucial in this age group, where an understanding of organ maturation and metabolic enzyme activity is required to determine a safety risk.[42] DTG is primarily metabolized in the liver by uridine diphosphate glucuronosyltransferase 1A1 (UGT1A1), which is also responsible for the conjugation of bilirubin with glucuronic acid.[43] UGT1A1 enzyme activity is typically slow at birth but rapidly increases. Between 30 and 40 w of gestational age, UGT1A1 is expressed at 1% of adult levels, reaching comparable adult levels by 14 w of chronologic age.[44] A potential concern of administrating DTG to neonates is the risk of severe jaundice with bilirubin neurotoxicity. INSTIs can increase concentrations of free bilirubin through displacement of bilirubin from albumin. *In vitro* studies of DTG have demonstrated displacement of bilirubin from albumin; however, at therapeutic plasma concentrations these findings were unlikely of clinical significance.[45] As DTG is being studied and rolled out in younger infants, the additional safety data on jaundice should be collected.

Antiretroviral Dosing Guidance for Term Neonates Requiring Treatment for Human Immunodeficiency Virus

To simplify ARV administration, the WHO recommends weight-band ARV dosing for infants less than 4 w of life,[37] compared to many resource-rich settings that prefer to administer an exact milligram per kilogram dose, which are more precise but are more time-consuming and prone to dosing errors.[19] Each of these strategies has its advantages and disadvantages. Weight-band dosing may be more pragmatic to implement in low-resource settings, but neonates at the lowest and highest range of the weight band risk high or low drug exposures, respectively. **Table 3** summarizes the literature describing weight-band dosing for ARV liquid and solid formulations and per kilogram dose for ARV liquid formulations.[19,34,37]

NEW DEVELOPMENTS (3)

Current WHO HIV treatment guidelines recommend a combination of 3 ARV agents.[19] However, concerns about the long-term side effects of a multi-drug regimen,

Table 3
Treatment dosing in term neonates (0-4 wk) using oral antiretroviral liquid solutions, granules and dispersible tablets[32,34,37]

	NVP 10 mg/mL	ZDV 10 mg/mL	LPV/r[a] 80/20 mg/mL	LPV/r 40/10 mg (1 Sachet)	ABC/3 TC[b] 120/60 mg (1 Tablet)	ABC 20 mg/mL	3 TC 10 mg/mL	MVC 20 mg/mL	RAL[c] 100 mg (1 Sachet)	
Age in Weeks	0–4	0–4	2–4	0–4	0–4	0–4	0–4	0–4	0–1	1–4
Frequency	BID	BID	BID	BID	OD	BID	BID	BID	OD	BID
Dose	6 mg/kg	4 mg/kg	300 mg/75 mg per m^2			2 mg/kg	2 mg/kg			
≥ 2 to < 3 kg	1.5 mL	1 mL	0.6 mL	2x sachets	1/4 tablet	0.4 mL	0.5 mL	1.5 mL	0.4 mL	0.8 mL
≥ 3 to < 4 kg	2 mL	1.5 mL	0.8 mL	2x sachets	1/4 tablet	0.5 mL	0.8 mL	1.5 mL	0.5 mL	1 mL
≥ 4 to < 5 kg	3 mL	2 mL	1 mL	-	-	0.6 mL	1 mL	-	0.7 mL	1.5 mL

All ARV drugs should be dosed based on the weight when treatment starts and maintained until 4 wk of age.

Abbreviations: 3 TC, lamivudine; ABC, abacavir; BID, twice-daily dosing; kg, kilograms; LPV/r, lopinavir/ritonavir; MVC, maraviroc; NVP, nevirapine; ZDV, zidovudine;

[a] LPV/r 80/20 mg solution should only be given from 2 wk of age;

[b] ABC/3 TC 120/60 mg is a double scored dispersible tablet;

[c] RAL granules should be administered once a day during the first week of life and twice daily afterward.

cumulative lifetime exposure together with improved safety and potency of newer ART formulations have shifted the focus to regimens with fewer drugs.[46] In addition, the burden of daily administration of oral medications associated with pill fatigue makes the case for long-acting formulations. These therapies can improve adherence through less frequent dosing, potentially enhancing clinical outcomes, especially for individuals facing challenges with daily oral medications.[47]

Two-Drug Regimens

While 2-drug daily oral regimens have been extensively studied in adults, resulting in the inclusion of these regimens in several national guidelines, there are limited studies in children and adolescents.[48]

For treatment-naïve adults with HIV, combinations of LPV/r+3 TC and DRV+3 TC have shown non-inferiority to 3 drug regimens; however, they are associated with gastrointestinal adverse effects and increased dosing frequency. Currently, the only recommended 2-drug regimen for treatment-naïve adults is DTG+3 TC. However, very high HIV viral loads (>500 000c/mL and low CD4 counts) are associated with more frequent virologic failure and the emergence of HIV drug resistance. In addition, hepatitis B co-infection is a contraindication for 2-drug regimens due to the absence of adequate anti-Hepatitis B activity.

For stable virologically suppressed adults, several guidelines include DTG+3 TC, DTG + rilpivirine (RPV), and ATV/r+3 TC as alternative 2-drug regimens, which can reduce the cumulative drug exposure, cost of the regimen and reduce the impact on the bone, cardiovascular and renal systems. Similarly, the SMILE/PENTA 17/ ANRS 152 trial showed non-inferiority when using a 2-drug regimen of an INSTI + Darunavir/Ritonavir in stable virologically suppressed children 6 to 18 y.

For children and adolescents, an ongoing study (PENTA21/d3) is evaluating DTG+3 TC in ART naïve and treatment children and adolescents, with results expected in 2025.

New Classes of Antiretroviral Drugs

Several new classes of drugs are under evaluation in adults and children. The sites of action and examples of these classes are shown in **Fig. 1**. These new classes include:

HIV maturation inhibitors (MIs) target the final stages of the HIV life cycle by interfering with the proteolytic processing of the viral Gag polyprotein into its domains.[49–53]

Capsid Inhibitors disrupt the functioning of the HIV capsid protein across various stages in the viral life cycle.[54,55]

Attachment inhibitors target various stages of the HIV entry process, including virus internalization, membrane fusion, and antibody interactions.

Long-Acting Injectable Formulations

Long-acting injectable (LAI) formulations offer people living with HIV the opportunity to reduce the burden of administering daily oral ART, potentially improving patient satisfaction and adherence.[46,56,57] Increasing the duration of action can be achieved by changing the chemical structure of drugs, which alters the elimination of drugs, using novel drug formulations with very long half-lives, or using novel delivery mechanisms. Developing LAI formulations for children and adolescents has additional challenges, including incorporating changing weight of children, differences in body composition, especially related to fat and muscle composition, and developmental changes in metabolic rates. Several formulations are in various stages of clinical development.

LAI cabotegravir (CAB) and RPV is a 2-drug combination regimen for the treatment of people living with HIV. The current registration of the product is for the treatment of

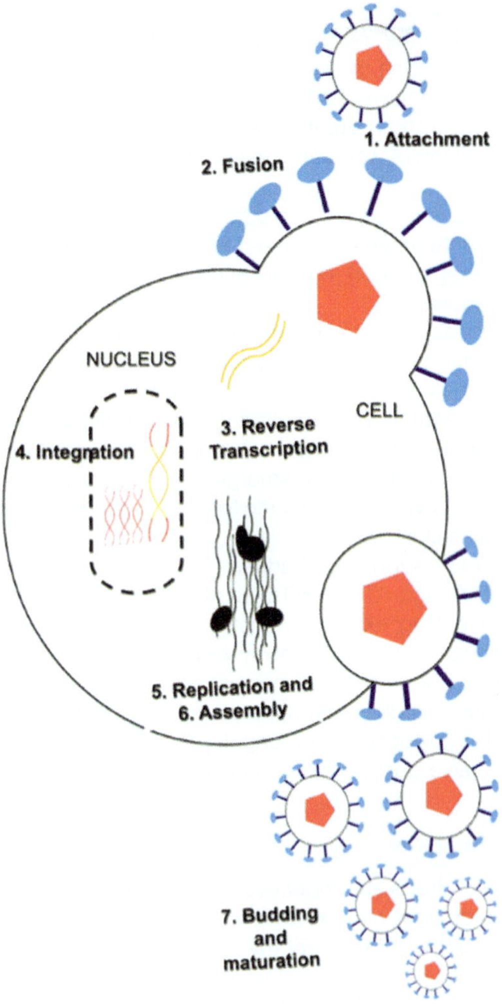

Fig. 1. New classes of drugs.

virally suppressed adults and adolescents on ART. The regimen is administered intramuscularly as 2 separate injections in the lateral gluteal muscle with or without a 4-week oral lead-in of oral CAB and RPV every 4 to 8 weeks. The need for refrigeration of injectable RPV, the cost of administration, and the cost of the medication are barriers to using the product in LMICs. The MOCHA trial established the appropriate dose of CAB/RPV and found that the combination was effective and safe in treating virally suppressed adolescents living with HIV. The regimen was found to be highly acceptable to both adolescents and their caregivers. A phase 3 study comparing CAB/RPV to standard-of-care in adolescents is ongoing. In the CRAYON study, injectable CAB/RPV is being evaluated in children 2 to 12 y old. Additional studies are being planned to evaluate the regimen in pregnant persons (IMPAACT P2040: CREATE study) and adolescents living with HIV with non-adherence.

Lenacapavir is approved as daily oral tablets and 6-monthly subcutaneous injections for the treatment of highly treatment-experienced adults with HIV in combination with an optimized background regimen and for PrEP. In the trial in highly treatment-experienced adults, 78% of participants maintained viral suppression for 52 w. Clinical trials for the treatment of adolescents and children living with HIV are being planned.

Broadly neutralizing anti-HIV-1 antibodies (bNAbs) are a new class of antiviral agents that neutralize HIV-1 and target infected cells for destruction by attaching to components of infected cells. The number determines the potency of bNAb strains of HIV that can be neutralized, the duration of neutralization, and the plasma concentrations required for neutralization. Due to a single individual's highly divergent viral populations, resistance to bNAb is the primary reason for treatment failure in clinical trials. The use of either combination of multiple bNAbs or bNAbs in combination with ARV drugs can overcome these issues. Modifications to the structure of the bNAbs can prolong the formulation's half-life when given intravenously or subcutaneously up to every 6 mo.

Long-acting Drug Delivery Systems

Several long-acting drug delivery systems of existing or new drug formulations are under evaluation.[58] Microarray patches (MAPs) are intradermal delivery devices that provide needleless drug delivery and can address the challenges of poor adherence in children.[58] Several drugs, including RPV and CAB nanosuspensions, are being evaluated for potential delivery via MAPs. MAPs are applied firmly as a patch on the skin for 5 to 10 mins and removed, leaving behind embedded microneedles in the dermis.[59]

SUMMARY

It is critical to manage pediatric HIV effectively by administering ART consistently and promptly to ensure better outcomes for children who are infected. Recent advancements in pediatric HIV care, such as early diagnosis and personalized ART, have significantly improved the overall quality of life for children affected by HIV. However, challenges such as medication adherence and potential long-term side effects still exist, highlighting the need for comprehensive healthcare strategies. To address these challenges and improve the long-term well-being of all children living with HIV, healthcare providers, caregivers, and communities must work together. Continued research and advocacy are crucial in advancing pediatric HIV care and maximizing the impact of ARV interventions.

Best Practices

What is the current practice for?

Treatment of HIV infection in children and youth

- Initiate ART promptly in children living with HIV, regardless of disease progression or immunologic status, to improve virologic control, reduce disease progression, diminish HIV reservoirs, and enhance long-term outcomes.
- Select ART regimens based on viral suppression rates, immunologic enhancement, toxicity profiles, availability of child-friendly formulations, dosing convenience, and limited drug interactions.
- Prioritize immediate initiation of combination ART (cART) for neonates (<28 day old) to mitigate mortality and morbidity risks associated with HIV infection.
- Ensure timely access to early infant HIV diagnosis through NAT, particularly in resource-constrained settings, to facilitate early initiation of cART.
- Develop and utilize age-appropriate ART formulations, considering PK differences and safety profiles in neonates.
- Implement dose adjustments based on rapid weight gain and developmental changes in neonates to optimize treatment efficacy and safety.

Bibliographic Source(s):
- Shiau S, Strehlau R, Technau KG, et al. Early age at start of antiretroviral therapy associated with better virologic control after initial suppression in HIV-infected infants. AIDS. 2017;31(3):355 to 364. https://doi.org/10.1097/QAD.0000000000001312.
- Schomaker M, Leroy V, Wolfs T, et al. Optimal timing of antiretroviral treatment initiation in HIV-positive children and adolescents: a multiregional analysis from Southern Africa, West Africa and Europe. Int J Epidemiol. 2017;46(2):453 to 465. https://doi.org/10.1093/ije/dyw097.
- Violari A, Cotton MF, Gibb DM, et al. Early antiretroviral therapy and mortality among HIV-infected infants. N Engl J Med. 2008;359(21):2233 to 2244. https://doi.org/10.1056/NEJMoa0800971.
- Babiker A, Castro nee Green H, et al., PENPACT-1 (PENTA 9/PACTG 390) Study Team. First-line antiretroviral therapy with a PI versus nonnucleoside reverse transcriptase inhibitor and switch at higher versus low viral load in HIV-infected children: an open-label, randomized phase 2/3 trial. Lancet Infect Dis. 2011;11(4):273-283. https://doi.org/10.1016/S1473-3099(1070313-3).
- Ruel TD, Kakuru A, Ikilezi G, et al. Virologic and immunologic outcomes of HIV-infected Ugandan children randomized to lopinavir/ritonavir or nonnucleoside reverse transcriptase inhibitor therapy. J Acquir Immune Defic Syndr. 2014;65(5):535 to 541. https://doi.org/10.1097/QAI.0000000000000071.
- Amuge P, Lugemwa A, Wynne B, et al., ODYSSEY Trial Team. Once-daily dolutegravir-based antiretroviral therapy in infants and children living with HIV from age 4 weeks: results from the below 14 kg cohort in the randomized ODYSSEY trial. Lancet HIV. 2022 Sep;9(9):e638-e648. https://doi.org/10.1016/S2352-3018(2200163-1)
- Panel on Antiretroviral Guidelines for Adults and Adolescents. Guidelines for the Use of Antiretroviral Agents in Adults and Adolescents with HIV. Department of Health and Human Services. Available at https://clinicalinfo.hiv.gov/en/guidelines/adult-and-adolescent-arv. (Accessed 03 April 2024)

DECLARATIONS

Funding: Financial support was not received for the study.

Author contributions: M. Archary, K. Mochankana and A. Bekker drafted the article, and all authors provided critical revisions and editing. All authors reviewed the article.

Competing interests: The authors declare that they have no financial or personal relationships that may have inappropriately influenced them in writing this article.

ACKNOWLEDGMENTS

The authors would like to thank the patients and their parents/carers who contributed to the research, as well as Leora Sewnarain for formatting and editing.

DISCLOSURE

We wish to confirm that there are no known conflicts of interest associated with this publication, and there has been no significant financial support for this work that could have influenced its outcome.

REFERENCES

1. Joint United Nations Programme on HIV/AIDS. AIDSInfo, global data on HIV epidemiology and response. Available at: https://aidsinfo.unaids.org/. Accessed February 5, 2024.
2. Atalell KA, Alene KA. Poor treatment outcomes of children on highly active antiretroviral therapy: protocol for a systematic review and meta-analysis. BMJ Open 2020;10(12):e040161.

3. Van Dyke RB, Lee S, Johnson GM, et al. Reported adherence as a determinant of response to highly active antiretroviral therapy in children who have human immunodeficiency virus infection. Pediatrics 2002;109(4):e61.
4. Phelps BR, Ahmed S, Amzel A, et al. Linkage, initiation and retention of children in the antiretroviral therapy cascade: an overview. AIDS 2013;27(Suppl 2): S207–13, 0 2.
5. Chi BH, Stringer JS, Moodley D. Antiretroviral drug regimens to prevent mother-to-child transmission of HIV: a review of scientific, program, and policy advances for sub-Saharan Africa. Curr HIV AIDS Rep 2013;10(2):124–33.
6. Hill LM, Saidi F, Freeborn K, et al. Tonse Pamodzi: developing a combination strategy to support adherence to antiretroviral therapy and HIV pre-exposure prophylaxis during pregnancy and breastfeeding. PLoS One 2021;16(6):e0253280.
7. Wilcher R, Petruney T, Cates W. The role of family planning in elimination of new pediatric HIV infection. Curr Opin HIV AIDS 2013;8(5):490–7.
8. Morris JL, Kraus DM. New antiretroviral therapies for pediatric HIV Infection. J Pediatr Pharmacol Therapeut 2005;10(4):215–47.
9. Lyons C, Mushavi A, Ngobeni-Allen F, et al. Ending pediatric AIDS and achieving a generation born HIV-free. J Acquir Immune Defic Syndr 2012;60(Suppl 2): S35–8.
10. Shiau S, Strehlau R, Technau KG, et al. Early age at start of antiretroviral therapy associated with better virologic control after initial suppression in HIV-infected infants. AIDS 2017;31(3):355–64.
11. Schomaker M, Leroy V, Wolfs T, et al. Optimal timing of antiretroviral treatment initiation in HIV-positive children and adolescents: a multiregional analysis from Southern Africa, West Africa and Europe. Int J Epidemiol 2017;46(2):453–65.
12. Violari A, Cotton MF, Gibb DM, et al. Early antiretroviral therapy and mortality among HIV-infected infants. N Engl J Med 2008;359(21):2233–44.
13. Rajasingham R, Meya DB, Greene GS, et al. Evaluation of a national cryptococcal antigen screening program for HIV-infected patients in Uganda: a cost-effectiveness modeling analysis. PLoS One 2019;14(1):e0210105.
14. Strategic timing of antiretroviral treatment – the START study. Available at: https://clinicaltrials.gov/study/NCT00867048. Accessed February 5, 2024.
15. Kay A, Mendez-Reyes J, Devezin T, et al. Optimal timing of antiretroviral therapy initiation in children and adolescents with human immunodeficiency virus-associated pulmonary tuberculosis. Clin Infect Dis 2023;76(1):10–7.
16. Ssebunya R, Wanyenze RK, Lukolyo H, et al. Antiretroviral therapy initiation within seven days of enrolment: outcomes and time to undetectable viral load among children at an urban HIV clinic in Uganda. BMC Infect Dis 2017;17(1):439.
17. Waalewijn H, Turkova A, Rakhmanina N, et al. Optimising pediatric dosing recommendations and treatment management of antiretroviral drugs using therapeutic drug monitoring data in children living with HIV. Ther Drug Monit 2019;41(4): 431–43.
18. Feng Q, Zhou A, Zou H, et al. Quadruple versus triple combination antiretroviral therapies for treatment naive people with HIV: systematic review and meta-analysis of randomised controlled trials. BMJ 2019;366:l4179.
19. Panel on antiretroviral therapy and medical management of children living with HIV. *Guidelines for the Use of antiretroviral Agents in pediatric HIV infection.* Department of health and human services. Year. Available at: https://clinicalinfo.hiv.gov/en/guidelines/pediatric-arv. Accessed March 27, 2024.
20. World Health Organization (WHO). Updated recommendations on HIV prevention, infant diagnosis, antiretroviral initiation and monitoring. 2021. Available at:

https://iris.who.int/bitstream/handle/10665/340190/9789240022232-eng.pdf?sequence=1. Accessed June 29, 2024.
21. Violari A, Lindsey JC, Hughes MD, et al. Nevirapine versus ritonavir-boosted lopinavir for HIV-infected children. N Engl J Med 2012;366(25):2380–9.
22. Babiker A, Castro nee Green H, Compagnucci A, et al. PENPACT-1 (PENTA 9/PACTG 390) Study Team. First-line antiretroviral therapy with a protease inhibitor versus non-nucleoside reverse transcriptase inhibitor and switch at higher versus low viral load in HIV-infected children: an open-label, randomised phase 2/3 trial. Lancet Infect Dis 2011;11(4):273–83.
23. Ruel TD, Kakuru A, Ikilezi G, et al. Virologic and immunologic outcomes of HIV-infected Ugandan children randomised to lopinavir/ritonavir or non-nucleoside reverse transcriptase inhibitor therapy. J Acquir Immune Defic Syndr 2014;65(5):535–41.
24. Amuge P, Lugemwa A, Wynne B, et al. ODYSSEY Trial Team. Once-daily dolutegravir-based antiretroviral therapy in infants and children living with HIV from age 4 weeks: results from the below 14 kg cohort in the randomised ODYSSEY trial. Lancet HIV 2022;9(9):e638–48.
25. Clinton health access initiative (CHAI). 2023 HIV market report: the state of the HIV market in low- and middle-income countries. 2023. Available at: https://chai19.wpenginepowered.com/wp-content/uploads/2023/11/2023-HIV-Market-Report_11.17.23.pdf. Accessed April 3, 2024.
26. Symonds W, Cutrell A, Edwards M, et al. Risk factor analysis of hypersensitivity reactions to abacavir. Clin Therapeut 2002;24(4):565–73.
27. Ventosa-Cubillo J, Pinzón R, González-Alba JM, et al. Drug resistance in children and adolescents with HIV in Panama. J Antimicrob Chemother 2023;78(2):423–35.
28. Prendergast AJ, Szubert AJ, Pimundu G, et al. The impact of viraemia on inflammatory biomarkers and CD4+ cell subpopulations in HIV-infected children in sub-Saharan Africa. AIDS 2021;35(10):1537–48.
29. World Health Organization (WHO). WHO recommendations on the diagnosis of HIV infection in infants and children – guideline. 2010. Available at: https://www.who.int/publications/i/item/9789241599085. Accessed February 5, 2024.
30. Meggi B, Vojnov L, Mabunda N, et al. Performance of point-of-care birth HIV testing in primary health care clinics: an observational cohort study. PLoS One 2018;13(6):e0198344.
31. Mwenda R, Fong Y, Magombo T, et al. Significant patient impact observed upon implementation of point-of-care early infant diagnosis technologies in an observational study in Malawi. Clin Infect Dis 2018;67(5):701–7.
32. U.S. Department of Health and Human Services. FDA-approved HIV medications. Available at: https://hivinfo.nih.gov/understanding-hiv/fact-sheets/fda-approved-hiv-medicines. Accessed June 29, 2024.
33. FDA Drug Safety Communication. Serious health problems seen in premature babies given Kaletra (lopinavir/ritonavir) oral solution. Available at: https://www.fda.gov/drugs/drug-safety-and-availability/fda-drug-safety-communication-serious-health-problems-seen-premature-babies-given-kaletra. Accessed June 29, 2024.
34. Bekker A, Salvadori N, Rabie H, et al. PETITE-ABC/3TC-LPVr Study Team. Paediatric abacavir-lamivudine fixed-dose dispersible tablets and ritonavir-boosted lopinavir granules in neonates exposed to HIV (PETITE study): an open-label, two-stage, single-arm, phase 1/2, pharmacokinetic and safety trial. Lancet HIV 2024;11(2):e86–95.

35. Bekker A, Capparelli EV, Violari A, et al. IMPAACT P1106 team. Abacavir dosing in neonates from birth to 3 months of life: a population pharmacokinetic modelling and simulation study. Lancet HIV 2022 Jan;9(1):e24–31.
36. Rosebush JC, Best BM, Chadwick EG, et al. for the IMPAACT 2007 Study Team. Pharmacokinetics and safety of maraviroc in neonates. Pharmacokinetics and safety of maraviroc in neonates. AIDS 2021;35(3):419–27.
37. World Health Organization (WHO). Consolidated guidelines on HIV prevention, testing, treatment, service delivery and monitoring: recommendations for a public health approach, 16 July 2021. Available at: https://iris.who.int/bitstream/handle/10665/342899/9789240031593-eng.pdf?sequence=1. Accessed June 29, 2024.
38. Clarke DF, Lommerse J, Acosta EP, et al. Impact of low birth weight and prematurity on neonatal raltegravir pharmacokinetics: impaact P1097. J Acquir Immune Defic Syndr 2020;85(5):626–34.
39. Bekker A, Salvadori N, Rabie H, et al. *Single-dose PK/Safety of DTG-dispersible Tablets in neonates supports multi-dosing: PETITE-DTG study* (abstract #941). Denver, Colorado, USA: CROI; 2024. March 3-6.
40. Capparelli EV, Mirochnick M, Dankner WM, et al. Pediatric AIDS clinical trials group 331 investigators. Pharmacokinetics and tolerance of zidovudine in preterm infants. J Pediatr 2003;142(1):47–52.
41. RETROVIR® (zidovudine) package insert. Available at: https://www.accessdata.fda.gov/drugsatfda_docs/label/2008/019910s033lbl.pdf. Accessed April 3, 2024.
42. Piscitelli J, Nikanjam M, Best BM, et al. Optimising dolutegravir initiation in neonates using population pharmacokinetic modeling and simulation. J Acquir Immune Defic Syndr 2022;89(1):108–14.
43. U.S. Department of health and human services. FDA package insert for dolutegravir. Available at: https://www.accessdata.fda.gov/drugsatfda_docs/label/2020/213983s000lbl.pdf. Accessed June 29, 2024.
44. Kawade N, Onishi S. The prenatal and postnatal development of UDP-glucuronyltransferase activity towards bilirubin and the effect of premature birth on this activity in the human liver. Biochem J 1981;196(1):257–60.
45. Schreiner CN, Ahlfors CE, Wong RJ, et al. In vitro study on the effect of maraviroc or dolutegravir on bilirubin to albumin binding. Pediatr Infect Dis J 2018;37(9):908–9.
46. Nachman S, Townsend CL, Abrams EJ, et al. Long-acting or extended-release antiretroviral products for HIV treatment and prevention in infants, children, adolescents, and pregnant and breastfeeding women: knowledge gaps and research priorities. Lancet HIV 2019;6(8):e552–8.
47. Temereanca A, Ruta S. Strategies to overcome HIV drug resistance-current and future perspectives. Front Microbiol 2023;14:1133407.
48. Gibas KM, Kelly SG, Arribas JR, et al. Two-drug regimens for HIV treatment. Lancet HIV 2022;9(12):e868–83.
49. Sarkar S, Zadrozny KK, Zadorozhnyi R, et al. Structural basis of HIV-1 maturation inhibitor binding and activity. Nat Commun 2023;14(1):1237.
50. Pak AJ, Purdy MD, Yeager M, et al. Preservation of HIV-1 Gag helical bundle symmetry by bevirimat is central to maturation inhibition. J Am Chem Soc 2021;143(45):19137–48.
51. Dicker I, Jeffrey JL, Protack T, et al. GSK3640254 is a novel HIV-1 maturation inhibitor with an optimised virology profile. Antimicrob Agents Chemother 2022;66(1):e0187621.

52. Spinner CD, Felizarta F, Rizzardini G, et al. Phase IIa proof-of-concept evaluation of the antiviral efficacy, safety, tolerability, and pharmacokinetics of the next-generation maturation inhibitor GSK3640254. Clin Infect Dis 2022;75(5):786–94.
53. Wen B, Zhang Y, Young GC, et al. Investigation of clinical absorption, distribution, metabolism, and excretion and pharmacokinetics of the HIV-1 maturation inhibitor GSK3640254 using an intravenous microtracer combined with enterotracker for biliary sampling. Drug Metab Dispos 2022;50(11):1442–53.
54. Sornsuwan K, Thongkhum W, Pamonsupornwichit T, et al. Performance of affinity-improved DARPin targeting HIV capsid domain in interference of viral progeny production. Biomolecules 2021;11(10):1437.
55. Kobayakawa T, Yokoyama M, Tsuji K, et al. Small-molecule anti-HIV-1 agents based on HIV-1 capsid proteins. Biomolecules 2021;11(2):208.
56. Brizzi M, Pérez SE, Michienzi SM, et al. Long-acting injectable antiretroviral therapy: will it change the future of HIV treatment? Ther Adv Infect Dis 2023;10. https://doi.org/10.1177/20499361221149773. 20499361221149773.
57. Lorenzetti L, Dinh N, van der Straten A, et al. Systematic review of the values and preferences regarding the use of injectable pre-exposure prophylaxis to prevent HIV acquisition. J Int AIDS Soc 2023;26(Suppl 2):e26107.
58. Flexner C, Owen A, Siccardi M, et al. Long-acting drugs and formulations for the treatment and prevention of HIV infection. Int J Antimicrob Agents 2021;57(1):106220.
59. Moffatt K, Tekko IA, Vora L, et al. Development and evaluation of dissolving microarray patches for co-administered and repeated intradermal delivery of long-acting rilpivirine and cabotegravir nanosuspensions for paediatric HIV antiretroviral therapy. Pharm Res (N Y) 2023;40(7):1673–96.

Prevention, Diagnosis, and Treatment of Tuberculosis in Children with Human Immunodeficiency Virus

Charles D. Mitchell, MD, MS

KEYWORDS

• Tuberculosis • Pediatrics • Diagnosis • Prevention and treatment

KEY POINTS

- The prevention of tuberculosis (TB) infection and disease is hindered by the high prevalence of latent TB infection (LTBI) in TB-endemic countries where the majority of children coinfected with TB and human immunodeficiency virus (HIV) reside.
- Isoniazid can prevent the majority of cases of LTBI from progressing to active TB disease but appears to not be effective in preventing primary TB infection and progression to active disease in infants and young children.
- The diagnosis of TB in children can be problematic especially in children living with HIV because of the paucibacillary nature of pulmonary TB in young children.
- While the majority of tuberculosis cases are treatable, drug resistance is common in many TB-endemic countries.

INTRODUCTION

Mycobacterium tuberculosis (MTB) has coevolved with humans. As early hominids migrated out of Africa and spread across the globe,[1] they carried with them the progenitors of what would become MTB. As a disease, tuberculosis is an ancient malady. MTB DNA has been detected in a 39,000 year old Neanderthal skeletal remains from a cave in Hungary[2]; as well as more recently in a vertebrate from Pompeii (79AD).[3] Classical pathologic findings of Pott's disease have also been documented in Egyptian mummies from 2400 BC.[4] Hence, as mankind has evolved and human civilizations developed, MTB and tuberculosis have been a constant companion. Human immunodeficiency virus (HIV) as a human pathogen and HIV-associated disease and acquired immune deficiency syndrome in contrast emerged relatively recently most likely within

Division of Pediatric Infectious Diseases and Immunology, Batchelor Childrens Research Institute, University of Miami Miller School of Medicine, 1580 Northwest 10th Avenue, Miami, FL 33133, USA
E-mail address: Cmitchel@med.miami.edu

Clin Perinatol 51 (2024) 833–847
https://doi.org/10.1016/j.clp.2024.08.012 **perinatology.theclinics.com**

the last century. It is interesting to compare and contrast the respective ages of these 2 agents with the respective progress made in their diagnosis and their clinical management. While significant progress has been made in treating TB and HIV within the last 50 years, the diagnosis of HIV infection is straightforward, while the confirmation of MTB disease can be problematic.

PREVENTION OF TUBERCULOSIS INFECTION AND DISEASE IN CHILDREN LIVING WITH HUMAN IMMUNODEFICIENCY VIRUS

In both the United States and the developing world, prevention of TB infection and TB disease in children living with HIV (CLWH) should be a high priority as the risk of latent TB progressing to active TB is 8 to 10 fold higher among patients living with HIV when compared with those without HIV.[5] TB infection control should be routinely practiced in the clinical setting and patients should be asked about possible exposure to infectious TB (especially within their own household) at each encounter and cautioned to avoid any known contacts. Antiretroviral therapy should be started early in CLWH to optimize HIV viral suppression and minimize HIV-mediated immunosuppression.[6] Annual screening should be done consistently to insure prompt detection of latent TB infection (LTBI).The value of this approach will vary depending upon the local TB prevalence, the patients' birth country, travel history of the patient or household members who may have recently returned from a TB-endemic area, or residence in congregate settings (ie, recent stays in migrant camps in Texas after immigrating from Mexico). All children with a positive tuberculin skin test (TST)/interferon-gamma release assay (IGRA) or who are known to have had close contact with an infectious case should be given preventive therapy after ruling out active disease. The risk of progression from latent to active disease is increased 26 to 31 fold in CLWH.[5] TB reactivation rates can be substantially reduced by 60% to 90% by preventative therapy employing isoniazid (INH) alone or in combination with rifampin or other drugs.[7,8]

In CLWH aged 2 years and older, a once-weekly combination therapy consisting of once weekly INH and rifapentine (3HP) is as safe and effective as 9 months of INH.[9,10] This regimen has acceptable drug–drug interaction between antiretroviral therapy (ART) and rifapentine and superior rates of adherence.[11] Alternative acceptable treatment regimens for children of all ages who have LTBI include 4 months of daily rifampin (used when a known contact has INH-resistant MTB), or 3 months of daily INH and rifampin. Directly observed therapy (DOT) may be utilized when adherence is questionable. The dosing of both dolutegravir and raltegravir may have to be adjusted with these latter regimens (**Table 1**).

A drug interaction has been studied in adults and not children, applies to adults taking DTG or RAL only

While the efficacy of secondary INH prophylaxis to prevent TB reactivation is accepted,[8] the use of INH as primary prophylaxis to prevent initial or primary MTB infection is questionable. The World Health Organization (WHO) has continued to recommend that HIV infected children aged over 1 year in high TB-incidence settings should receive INH preventive therapy if there is no contraindications and they have a negative symptom screen whether they are on ART or not.[12] A phase III, prospective double blind placebo controlled trial (PACTG/IMPAACT 1041) of primary INH prophylaxis in southern Africa in both HIV perinatally exposed HIV infected and uninfected infants and young children given from 3 to 27 months of age found that there was no reduction in active TB disease in the INH treatment groups.[13] A subsequent Cochrane review was designed to address a similar question; whether TB preventative therapy (IPT) was efficacious in reducing active TB, death, and reported adverse effects in

Table 1
Tuberculosis prevention treatment options

Medicines	Isoniazid (H)	Isoniazid (H) and Rifapentine (P)	Isoniazid and Rifampicin (R)	Rifampicin (R)	Isoniazid (H) and Rifapentine (P)
Duration (months)	6	3	3	4	1
Interval/Frequency	Daily	Weekly	Daily	Daily	Daily
Children[a]	All ages, child-friendly formulation available; preferred in CLWHIV on LPV-RTV, NVP or DTG	≥ 2 y. No child-friendly formulation available	All ages, child-friendly (dispersible) formulation available and recommended up to 25 kg weight	All ages, no child-friendly formulation available, no formulation available for infants <8 kg weight Useful where index has INH-resistant MTB	
Interactions with ART[a,b]	No restriction	Contraindicated: All PIs, NVP/NNRTIs, TAF Use: TDF, EFV (600 mg), DTG[a], RAL[a]	Contraindicated: All PIs, NVP/most NNRTIs Use with caution TAF Adjust dose: DTG, RAL Use: TDF, EFV (600 mg)	Contraindicated: All PIs, NVP/most NNRTIs, TAF Adjust dose: DTG, RAL Use: TDF, EFV (600 mg)	Contraindicated: All PIs, NVP/most NNRTIs, TAF Use: TDF, EFV (600 mg), DTG[a], RAL[a]

[a] DTG, dolutegravir; EFT, efavirenz; LPV-RTV, lopinavir-ritonavir; NNRTI, non-nucleoside reverse transcriptase inhibitors; NVP, nevirapine; PIs, protease inhibitors; RAL, raltegravir; TAF, tenofovir alafenamide; TDF, tenofovir disoproxil fumarate.
[b] A drug interaction has been studied in adults and not children, applies to adults taking DTG or RAL only.
Adapted from WHO operational handbook on tuberculosis. Module 1: Prevention Tuberculosis preventive treatment 2020.

CLWH.[14] In this later case, the ability of IPT to prevent both primary disease resulting from initial infection and secondary TB disease following reactivation was being assessed in a controlled trial of INH versus placebo in CLWH. In CLWH not on ART, INH reduced the number of children developing TB by 69% and death by 54% (both with low certainty evidence). The number of adverse effects was similar in the 2 groups. In the one study of CLWH on ART, there was no apparent benefit or harm of INH (very low certainty evidence). A more recent systematic review and meta-analysis found that INH did not reduce the incidence of TB in CLWH[5] but did not address whether INH was effective in CLWH not receiving ART.

The live bacterial vaccine, Bacillus Calmette Guerin (BCG), is the only TB vaccine licensed for clinical use. It is routinely used in TB-endemic areas as a neonatal vaccine to reduce the risk of disseminated TB but it is not thought to protect against pulmonary TB.[15] The WHO has recommended delaying BCG vaccination until an HIV-infected infant is stable on ART. In practice, however, BCG is usually given during the neonatal period unless there is clinical evidence of HIV infection. The Red Book recommends that its use in the United States be limited to select circumstances, that is, repeated MTB exposures or failure of other control measures. It is not routinely recommended for CLWH in the United States because of the local epidemiology of TB in the United States and the risk of complications, that is, BCG lymphadenitis.

DIAGNOSIS OF TUBERCULOSIS INFECTION

Diagnosis of Latent Tuberculosis Infection

Approximately, 25% to 30%[16] of the world's population is infected with MTB with the greater majority having latent TB. Most live in developing countries. Because of the high rate of progression to clinical TB disease following primary infection in younger children (ie, 50% of infants without HIV in the first year of life progress to TB disease) and the increased risk of progression in people with both TB and HIV,[17] screening for LTBI in CLWH should be started between 3 and 12 months of age and then repeated annually. Because of this appreciable risk, HIV-infected children should be frequently asked about possible TB exposures.[7]

Both of the methods used to diagnose latent TB (Mantoux or TST and the IGRA), rely upon detecting a T cell-immune response to MTB antigens. Both might be impaired in immunosuppressed CLWH although as per Center for Disease Control and Prevention (CDC) guidelines, they can be used in sufficiently nourished children aged 5 years or more with well-controlled HIV infection.[11,18] The Food and Drug Administration (FDA) has approved the QuantiFERON-TB Gold (QFT), the QFT-Plus (Cellestis Limited, Valencia, Ca.), and T SPOT@.TB assay (Oxford Immunotec, Marlborough, Massachusetts). Interpretation of the results of both the TST and the IGRA must include consideration of epidemiologic (ie, contact history, country of origin), and medical factors (concomitant diagnoses). The American Academy of Pediatrics Red Book Committee on Infectious Diseases[15] has recommended that the IGRA can be used in children aged 2 years or more although the CDC still recommends that the TST be used between ages 2 and 5 years. The IGRA is preferred for screening BCG-vaccinated patients because of the possible cross-reactivity between TST and BCG, and those not likely to return in 2 days for the reading of a TST.[19] While the IGRA can be performed in 1 day, in many centers, it may take 24 to 48 hours to get the results because of the need to do batch testing.

Nguyen and colleagues reported the results of QFT-Plus testing in Vietnamese children with TB. Using multiple logistic regression modeling, they noted that age, a history of TB, or having confirmed TB were significantly associated with having a positive

QFT-Plus. The sensitivity of the QFT-Plus in children with pulmonary TB (PTB; 84.2%) was superior to that in children with extrapulmonary TB (EPTB; 14.3%) or PTB and EPTB [14.3%]. The overall sensitivity of the QFT-Plus assay in children in this study was 54.5%.[20] None of the children tested for HIV (27.5% of the study population of 222) were found to have HIV. Further studies need to be done to generate additional data regarding sensitivity and specificity of the IGRA in CLWH and young children aged under 2 years.

Simultaneous performance of both assays may increase the sensitivity of detecting latent TB, but if done, the IGRA should be drawn before placing the TST. A positive result from either one is diagnostic of LTBI. Following initial MTB infection, TST reactivity may develop before the IGRA becomes positive (personal communication: Edward Graviss). Neither the TST nor the IGRA can be construed to definitely exclude TB infection or disease in a child living with HIV.[11]

The traditional Mantoux test or the TST involves injecting 0.1 mL of purified protein derivative (PPD) solution intradermally in the left arm. PPD that is, in fact, not purified contains a complex mixture of MTB-derived proteins some of which may cross-react with other non-tuberculose mycobacterium. The TST should not be read until 48 hours postinjection and the interpretation should be based upon the degree of induration at the injection site. The administration and interpretation of the TST should be done by trained personnel preferably with experience in its performance. The use of control antigens is no longer recommended. As the TST may be adversely affected by severe malnutrition and measles, or live virus vaccinations, the timing of the latter should be done at the same time or delayed for 4 weeks following vaccination.[15] Two step TST testing may elicit a positive response in patients who have some prior sensitization but will not induce a false-positive response. This phenomenon has not been well studied in children or in people living with HIV.[19]

A positive TST test in PLWH is indicated by 5 mm or greater of induration at 48 hours postinjection but the TST in this population may lack sensitivity. A positive response in a person not living with HIV is traditionally thought of as 10 or more mm of induration. The determination of the cutoffs for a positive reaction in these latter patients may be influenced by other epidemiologic, medical, or timing factors. A further discussion of this can be found in reference.[15]

The IGRA is a blood test that involves in vitro incubation of the lymphocytes in the presence of TB antigens followed by measurement of extracellular production of gamma interferon (IFN©). Two diagnostic TB IGRA assays are currently FDA approved for use in the United States, the QuantiFERON-TB Gold Plus (QFT-Plus), and the T-SPOT.TB test (T-Spot; CDC Web site). The T-SPOT is somewhat different as it detects the number of immunoreactive T cells that produce IFN©. The results of the IGRA can be reported as being either positive, negative, or indeterminate. An indeterminate result usually occurs when the positive control does not work thus impairing the interpretation of the assay. If there is a strong suspicion of TB infection, then it should be repeated recognizing that if the patient is malnourished, or immunosuppressed, the same result may occur. While a TST that may show some degree of cross-reactivity with BCG following vaccination, the IGRA will not; hence, a positive IGRA reaction suggests MTB infection. Neither the TST nor the IGRA can distinguish latent from active TB infection.[7]

If either the TST or the IGRA is positive, then the patient should have a chest radiograph and clinical evaluation to exclude active clinical disease.

Diagnosis of Active Tuberculosis Disease

The diagnosis of TB disease is similar in all children regardless of HIV status; although the diagnosis in infected children may be problematic because they may have a lower pathogen load. The constellation of symptoms that a child with TB presents with may be helpful in making the diagnosis but they are nonspecific. They include the following signs or symptoms of TB: cough greater than 14 days, documented weight loss in past 3 months or failure to thrive, anorexia, persistent lethargy, or fever.[21] A refined symptom-based approach proved useful in diagnosing PTB in all children but less useful in immunocompromised CLWH. Clinical case definitions for classifications of intrathoracic TB in children were developed in an attempt to standardize the diagnosis of PTB and include the designations of confirmed PTB (based upon a detecting MTB on culture or Polymerase Chain Reaction (PCR) in sputum), unconfirmed PTB (based upon a constellation of clinical findings without microbiological confirmation), and unlikely TB (without either microbiological or compatible clinical findings).[22] Similarly, there are no findings on clinical examination that are specific for TB but there are certain signs that are highly suggestive of EPTB (recent onset gibbus resulting from vertebral TB, non-painful enlarged cervical lymphadenopathy). The term paucibacillary, often used to describe PTB in young children in general, refers to the low rate of positive MTB cultures obtained from sputum or gastric wash specimens from these patients. The exact cause of this is unclear. It may be that in an immunologically immature host, that is, a child aged under 1 to 2 years or with HIV coinfection, the risk of active TB disease may result from even a lower inoculum of the TB bacilli.

A chest radiograph is required to document the classical findings of PTB: perihilar/peritracheal lymphadenopathy, peripheral pulmonic focus, consolidation, cavitations, and atelectasis.[23] A chest radiograph may also reveal miliary TB (diffuse reticular nodular lesions in both lung fields) suggestive of disseminated TB. A miliary pattern in a child who acquired HIV perinatally not yet on ART, however, may be secondary to lymphoid interstitial pneumonitis and not miliary TB (personal experience by the author).

The direct methods to confirm a microbiological diagnosis of TB include acid-fast bacillus (AFB) microscopy, nucleic acid amplification tests (NAATs), and AFB culture. The sensitivity of these assays, however, is limited in all young children (both living with and without HIV) because of the paucibacillary nature of their TB lung disease and their inability to expectorate.[15] The NAAT has replaced the use of AFB microscopy in many centers likely because of its enhanced sensitivity and the possibility that a positive AFB smear may be detecting non-TB Mycobacterium (NTM), that is, *Mycobacterium avium*, or *Mycobacterium fortuitum* and not MTB. While NTM may be pathogenic in immunosuppressed children, they are usually commensal organisms. There are 2 FDA-approved NAATs: the Amplified Mycobacterium Tuberculosis Direct Test (Gen-Probe) and the Xpert MTB/RIF (Xpert, Cepheid) that can detect rifampin but not INH resistance in sputum samples. The Xpert MTB/RIF has been endorsed by WHO for testing of sputum specimens from children as well as extrapulmonary specimens.[24] A systematic review and meta-analysis of the sensitivities of the Xpert MTB/RIF and culture of respiratory specimens found that they were similar (approximately 62% for expectorated/induce sputum and 66% for gastric wash samples).[25] A recent Cochrane Review (2022) found that the respective sensitivities of NAAT to culture for extrapulmonary samples varied by specimen type.[26] There have been various methods attempted to expedite the detection of MTB on culture, and while these have been helpful, they have not appreciably improved the sensitivity of culture.

Given the difficulties of confirming a TB diagnosis in children, there have been efforts at making a diagnosis based upon non-sputum-based testing. The urinary excretion of lipoarabinomannan (LAM, an MTB virulence factor that protects the bacilli against oxidative radical mediated killing) has been shown in a prospective study to lack sensitivity (<50%) and specificity (~60%) for diagnosing TB in both HIV-infected and uninfected children.[27,28]

Xpert has also been used to detect MTB in stool samples from children both living with HIV and without but the sensitivity was suboptimal and lower than Xpert testing of respiratory specimens reported in this same study.[29] Whole blood gene expression has been shown to have promise diagnosing TB in adults, but this is not approved for routine use, is not a point-of-care (POC) test, and is not well studied in children with HIV.[30]

More recently, Mao and colleagues reported preliminary data of a blood-based assay that detects the MTB Culture Filtrate Protein (CFP)-10 virulence factor peptides employing nanotechnology and matrix-assisted laser desorption ionization time-of-flight mass spectrometry. In HIV-infected infants, CFP-10 signal had 100% sensitivity for confirmed TB (5 out of 5, 95% confidence interval [CI], 47.8–100) and 83.7% sensitivity for unconfirmed TB (36 out of 43, 95% CI 69.3–93.2), with 93.1% specificity (203 out of 218, 95% CI 88.9–96.1). In HIV-uninfected infants, CFP-10 signal detected a single confirmed TB case and 75.0% of unconfirmed TB cases (15 out of 20; 95% CI 50.9–91.3), with 96.2% specificity (177 out of 184, 95% CI, 92.3–98.5). Both CFP-10-positivity and concentration declined following anti-TB therapy initiation. As this was a retrospective analysis of prospectively collected samples and the number of cases was limited, further discussion on this assay must await additional data.[31] This would not be a POC assay but this same group is investigating the potential of using Clustered Regularly Interspaced Short Palidromic Repeats; a gene editing tool (CRISPR) PCR technology for diagnosing TB as a POC blood-based assay.[32]

TREATMENT OF ACTIVE TUBERCULOSIS IN CHILDREN LIVING WITH HUMAN IMMUNODEFICIENCY VIRUS

Treatment of Drug-susceptible Tuberculosis Disease in Children Living with Human Immunodeficiency Virus

TB molecular and phenotypic drug susceptibility testing (DST) should be done on all patient MTB isolates. Alternatively, if available, the DST pattern of an adult TB contact can be used to guide therapy.[18] The treatment of TB disease in CLWH should be conducted under DOT to insure adherence and prevent treatment failure and/or the development of resistance.[7] Treatment of TB is similar in CLWH and children living without HIV but may be complicated by ART and TB drug interactions and their associated toxicities. The assistance of an expert with prior experience in managing these cases is recommended. The minimum total duration in patients with pulmonary disease is 6 months and traditionally involves the 4 drug regimen of once-daily INH, rifampin, pyrazinamide, and ethambutol for the first 2 months followed by the continuation of both INH and rifampin for 4 months ("4 for 2 followed by 2 for 4").[7] In cases with known drug-susceptible TB, INH, rifampin, and pyrazinamide may be used as a 3 drug regimen for the first 2 months with the first 2 being used for the final 4 months.[18]

Drug dosing for each of the anti-TB agents is listed in the Red Book.[15]

For CLWH with EPTB disease (TB meningitis, osteoarticular disease, or miliary disease), treatment should be continued for 12 months (2 month intensive phase followed by a 10 months continuation phase) in those cases with a fully susceptible isolate. For TB meningitis, ethionamide or an aminoglycoside should replace ethambutol because of their ability to achieve higher cerebrospinal fluid levels.[33] Details are provided in **Table 2**.

All CLWH already on ART-containing nevirapine and/or protease inhibitors who are starting TB therapy should have rifampin replaced by rifabutin as the former is a potent

Table 2
Tuberculosis treatment recommendations

Age	Severity of TB	Total Treatment Duration (months)	Intensive Phase months/Regimen	Continuation Phase Months/Regimen
Drug-sensitive pulmonary TB				
<3 mo or weighing <3 kg	Pulmonary TB of any severity	6	2/HRZE[b]	4/HR
3 mo to <12 y	Non-severe pulmonary TB[a]	4	2/HRZE[b]	2/HR
	Severe pulmonary TB	6	2/HRZE[b]	4/HR
12 to <16 y	Non-severe pulmonary TB	4	2/HRZE[b]	4/HR
	Severe pulmonary TB	6	2/HRZE[b]	4/HR
	Pulmonary T of any severity	4	2/HPZM	2/HPM
16 to <20 y	Pulmonary TB of any severity	6	2/HRZE[b]	4/HR
	Pulmonary TB of any severity	4	2/HPZM	2/HPM
Drug-sensitive extrapulmonary TB				
<3 mo or weighing <3 kg	Peripheral lymph node TB	6	2/HRZE[b]	4/HR
3 mo to <16 y	Peripheral lymph node TB	4	2/HRZE[b]	2/HR
>16 y	Peripheral lymph node TB	6	2/HRZE[b]	4/HR
0–19 y	Extrapulmonary TB	6	2/HRZE	4/HR
	TB meningitis	12	2/HRZEto	10/HR
	Osteoarticular TB	12	2/HRZE	10/HR

H isoniazid, R rifampicin, Z pyrazinamide, E ethambutol, HPZM—isoniazid, rifapentin, moxifloxacin, pyrazinamide, HPM—isoniazid, rifapentin, moxifloxacin, HRZEto—isoniazid, rifampicin, pyrazinamide, ethionamide.

[a] Non-severe pulmonary TB defined as peripheral lymph node TB, intrathoracic lymph node TB without airway obstruction, uncomplicated TB pleural effusion or paucibacillary, non-cavitatory disease confined to one lobe of the lungs, and without a military pattern.

[b] The use of ethambutol is recommended in Children Living with HIV (CLHIV) or high HIV prevalence settings or isoniazid resistance.

Adapted from WHO operational handbook on tuberculosis. Module 5: Management of tuberculosis in children and adolescents 2022)

CYP3A enzyme system inducer and can result in reduced plasma drug concentrations. Rifabutin exhibits minimal CYP3A drug interactions.[15] Rifampin has minimal drug interaction with efavirenz; hence, regimens containing this agent are preferable. If not feasible, other options include the following: nevirapine with a dose adjustment (200 mg/m3); ritonavir-boosted PI-based regimens; or a temporary triple nucleoside reverse transcriptase inhibitor regimen (ie, abacavir–emtricitabine–zidovudine) in children who are virologically suppressed. There are only limited data at present on the use of an integrase-based regimen in combination with rifampin-based treatment. In CLWH greater than 20 kg, twice daily dolutegravir achieves adequate pharmacokinetic levels when used in conjunction with rifampin, while raltegravir dosing of 12 mg/kg twice daily in children less than 20 kg on rifampin achieves targeted levels.[7]

For ART naïve children on TB therapy, ART should be started within 2 to 8 weeks of starting TB treatment as both adult and pediatric data suggest that early ART therapy is associated with reduced mortality in profoundly immunosuppressed patients despite the risk of immune response inflammatory syndrome (IRIS). ART initiation in such children within 2 weeks of starting TB therapy would be indicated if there is severe HIV disease.[34] CLWH who are not severely ill should have their ART started within 8 weeks. The CLWH with TB meningitis should be evaluated for early ART initiation but this option should be weighed against the fact that the optimal time for starting ART in patients with central nervous system (CNS) TB remains controversial because of the potential severe effects of CNS IRIS.[35]

Treatment of Drug-resistant Tuberculosis in Children Living with Human Immunodeficiency Virus

Drug-resistant TB should be suspected when (1) there is a history of inadequate prior TB treatment or the index case has such a history; (2) the index case is known to have drug-resistant TB; (3) residence in or travel to regions or setting with a high prevalence of drug-resistant TB; (4) putative source case has positive AFB smears or cultures 2 or more months after starting TB therapy; (5) relapse of TB following completion of TB therapy; and/or (6) failure to respond to adequate TB therapy.[7]

The fundamental principle in proscribing a regimen in these children is that the regimen be individualized based on the resistance pattern of the *MTB* isolate, the prior treatment history of the patient, and the susceptibility pattern of the isolate from a likely contact source if one is available. Additional considerations should be given the following: the relative activities of each drug (ie, bacteriocidal vs bacteriostatic), then extent of disease, and any comorbid conditions.

In cases with isolated INH resistance,[18] the INH should be discontinued and the child treated for 6 to 9 months with a rifampin-based regimen in combination with pyrazinamide and ethambutol. Recent reports also suggest that a late-generation fluoroquinolone be added for the duration of therapy. Detection of rifampin resistance by a rapid test suggests that the isolate is multidrug-resistant as 70% of these isolates are multidrug-resistant TB (MDR-TB). Phenotypic testing (DST) for both INH and rifampin should be done to confirm susceptibility or resistance to these agents.

The treatment of children with multidrug-resistant tuberculosis should be based on DST to optimize the treatment response. Continued use of agents to which the MDR isolate is resistant is associated with treatment failure, the development of additional drug resistance, and toxicity. The results of susceptibility testing of an MDR isolate from a known source case can be used to guide therapy when the child's isolate is not available. A minimum regimen of 5 active drugs should be used (2 or more of which should be bactericidal).[18,33,36,37] A full discussion of the treatment of multidrug-resistant tuberculosis is beyond the scope of this monograph, but the *WHO*

Operational Handbook on Tuberculosis, Module 4 Treatment, Drug-resistant Tuberculosis Treatment contains a full discussion of the treatment of MDR-TB and extensively drug-resistant TB (XDR-TB[38]; see also **Tables 3** and **4**).

Treatment of Extensively Drug-resistant Tuberculosis

The management of extensively drug-resistant TB should be performed in concert with an expert experienced in treating these patients. Both the WHO and CDC have recently updated their definition of XDR-TB. The WHO defines XDR-TB as any isolate that is MDR/RR-TB and resistant to both any fluoroquinolone and one additional WHO-defined Group A drug (eg, bedaquiline or linezolid).[39] The WHO Grouping (A, B, and C) of anti-TB agents recommended for use in longer MDR-TB and MDR/RR-TB regimens can be found in the WHO Handbook and in reference 39. The US-CDC definition of XDR-TB describes XDR-TB as those strains that are resistant to INH, rifampin, a fluoroquinolone, and either (1) resistant to a second-line injectable agents such as amikacin, capreomycin, and kanamycin; or (2) resistant to bedaquiline or linezolid.[40]

This table is intended to guide the design of individualized, longer MDR-TB regimens. Medicines in Group C are ranked by decreasing order of usual preference for us, subject to other considerations.

Adjunctive Therapy

Corticosteroids should be used as adjunctive therapy for CLWH who have TB meningitis, severe IRIS or TB bronchial compression, pleural effusion, or TB pericarditis as they have been shown to reduce complications and are associated with more rapid symptom resolution.[7]

Pyridoxine (1–2 mg/kg body weight/day usually given as 25–50 mg tablets) should be given as concomitant therapy to prevent the occurrence of INH or cycloserine-associated peripheral neuropathy in CLWH especially those with nutritional deficiency.

Monitoring for Clinical Response and Adverse Events

Continued clinical monitoring during DOT should be done to identify adverse effects and document that a clinical response (ie, bacteriologic conversion, symptom resolution, weight gain) or treatment failure has occurred. DOT should eliminate nonadherence as a factor but treatment failure could be due to poor drug absorption or drug resistance. The latter should be suspected whether an AFB culture or smear is still positive after 2 months of therapy. It is uncertain whether the same is true for a persistently positive NAAT as this could represent residual MTB genomic material.

Radiologic changes (ie, hilar adenopathy, infiltrates) may lag behind clinical improvement; hence, a repeat chest radiograph should not be done for at least 2 months after the start of treatment.[23]

INH may be associated with gastric upset and/or subclinical transient elevations in serum transaminases occurring in 3% to 10% of children. Administration with food will prevent the former. The latter may resolve spontaneously on continued therapy usually when the liver enzymes are less than 5 times the upper limit of normal (ULN). If the transaminases exceed 5 times the ULN or 3 times the ULN in a patient who becomes symptomatic and jaundiced that suggest clinical hepatitis (<1 % of children), INH treatment must be stopped until the liver enzymes return to normal. Continued therapy has rarely been associated with drug-induced liver failure. In many cases, the liver enzymes will normalize and the patient will tolerate restarting INH therapy.[7]

The risk of hepatoxicity is a major concern in CLWH on ART starting combination treatment of TB disease as rifampin and other first-line TB drugs may also be

Table 3
Regimen options and factors to be considered for the selection of treatment regimens for patients with multidrug or rifampicin-resistant tuberculosis

Regimen	MDR/RR-TB Fluoroquinolone Susceptible	Pre-XDR-TB	XDR-TB	Extensive Pulmonary Tb	Extrapulmonary TB	Age <14 y
6 mo BPaLM/BPaL	Yes (BPaLM)	Yes (BPaL)	No	Yes	Yes—except TB involving CNS, military TB, and osteoarticular TB	No
9 mo all oral	Yes	no	No	No	Yes—except TB meningitis, military TB, osteoarticular TB, and pericardial TB	Yes
Longer individualized 18 mo	Yes[a]/No	Yes[a]/No	No	Yes	No	Yes
Additional factors to be considered if several regimens are possible	Drug intolerance or adverse events Treatment history, previous exposure to regimen component drugs or likelihood of drug effectiveness Patient or family preference Access to and cost of regimen component drugs					

Abbreviations: BPaL, bedaquiline, pretomanid, and linezolid; BPaLM, bedaquiline, pretomanid, linezolid, and moxifloxacin; CNS, central nervous system; MDR/RR-TB, multidrug or rifampicin-resistant TB; TB, tuberculosis; XDR-TB, extensively drug-resistant TB.

[a] When 6 mo BPALM/BP{aL and 9 mo regimens could not be used.

From WHO operational handbook on tuberculosis Module 4Treatment Drug-resistant Tuberculosis treatment 2022.

Table 4
Grouping of medicines recommended for use in longer multidrug-resistant TB regimens

Groups and Steps	Medicine	Abbreviation
Group A Include all 3 medicines	Levofloxacin or Moxifloxacin	Lfx Mfx
	Bedaquiline	Bdq
	Lenozelid	Lzd
Group B Add one or both medicines	Clofazimine	Cfz
	Cycloserine or terizidone	Cs Trd
Group C Add to complete the regimen, and when medicines from Groups A and B cannot be used	Ethambutol	E
	Delaminid	Dlm
	Pyrazinamide	Z
	Imipenem-cilastin or meropenem	Ipm-Cln Mpm
	Amikacin or Streptomycin	AM S
	Ethonamide or priothionamide	Eto Pto
	P-aminosalicylic acid	PAS

a38

hepatotoxic. Routine monitoring of liver enzymes should be done at baseline and after 2, 4, and 8 weeks of therapy. Routine monitoring should be done every 2 to 3 months thereafter. TB therapy should be halted immediately if clinical hepatitis and/or serum transaminases exceed 5 times the ULN.

Patients should be advised that rifampin will cause their urine and secretions to turn orange and may discolor contact lenses. Ethambutol may induce optic neuritis that may present with visual blurring, central scotomata, and red–green color blindness. All children old enough to cooperate should be screened for color blindness prior to starting ethambutol using Ishihara Color Plates. While ethambutol-induced optic neuritis is less common in children versus adults and may be reversible, it may result in long-term damage hence the need to periodically recheck the patient's color vision. Ethambutol use in very young children whose color vision cannot be assessed is still recommended. The family, however, should be advised about this potential toxicity despite its rarity. Intermittent dosing of ethambutol (ie, 2 or 3 times weekly) in children is not recommended. Additional adverse effects that may occur include the following: hypothyroidism secondary to ethionamide, or 4(para)-aminosalicylic acid, nephrotoxicity and/or ototoxicity associated with aminoglycosides (the latter may progress for several months posttreatment), QT interval on the EKG (QT) prolongation secondary to bedaquiline, delamanid, clofazimine, or fluoroquinolones (regular Electrocardiogram (EKG) monitoring is recommended when these are used in combination), and cytopenia associated with prolonged linezolid use.

TB IRIS in children is seen in (1) patients with occult TB before starting ART that is "unmasked" following immunoreconstitution (unmasking or incident IRIS) usually within 3 months of starting ART or (2) in patients with paradoxic clinical worsening of TB disease IRIS following ART initiation.[35] In prospective observational studies, IRIS was reported in 5% to 10% of CLWH within 4 weeks of starting ART secondary to MTB, atypical mycobacteria, as well as BCG in previously BCG-vaccinated infants.

Reoccurrence of active TB disease may rarely occur in patients with profound immunosuppression following completion of recommended therapy. If it occurs within

6 to 12 months, then it likely represents treatment failure and efforts made to identify its cause. If it occurs after 6 to 12 months, then it probably represents a reinfection.

FUTURE DIRECTIONS

While progress has been made in the treatment of childhood tuberculosis, the spread of both MDR and XDR-TB remains major stumbling blocks in global regions where the majority of CLWH co-infected with TB reside. Recent advances in developing blood-based assays that can detect and quantitates molecular elements of MTB may facilitate both the diagnosis and clinically monitoring of PTB and EPTB. Modifications of these same approaches for POC use may significantly improve our ability to diagnose and respond to this ancient malady.

Best Practices

- Effective prevention of TB in children with HIV is hampered by the local prevalence of LTBI in global regions where both HIV and TB are endemic.
- The problematic confirmation of a diagnosis of TB in children may be aided by the recent development of blood-based assays that directly detect specific molecular components of MTB.
- The treatment of TB in children with HIV should involve DOT and the DST of every isolate of MTB.

DISCLOSURE

The author has nothing to disclose. Nanopin Biotechnologies: Research funding.

REFERENCES

1. Hershberg R, Lipatov M, Small PM, et al. High functional diversity in Mycobacterium tuberculosis driven by genetic drift and human demography. PLoS Biol 2008;6(12):e311.
2. Palfi G, Molnar E, Bereczki Z, et al. Re-examination of the Subalyuk Neanderthal remains uncovers signs of probable TB infection (Subalyuk Cave, Hungary). Tuberculosis 2023;143S:102419.
3. Scorrano G, Viva S, Pinotti T, et al. Bioarchaeological and palaeogenomic portrait of two Pompeians that died during the eruption of Vesuvius in 79 AD. Sci Rep 2022/05/26 2022;12(1):6468.
4. Donoghue HD, Lee OY, Minnikin DE, et al. Tuberculosis in Dr Granville's mummy: a molecular re-examination of the earliest known Egyptian mummy to be scientifically examined and given a medical diagnosis. Proc Biol Sci 2010;277(1678):51–6.
5. Charan J, Goyal JP, Reljic T, et al. Isoniazid for the prevention of tuberculosis in HIV-infected children: a systematic review and meta-analysis. Pediatr Infect Dis J 2018;37(8):773–80.
6. Violari A, Cotton MF, Gibb DM, et al. Early antiretroviral therapy and mortality among HIV-infected infants. N Engl J Med 2008;359(21):2233–44.
7. HIV.gov CI. Guidelines for the prevention and treatment of opportunistic infections in children with and exposed to HIV. 3/15/24. Available at: https://clinicalinfo.hiv.gov/en/guidelines/pediatric-opportunistic-infection. Accessed March 15, 2024.
8. Getahun H, Matteelli A, Abubakar I, et al. Management of latent Mycobacterium tuberculosis infection: WHO guidelines for low tuberculosis burden countries. Eur Respir J 2015;46(6):1563–76.

9. Sterling TR, Villarino ME, Borisov AS, et al. Three months of rifapentine and isoniazid for latent tuberculosis infection. N Engl J Med 2011;365(23):2155–66.
10. Villarino ME, Scott NA, Weis SE, et al. Treatment for preventing tuberculosis in children and adolescents: a randomized clinical trial of a 3-month, 12-dose regimen of a combination of rifapentine and isoniazid. JAMA Pediatr 2015; 169(3):247–55.
11. Sterling TR, Njie G, Zenner D, et al. Guidelines for the treatment of latent tuberculosis infection: recommendations from the National Tuberculosis Controllers Association and CDC, 2020. MMWR Recomm Rep (Morb Mortal Wkly Rep) 2020; 69(1):1–11.
12. GTB) GTP. Module 1: prevention - Infection prevention and control. In: Organization WH, editor. WHO consolidated guidelines on tuberculosis. WHO Guidelines Approved by the Guidelines Review Committee; 2022.
13. Madhi SA, Nachman S, Violari A, et al. Primary isoniazid prophylaxis against tuberculosis in HIV-exposed children. N Engl J Med 2011;365(1):21–31.
14. Zunza M, Gray DM, Young T, et al. Isoniazid for preventing tuberculosis in HIV-infected children. Cochrane Database Syst Rev 2017;8(8):CD006418.
15. Committee on Infectious Diseases AAoP. Tuberculosis. Red Book: 2021–2024 Report of the Committee on Infectious Diseases. 32 ed. 786-814.
16. Pai M, Behr MA, Dowdy D, et al. Tuberculosis. Nat Rev Dis Primers 2016;2:16076.
17. Marais BJ, Gie RP, Schaaf HS, et al. The natural history of childhood intra-thoracic tuberculosis: a critical review of literature from the pre-chemotherapy era. Int J Tubercul Lung Dis 2004;8(4):392–402.
18. Nahid P, Dorman SE, Alipanah N, et al. Official American thoracic society/Centers for disease control and prevention/infectious diseases society of America Clinical Practice Guidelines: treatment of drug-susceptible tuberculosis. Clin Infect Dis 2016;63(7):e147–95.
19. Mazurek GH, Jereb J, Vernon A, et al. Updated guidelines for using interferon gamma release assays to detect mycobacterium tuberculosis infection - United States, 2010. MMWR Recomm Rep (Morb Mortal Wkly Rep) 2010;59(RR-5):1–25.
20. Nguyen DT, Phan H, Trinh T, et al. Sensitivity and characteristics associated with positive QuantiFERON-TB Gold-Plus assay in children with confirmed tuberculosis. PLoS One 2019;14(3):e0213304.
21. Beneri CA, Aaron L, Kim S, et al. Understanding NIH clinical case definitions for pediatric intrathoracic TB by applying them to a clinical trial. Int J Tubercul Lung Dis 2016;20(1):93–100.
22. Marcy O, Goyet S, Borand L, et al. Tuberculosis diagnosis in HIV-infected children: comparison of the 2012 and 2015 clinical case definitions for classification of intrathoracic tuberculosis disease. J Pediatric Infect Dis Soc 2022;11(3): 108–14.
23. Andronikou S. Radiology of childhood tuberculosis. Handbook of child & AAdolescent tuberculosis. Oxford; 2016. p. 109–46, chap 8.
24. Organization WH. Policy statement: automated real-time nucleic acid amplification technology for rapid and simultaneous detection of tuberculosis and rifampicin resistance: Xpert MTB/RIF system. Available at: http://apps.who.int/iris/bitstream/10665/44586/1/9789241501545_eng.pdf. Accessed March 24, 2024.
25. Detjen AK, DiNardo AR, Leyden J, et al. Xpert MTB/RIF assay for the diagnosis of pulmonary tuberculosis in children: a systematic review and meta-analysis. Lancet Respir Med 2015;3(6):451–61.

26. Kay AW, Gonzalez Fernandez L, Takwoingi Y, et al. Xpert MTB/RIF and Xpert MTB/RIF ultra assays for active tuberculosis and rifampicin resistance in children. Cochrane Database Syst Rev 2020;8(8):CD013359.
27. Nicol MP, Allen V, Workman L, et al. Urine lipoarabinomannan testing for diagnosis of pulmonary tuberculosis in children: a prospective study. Lancet Global Health 2014;2(5):e278–84.
28. Nkereuwem E, Togun T, Gomez MP, et al. Comparing accuracy of lipoarabinomannan urine tests for diagnosis of pulmonary tuberculosis in children from four African countries: a cross-sectional study. Lancet Infect Dis 2021;21(3): 376–84.
29. Walters E, Scott L, Nabeta P, et al. Molecular detection of mycobacterium tuberculosis from stools in young children by use of a novel centrifugation-free processing method. J Clin Microbiol 2018;56(9).
30. Vonasek BJ, Rabie H, Hesseling AC, et al. Tuberculosis in children living with HIV: ongoing progress and challenges. J Pediatric Infect Dis Soc 2022; 11(Supplement_3):S72–8.
31. Mao L, LaCourse SM, Kim S, et al. Evaluation of a serum-based antigen test for tuberculosis in HIV-exposed infants: a diagnostic accuracy study. BMC Med 2021;19(1):113.
32. Huang Z, LaCourse SM, Kay AW, et al. CRISPR detection of circulating cell-free Mycobacterium tuberculosis DNA in adults and children, including children with HIV: a molecular diagnostics study. Lancet Microbe 2022;3(7):e482–92.
33. (GTB) GTP. Module 5: management of tuberculosis in children and adolescents. In: Organization WH, editor. WHO operational handbook on tuberculosis. 2022.
34. Abdool Karim SS, Naidoo K, Grobler A, et al. Timing of initiation of antiretroviral drugs during tuberculosis therapy. N Engl J Med 2010;362(8):697–706.
35. Link-Gelles R, Moultrie H, Sawry S, et al. Tuberculosis immune reconstitution inflammatory syndrome in children initiating antiretroviral therapy for HIV infection: a systematic literature review. Pediatr Infect Dis J 2014;33(5):499–503.
36. Al-Dabbagh M, Lapphra K, McGloin R, et al. Drug-resistant tuberculosis: pediatric guidelines. Pediatr Infect Dis J 2011;30(6):501–5.
37. Schaaf HS, Marais BJ. Management of multidrug-resistant tuberculosis in children: a survival guide for paediatricians. Paediatr Respir Rev 2011;12(1):31–8.
38. GTB) GTP. Module 4: treatment drug-resistant tuberculosis treatment. In: Organization WH, editor. WHO operational handbook on tuberculosis. 2020.
39. World Health Organization. Meeting report of the WHO expert consultation on the definition of extensively drug-resistant tuberculosis. Available at: https://www.who.int/publications/i/item/meeting-report-of-the-who-expert-consultation-on-the-definition-of-extensively-drug-resistant-tuberculosis. Accessed March 25, 2024.
40. Centers for Disease Control and Prevention. Surveillance definitions for extensively drug resistant (XDR) and pre-XDR tuberculosis. 2022. Available at: https://www.cdc.gov/tb/publications/letters/2022/surv-def-xdr.html; https://www.cdc.gov/tb/publications/letters/2022/surv-def-xdr.html. Accessed March 25, 2024.

The Long-Term Health Outcomes of People Living with Perinatal Human Immunodeficiency Virus

A Scoping Review

Scarlett Bergam, MPH[a,1], Whitney Puetz, MPH[b,1],
Brian C. Zanoni, MD, MPH[c,d,e,*]

KEYWORDS

- Growth and development • HIV • Long-term health outcomes • Perinatal HIV
- Reproductive health • Psychosocial and behavioral health • Immunologic outcomes
- Antiretroviral treatment resistance

KEY POINTS

- Perinatally acquired human immunodeficiency virus (HIV) can lead to delayed pubertal onset and growth deficiencies in youth.
- Youth with perinatal HIV (PHIV) are at risk for a range of neurologic challenges, including cognitive deficits and an increased long-term risk of stroke.
- In addition, they face a range of psychosocial and behavioral health challenges, including higher rates of behavioral risks, learning disabilities, substance use disorders, and psychiatric issues.
- People with PHIV are at risk for cardiac abnormalities, including left ventricular dysfunction and systemic hypertension.

Funding: S. Bergam was funded by the George Washington School of Medicine and Health Sciences 2023 Health Services Scholarship. W. Puetz was funded by Emory University's 2023 Global Field Experience Financial Award (GFEFA) and the Boozer Noether Internships in Social Ethics and Community Service scholarship.

[a] Department of Behavioral and Social Sciences, George Washington University of Medicine and Health Sciences, Washington, DC, USA; [b] Department of Behavioral, Social and Health Education Sciences, Emory University Rollins School of Public Health, Atlanta, GA, USA; [c] Department of Medicine, Emory University School of Medicine, Atlanta, GA, USA; [d] Department of Pediatric Infectious Diseases, Emory University School of Medicine, Atlanta, GA, USA; [e] Children's Healthcare of Atlanta, Atlanta, GA, USA

[1] Co-first authors: S. Bergam and W. Puetz contributed equally to the creation of this article.

* Corresponding author. Emory University School of Medicine, 2015 Uppergate Drive, Atlanta, GA 30322.

E-mail address: bzanoni@emory.edu

Clin Perinatol 51 (2024) 849–864
https://doi.org/10.1016/j.clp.2024.08.005 **perinatology.theclinics.com**

INTRODUCTION

Perinatal transmission of human immunodeficiency virus (HIV) occurs when HIV is transmitted from a pregnant person to their child in pregnancy or while breastfeeding. The first reported cases of HIV infection in children and infants occurred in 1982 in the United States.[1] Although rates of perinatal transmission have declined in recent years due to widespread prenatal testing and treatment of pregnant people, as well as increasing rates of scheduled cesarean delivery, perinatal transmission persists, especially in resource-poor settings.[2] Of the 39 million people living with HIV across the globe in 2023, 2.9 million were children and adolescents younger than 19 years.[3] Globally, only half (52%) of children with HIV—compared with three-quarters of adults with HIV—are receiving ART.[4] Although there were still an estimated 130,000 perinatal HIV (PHIV) infections around the world in 2022, the scale up in access to ART has significantly reduced the rates of perinatal transmission from peak rates in the mid 1990s.[4] With access to ART, people with PHIV have lived for decades, with the oldest cohort approaching 40 years of age.

Thanks to widespread access to ART regimens, virologic and other health outcomes have improved dramatically in people with PHIV. However, lifelong HIV and ART can negatively affect body systems, affecting pubertal development and sexual maturation, growth in weight and height, bone metabolism, metabolic functions, brain development, mental health, and reproductive health.[5] The aim of this scoping review is to synthesize the existing evidence on the long-term health outcomes of people with PHIV.

METHODOLOGY

Data Sources and Search Strategy

The authors conducted a scoping review of PubMed and Google Scholar for any published observational study, randomized control trial, systematic review, or meta-analysis with data on long-term outcomes of PHIV. The reference lists of publications found were also reviewed for further evidence. Initial keywords used in the searches included "HIV/AIDS," "perinatal," "MTCT," "mother-to-child transmission," "vertical transmission," and "long-term outcomes." Additional keywords used in a second search included "growth," "development," "puberty," "pregnancy," "psychosocial," "behavioral," "neurologic," "immunologic," and "cardiovascular." Results were restricted to English language studies. In addition to screening articles, the authors consulted with experts working in PHIV medical care, research, and programming in both South Africa and the United States.

Eligibility Criteria

To identify relevant publications collected through online searches and consultations with experts, the following criteria were used: (1) included data from people with confirmed or suspected PHIV, (2) assessed health outcomes in adolescence or adulthood, (3) were published between January 2000 and June 2023. The final inclusion criterion was to ensure that studies evaluated the population who had access to effective and available ART throughout their lifetimes.

Data Extraction

Two authors (SB and WP) screened all search results, reviewed all documents, and summarized data from the most relevant studies pertaining to long-term health outcomes in people with PHIV. The two coauthors worked together in person to capture similar types of data for each publication being analyzed. The most relevant and comprehensive articles for each section were included in analysis.

Data Synthesis

Review findings are presented as a narrative synthesis following a checklist for Preferred Reporting Items for Systematic reviews and Meta-Analyses extension for Scoping Reviews (PRISMA-ScR) (**Table 1**).[6] Literature was grouped by body system to provide a comprehensive overview of the state of the evidence of long-term health outcomes of PHIV.

RESULTS

Thirty-five articles were included in this analysis (**Fig. 1**). The studies included are presented in the following six health domains: (1) growth and development (six articles included), (2) neurologic outcomes (seven articles included), (3) cardiovascular health (five articles included), (4) psychosocial and behavioral health (seven articles included), (5) immunologic outcomes (two articles included), and (6) ART resistance (eight articles included).

Growth and Development

Pubertal onset has been shown to occur significantly later in those with PHIV than in perinatally HIV-exposed and uninfected (PHEU) youth and is even more delayed in severe cases of untreated HIV disease.[7] According to pooled data from two longitudinal cohort studies, age at sexual maturity was delayed by an average of 6 months in youth with PHIV compared with PHEU youth.[8] Much of this difference is attributable to growth deficiencies. In a cohort of 288 South African adolescents with PHIV between the ages of 13 and 18 years, 29.2% were underweight for age.[9] Poor growth was associated with being older at the initiation of ART.

Other metabolic considerations in children with PHIV include lipodystrophy, dyslipidemia, insulin resistance, bone loss, and lactic acidosis.[10] In a study comparing children with PHIV in Zimbabwe with age, sex, height, and puberty-matched PHEU youth, lumbar spine bone mineral apparent density (LS-BMAD) was significantly lower in children with PHIV.[11] For each year of ART delay, a 0.13 standard deviation reduction in LS-BMAD was observed, revealing ART's protective effect on bone health.

Severe endocrine dysfunction, including growth failure and pubertal delay in children, may be a sign of advanced HIV. Growth and pubertal delays can be ameliorated with screening and assessing underlying cause, continuous monitoring, and therapeutic measures by pediatric care providers and endocrinologists, including early initiation and adherence to antiretroviral treatment and treating hypogonadism when appropriate.[12]

Neurologic Outcomes

The neurologic outcomes of PHIV and ART have been well documented throughout the lifespan. Although preliminary data evaluating birth outcomes among ART-exposed infants in Botswana suggested a slight increased risk of neural tube defects in children born to mothers who used the integrase inhibitor dolutegravir in the first 6 weeks of pregnancy—0.30% compared with 0.08% in pregnancies with other types of ART exposure[13]—a larger, more recent study (2023) did not find an association between dolutegravir and increased risk of neural tube defects.[14]

After birth, the central nervous system is affected by early HIV disease progression, with impacts that endure into young adulthood.[15] ART early in infancy has a protective effect on neurologic outcomes of children with PHIV. Neurobehavioral characteristics of young adults living with PHIV, only 38% of whom had lifetime adherence with ART,

Table 1
Preferred reporting items for systematic reviews and meta-analyses extension for scoping reviews checklist

Section	Item	PRISMA-ScR Checklist Item	Reported on Page #
Title			
Title	1	Identify the report as a scoping review.	1
Abstract			
Structured summary	2	Provide a structured summary that includes (as applicable) background, objectives, eligibility criteria, sources of evidence, charting methods, results, and conclusions that relate to the review questions and objectives.	1
Introduction			
Rationale	3	Describe the rationale for the review in the context of what is already known. Explain why the review questions/objectives lend themselves to a scoping review approach.	3
Objectives	4	Provide an explicit statement of the questions and objectives being addressed with reference to their key elements (eg, population or participants, concepts, and context) or other relevant key elements used to conceptualize the review questions and/or objectives.	3
Methods			
Protocol and registration	5	Indicate whether a review protocol exists; state if and where it can be accessed (eg, a Web address); and if available, provide registration information, including the registration number.	3
Eligibility criteria	6	Specify characteristics of the sources of evidence used as eligibility criteria (eg, years considered, language, and publication status) and provide a rationale.	4
Information sources[a]	7	Describe all information sources in the search (eg, databases with dates of coverage and contact with authors to identify additional sources), as well as the date the most recent search was executed.	3
Search	8	Present the full electronic search strategy for at least one database, including any limits used, such that it could be repeated.	3

(*continued on next page*)

Table 1
(*continued*)

Section	Item	PRISMA-ScR Checklist Item	Reported on Page #
Selection of sources of evidence[b]	9	State the process for selecting sources of evidence (ie, screening and eligibility) included in the scoping review.	4
Data charting process[c]	10	Describe the methods of charting data from the included sources of evidence (eg, calibrated forms or forms that have been tested by the team before their use, and whether data charting was done independently or in duplicate) and any processes for obtaining and confirming data from investigators.	4
Data items	11	List and define all variables for which data were sought and any assumptions and simplifications made.	4
Critical appraisal of individual sources of evidence[d]	12	If done, provide a rationale for conducting a critical appraisal of included sources of evidence; describe the methods used and how this information was used in any data synthesis (if appropriate).	n/a
Synthesis of results	13	Describe the methods of handling and summarizing the data that were charted.	4
Results			
Selection of sources of evidence	14	Give numbers of sources of evidence screened, assessed for eligibility, and included in the review, with reasons for exclusions at each stage, ideally using a flow diagram.	4
Characteristics of sources of evidence	15	For each source of evidence, present characteristics for which data were charted and provide the citations.	4–15
Critical appraisal within sources of evidence	16	If done, present data on critical appraisal of included sources of evidence (see item 12).	n/a
Results of individual sources of evidence	17	For each included source of evidence, present the relevant data that were charted that relate to the review questions and objectives.	4–15
Synthesis of results	18	Summarize and/or present the charting results as they relate to the review questions and objectives.	4–15

(*continued on next page*)

Table 1
(*continued*)

Section	Item	PRISMA-ScR Checklist Item	Reported on Page #
Discussion			
Summary of evidence	19	Summarize the main results (including an overview of concepts, themes, and types of evidence available), link to the review questions and objectives, and consider the relevance to key groups.	15–16
Limitations	20	Discuss the limitations of the scoping review process.	16
Conclusions	21	Provide a general interpretation of the results with respect to the review questions and objectives, as well as potential implications and/ or next steps.	17
Funding			
Funding	22	Describe sources of funding for the included sources of evidence, as well as sources of funding for the scoping review. Describe the role of the funders of the scoping review.	17

Abbreviations: JBI, Joanna Briggs Institute; PRISMA-ScR, preferred reporting items for systematic reviews and meta-analyses extension for scoping reviews.

[a] Where sources of evidence (see second footnote) are compiled from, such as bibliographic databases, social media platforms, and Web sites.

[b] A more inclusive/heterogeneous term used to account for the different types of evidence or data sources (eg, quantitative and/or qualitative research, expert opinion, and policy documents) that may be eligible in a scoping review as opposed to only studies. This is not to be confused with information sources (see first footnote).

[c] The frameworks by Arksey and O'Malley (6) and Levac and colleagues (7) and the JBI guidance (4, 5) refer to the process of data extraction in a scoping review as data charting.

[d] The process of systematically examining research evidence to assess its validity, results, and relevance before using it to inform a decision. This term is used for items 12 and 19 instead of "risk of bias" (which is more applicable to systematic reviews of interventions) to include and acknowledge the various sources of evidence that may be used in a scoping review (eg, quantitative and/or qualitative research, expert opinion, and policy document).

From Tricco AC, Lillie E, Zarin W, O'Brien KK, Colquhoun H, Levac D, et al. PRISMA Extension for Scoping Reviews (PRISMAScR): Checklist and Explanation. Ann Intern Med. 2018;169:467–473. https://doi.org/10.7326/M18-0850.

showed a higher rate of psychiatric dysfunction, slower speed of information processing, worse working memory, and lower verbal fluency than age-matched peers.[16] Youth with PHIV have been found to have a worsened memory and executive functioning score than PHEU youth, although increased length of time and current adherence to an ART regimen were protective factors.[17] Among PHIV, better immunologic status is associated with verbal recall, recognition, and cognitive inhibition. Using four Delis-Kaplan Executive Function System subtests, PHIV youth—especially those who had previous AIDS-defining diagnoses—were significantly slower on the Inhibition and Color Naming/Reading tests, and made more mistakes on the Inhibition test, than PHEU youth.[18] Although the prevalence of HIV-associated cognitive impairment in youth with PHIV has declined on a population level since the rollout of ART, multifactorial reasons for continued neurologic deficits in many youth include neurotoxic effects of ART and irreversible brain injury due to untreated HIV before ART initiation.[19]

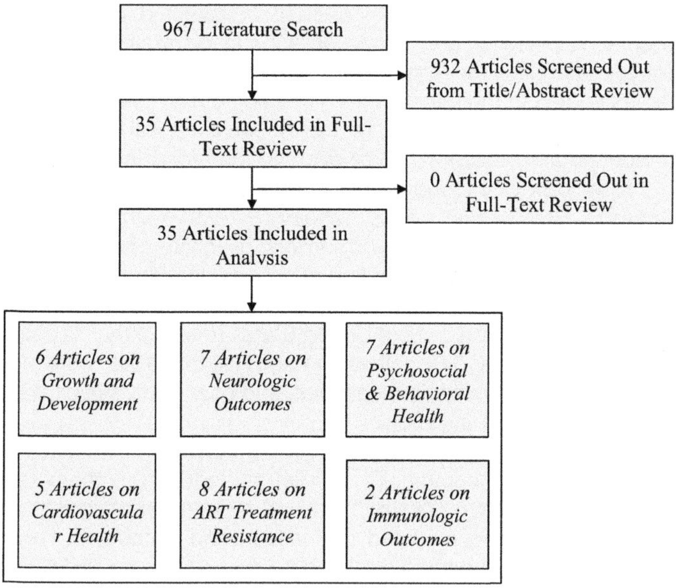

Fig. 1. Scoping review flowchart.

Cardiovascular Health

Numerous studies have shown cardiac abnormalities in people with PHIV. Cardiac manifestations of HIV have been studied in children with PHIV since 1989, showing that left ventricular dysfunction and increased left ventricular thickness are common and significant indicators for survival.[20] Youth with PHIV are at elevated risk for subclinical cardiovascular disease (CVD), such as carotid intima-media thickness, which can be measured with noninvasive methods such as pulse wave velocity.[21] Of 480 echocardiograms of children and adolescents with PHIV, 46 (31%) showed abnormalities that were frequently subclinical.[22] Common abnormalities included right ventricular dilation, left ventricular dilation, septal hypertrophy, and left ventricular hypertrophy. There is a correlation between poor immunologic status (low CD4 count) and a higher risk of cardiac imaging abnormalities. Further, according to a retrospective cohort study of adults with PHIV in the United States, 26.6% had systemic hypertension.[23] Specific prevention and treatment of HIV-related cardiovascular disease beyond adherence to ART has been understudied, but one study indicated that a standard vitamin D3 dose of 18,000 IU/month over 24 months significantly reduced carotid intima-media thickness in youth with PHIV.[24] Further, youth with PHIV have been found to have increased long-term risk for stroke.[24] Many cases of acute stroke in this population have been asymptomatic, suggesting the need for screening of asymptomatic patients for cerebrovascular accidents. Avoiding alcohol and maintaining normal systolic blood pressure may also help prevent premature cardiovascular disease in this population.[21] These cardiovascular implications reveal the research that needs to be done in understanding and preventing the systemic impacts of PHIV.

Psychosocial and Behavioral Health

Recent studies examining the emotional and behavioral development of people with PHIV have yielded mixed results. Overall, the current literature suggests an increased risk of behavioral health challenges in people with PHIV across the globe, including early sexual debut and pregnancy, higher rates of unprotected sex, decreased medication adherence, and higher prevalence of learning disabilities.[25] A study on the experience of young adults (18–24 years old) with PHIV in Washington, D.C. revealed common themes related to their challenges, including difficulties in self-care and caring for their families, limited education, restricted social capital, unemployment, and struggles to meet adult milestones.[26] However, a study focusing on children aged 9 to 16 years in New York City found that individuals with PHIV were able to achieve adult milestones.[27] Both young adults exposed to HIV—either infected or uninfected—had high rates of substance use disorders, psychiatric issues, and behavioral risks; this suggests that psychosocial factors may confound the impact that HIV status has alone. Severity of PHIV has been found to be associated with psychiatric outcomes. Another study conducted in the United States revealed that people with a severe HIV history, defined as a CD4+ cell percentage less than 15%, were more likely to have learning disabilities, psychiatric diagnoses, and psychiatric hospitalization, even after adjusting for age at ART initiation.[28]

Resilience, defined as positive development and adaptation in the face of adversity, has been studied to identify community, familial, and individual characteristics that promote positive psychological development and reduce the occurrence of mental health disorders. In a study conducted in Thailand and Cambodia, resilience was assessed in children with PHIV compared with children who were PHEU and children who were HIV-unexposed and uninfected (HUU).[29] The study found that children who were PHEU showed the highest level of resilience compared with those with PHIV or who were HUU. Factors associated with resilience included female sex, caregiver type, PHEU status, and higher household income. In addition, factors such as social support, access to health care services, and positive caregiver relationships were associated with better resilience outcomes.

Mental health is closely tied to ART adherence in people with PHIV. The impact of quality of life on ART adherence was assessed in a study involving youth in Thailand who started ART as children.[30] High levels of HIV adherence were associated with better quality of life. Male young adults with PHIV had lower quality of life and lower HIV adherence compared with women, with significant differences in psychological health scores. One potential reason for nonadherence, as suggested by current literature, is the increased responsibility for managing their own medication as children grow older.[25] In Spain, a study investigated the treatment gaps among people with PHIV, specifically focusing on mental health issues and their association with psychosocial risk factors. Psychosocial risk factors were prevalent among the study participants, with 32% having at least one risk factor.[31] Psychosocial risk factors were associated with mental health issues, as well as adherence problems, with a high prevalence of mental health issues (85.7%) and adherence issues (91.7%) among those with at least one psychosocial risk factor.

These findings underscore the need for a multidisciplinary approach that considers the social determinants of health and various factors affecting youth living with PHIV, with a specific focus on addressing psychological factors, especially in the Global South where research in this field is lacking.

Immunologic Outcomes

HIV targets and depletes CD4+ T cells, which are crucial for coordinating the immune response, leading to significant immune system impairment and increased susceptibility to various infections throughout an individual's life. HIV weakens the body's immune system and leads to premature immunosenescence and immune exhaustion, putting people living with HIV at increased risk of developing non-AIDS comorbidities such as metabolic syndrome (MetS) and CVD because of chronic immune activation and inflammation due to attacks on the gastrointestinal tract, thyroid, and lymphoid tissues, enhanced by opportunistic coinfections (ie, hepatitis C and B viruses, Epstein-Barr virus, cytomegalovirus). The risk of developing MetS and CVD, in some studies, increases more in women than men and in patients with PHIV more than in patients who are horizontally infected with HIV.[32] Immunologic dysfunction and premature immune senescence have also been associated with an increased risk of developing cancer in patients with PHIV.[32] Chronic immune activation and inflammation can result from several factors, including the disruption of the gastrointestinal mucosa, coinfections, and cumulative ART toxicity, which causes increased production of proinflammatory cytokines, thymic dysfunction, persistent antigen stimulation due to low residual viremia, microbial translocation, and dysbiosis.[32]

The most significant impact of HIV infection on the gastrointestinal tract is the tissue damage it causes and the imbalance in intestinal microbiota composition (dysbiosis), with studies showing an increase of proinflammatory bacteria (eg, some strains of Prevotella) and a decrease in Bacteroides that produce antiinflammatory cytokines and a significant depletion of memory CD4+ T cells. This imbalance can lead to the release of bacterial products into the circulation (microbial translocation) that induce immune activation and inflammation.[32] When lipopolysaccharides are released into the circulation and bind with CD14, they activate Toll-like receptor 4, producing proinflammatory cytokines and initiating a robust immune response that can result in persistent inflammation. Even with effective ART treatment, soluble CD14, a marker of microbial translocation, can remain high in people with HIV, leading to inflammation and vascular activation that increases the risk of developing CVD. Microbial translocation can be considered one of the significant drivers of morbidity and mortality in HIV infection due to its role in inducing and sustaining persistent inflammation.[32]

Other studies hypothesize that, even though ART can achieve viral suppression, immune activation may remain high due to the depletion of CD4 cells.[33] It is common for individuals with low CD4 counts to have increased levels of T cell activation, which is linked to higher levels of inflammation and coagulation (a condition referred to as residual immune dysregulation syndrome) and can thus contribute to the development of cardiovascular disease. In addition to contributing to cardiovascular disease, a study found that elevated T cell activation, despite viral suppression and improvement in the markers for inflammation over time, can worsen gastrointestinal integrity and fungal translocation.[34] This decrease in gastrointestinal barrier function can lead to long-term gastrointestinal comorbidities in people living with PHIV.

Immunologic outcomes can be influenced by ART initiation and interruption. Delayed ART initiation increases cytokines and chemokines compared with early ART initiation.[35] ART discontinuation for at least 3 months after 6 months of continuous use causes a decline in CD4 count.[36] Some have hypothesized that despite ART use in young people ($\geq$16 years old) living with PHIV, continuous immune activation reflected in a failure of CD4:CD8 ratio normalization may persist.[32] One study found that most (62.3%) of 115 participants had persistent immune activation despite ART use. The mechanism for this is not fully understood; however, it is hypothesized that because of an inverse relationship seen between the CD4:CD8 ratio and cytomegalovirus (CMV) immunoglobulin G titer, CMV and HIV coinfection may persistently activate the immune system.[33]

HIV infection during the perinatal period occurs during a critical time in the development of the immune system. Age-related differences in the immune system at the time of infection, the route of transmission, and the initiation of ART affect immune system development in people with PHIV. In the absence of ART, the disease progresses faster than in those who were horizontally infected with HIV due to their immature immune system, which results in elevated levels of HIV viremia. HIV viremia can decrease with the introduction of ART. However, cumulative exposure to HIV or ART before and after birth can cause chronic immune activation and persistent inflammation. High levels of viral replication can lead to higher expression of T-cell surface activation (CD38, HLA-DR, Ki67) and apoptosis marker CD95, and CD8 T-cell exhaustion, with a percentage of activated CD8 + CD38 and exhausted CD8+PD1+ T cells being negatively associated with telomere length, highlighting the connection between persistent immune activation and exhaustion with immune senescence.[32] Overall, the chronic immune activation and persistent inflammation caused by HIV, despite ART, contribute significantly to various comorbidities and immune system deterioration in affected individuals.

Antiretroviral treatment resistance

Infants can acquire drug resistanve to ART, either through failed antiretroviral prophylaxis or if the mother transmits a drug-resistant strain of the virus during pregnancy, or face challenges with ART adherence. Despite early initiation of ART, drug-resistant strains of HIV can persist in an infant's T cells and remain detectable for years. HIV drug resistance is associated with adverse clinical outcomes and reduced effectiveness of ART.

Pretreatment drug resistance has been observed to be increasing worldwide in recent years. A study published in 2016 examining pretreatment drug resistance in children with PHIV in Sub-Saharan Africa revealed a notable increase in pretreatment drug resistance prevalence, increasing from 0% in 2004 to 26.8% in 2013.[34] Infants are at risk of acquiring pretreatment drug resistance due to exposure to ART for preventing perinatal transmission of HIV. Interestingly, the study found that about one-third of children had pretreatment drug resistance to nonnucleoside reverse transcriptase inhibitors (NNRTIs) even if they were not exposed to PHIV prophylaxis. The World Health Organization (WHO) HIV Drug Resistance Report 2021, a survey conducted in 10 countries in Sub-Saharan Africa, found that almost half of infants newly diagnosed with HIV had pretreatment drug-resistant HIV (resistant to efavirenz, nevirapine, abacavir, and lamivudine).[35] A WHO report from 2017 highlighted an increase in HIV drug resistance prevalence among individuals initiating first-line ART, including children and adolescents with PHIV, particularly in southern and eastern Africa. Recent nationally representative surveys of 11 countries found that 7 of the 11 countries had a prevalence of pretreatment ART resistance at greater than 10% (Argentina, Guatemala, Mexico, Namibia, Nicaragua, Uganda, and Zimbabwe), including in children with PHIV.[36] As of 2024, the Panel on Antiretroviral Therapy and Medical Management of Children Living with HIV recommends integrase inhibitor–based first-line ART for infants younger than 3 years.[37]

In childhood and adolescence, treatment resistance is often a reason for ART failure. A literature review conducted in 2020 contrasted studies from both low-income and high-income countries.[38] In low-income countries, children failing first-line regimens exhibited high rates of viral resistance: 88% for NNRTIs, 80% for nucleoside reverse transcriptase inhibitors, and 54% for protease inhibitors, similar to rates found in European countries. The high prevalence of NNRTI resistance observed in pre-ART children in Sub-Saharan Africa can be attributed to drug exposure through efforts to prevent perinatal transmission. In adolescents with PHIV on lifetime ART in high-income countries, resistance rates varied between 73% and 82% for at least one drug class, with triple-class resistance ranging from 12% to 17%. The risk of developing resistance mutations increases when patients receive single or dual antiretrovirals (for infant prophylaxis) before starting combination ART. Multidrug resistance has been observed in both low- and high-income countries, with 90% of those who failed first-line ART showing resistance mutations.

Nonadherence also plays a role in the development of HIV drug resistance. A study based in Cameroon of individuals with PHIV found that about one-third of participants exhibited poor adherence to their NNRTI-based regimen, which resulted in both urban and rural settings showing a high prevalence of HIV drug resistance reaching 90%.[39]

Newer classes of ARV drugs, such as integrase inhibitors, have been introduced in recent years. These drugs have a higher genetic barrier to resistance compared with previous medications. In 2018, the WHO recommended dolutegravir-containing ART as the preferred first-line treatment of infants, children, adolescents, and adults.[40] In 2021, this guideline was extended to include children weighing 3 kg or more and age 4 weeks or older for dolutegravir (DTG) and children from birth if 2 kg or more for raltegravir.[37] Although countries with high levels of NNRTI use have been transitioning to these newer drugs due to their high barrier to resistance, the possibility of resistance to these drugs remains, although the exact risk is unknown. This concern was raised at a 2022 WHO meeting regarding the risk of DTG resistance development with the use of tenofovir disoproxil fumarate + lamivudine + dolutegravir in situations of poor adherence or suboptimal DTG regimens.[41] With HIV drug resistance on the increase and the potential for resistance to newer classes of ART, it is crucial to understand the causes of HIV drug resistance and how to mitigate its impact.

DISCUSSION

Future Directions and Research Gaps

With access to regular medical care and adherence to ART, people born with HIV can live just as long as their peers living without HIV. However, special considerations must be made for long-term health outcomes in this population (**Fig. 2**). Although access to ART has vastly improved health outcomes for people with PHIV, access is inequitable across the globe and within key populations. Ensuring continued access to free ART in low- and middle-income countries is key to removing one important barrier to ART treatment adherence. Early testing and treatment have reduced the number of infants born with HIV in the United States to less than 200 per year. However, in the Global South, the PHIV transmission rate persists and has created a second generation of youth with PHIV. A collaboration between infectious disease and obstetric health care workers is necessary to ensure that young women of reproductive age living with PHIV are virally suppressed and do not transmit HIV to their infants perinatally. Widespread testing, treatment, and population-wide education are still as needed as ever to reduce the burden of HIV on the next generation.

Continued research is needed in multiple comorbidities of PHIV. Studies on the psychosocial health of people with PHIV emphasize the need for further research to gain a better understanding of how to effectively address the neurocognitive, psychological, and behavioral challenges faced by children in this population. This research includes examining how HIV influences a child's psychosocial and behavioral well-being, as well as its effects on their resilience, ability to meet adult milestones, adherence to HIV treatment, and overall aspects of their life. In addition, even with viral suppression and early ART initiation, immune dysregulation can still occur in people with PHIV that can cause long-term immunologic comorbidities. The mechanisms of immunologic responses and disease pathways in people with PHIV must continue to be studied to better understand how to mitigate these poor health outcomes. With only 40 years

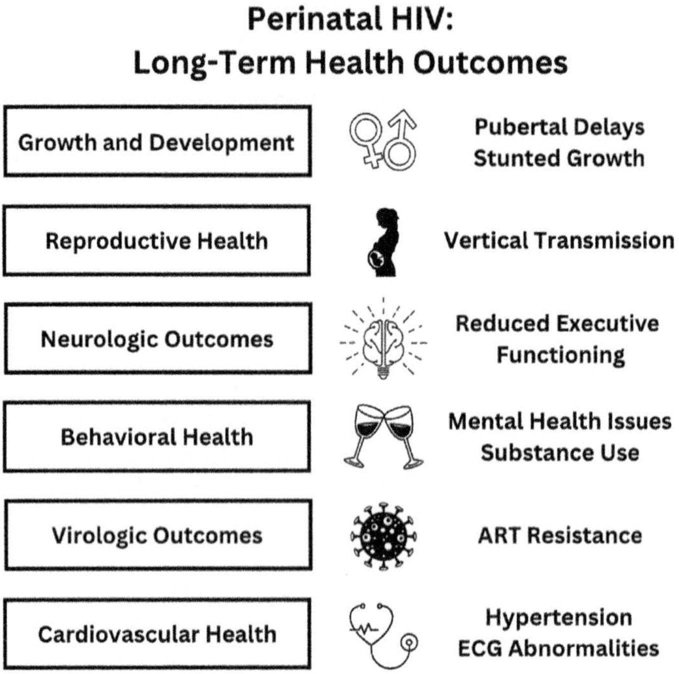

Fig. 2. Illustrated review of long-term health outcomes.

since the first case of PHIV, further areas for research and understanding include the risk of cancer, the impact of ART on aging, and the risk for frailty and cognitive decline even in people who are virally suppressed.

Physicians who treat people with PHIV must be aware of and regularly screen for systemic long-term health outcomes, including complete neurologic, cardiac, and psychiatric examinations and regular serologic testing. Virologic testing and adherence counseling are crucial to maintaining overall patient health and well-being.

Limitations

Although this scoping review aimed to provide a comprehensive overview of the available literature on the chosen topic, it is important to acknowledge several limitations that may have influenced the findings and interpretations. The use of specific keywords and databases may introduce a degree of selection bias, limiting the generalizability of the findings. Further, this scoping review was conducted in English, which may have resulted in the exclusion of studies published in other languages. In addition, there is a possibility of publication bias, as this scoping review was limited to published studies. Unpublished studies, gray literature, and ongoing research might have provided additional insights or different perspectives on the topic, which were not captured in this review. Unlike a systematic review, this scoping review did not include a formal quality assessment of the included studies. Although this approach allows for a broad exploration of the topic, it also means that the review does not account for variations in study quality, potentially affecting the reliability and validity of the findings.

SUMMARY

People born with PHIV are now able to lead long lives, thanks to advances in medical care. An overall decline of PHIV has occurred due to prenatal testing and treatment of pregnant people. Despite these achievements, PHIV remains a problem in resource-poor settings, and the increase in ART resistance may increase PHIV infections in the future. Thus, there is a need for providers to keep up to date on the long-term outcomes of PHIV in this constantly evolving field.

Various challenges are faced throughout the lifetime of individuals born with HIV, even with viral suppression from ART. These challenges include psychosocial and behavioral health issues, such as learning disabilities, psychiatric disorders, and substance use. Cardiovascular health problems, hypertension, and cardiac abnormalities have also been observed. In addition, immunologic outcomes are a concern, with ongoing immune activation even with ART use, leading to potential long-term health issues. To address these challenges, a multidisciplinary approach is necessary to provide effective life-long care and support for individuals living with PHIV. New evidence, interventions, or practices will continue to emerge after the publication of this review, and these developments should continue to be examined as we simultaneously work to reduce the incidence of PHIV.

Best Practices

What are the current practices for treating young adults living with perinatal HIV (PHIV)?

- The article highlights several current practices for treating young adults living with PHIV:
- *Antiretroviral Treatment (ART)*: the scale-up of ART has significantly reduced the rates of perinatal transmission of HIV. Most young PHIV have access to ART, which has promoted longevity. First-line treatment of PHIV is an integrase inhibitor–based ART. Genotypic resistance testing should be conducted in the case of treatment failure or if resistance is otherwise suspected.
- *Neurologic Outcomes:* the neurologic outcomes of PHIV are well documented, and ART early in infancy seems to have a protective effect. Clinicians should screen for neurologic disease throughout the lifespan, from executive functioning in adolescents with PHIV to stroke and dementia in adults with PHIV.
- *Cardiovascular Health:* cardiac abnormalities are observed in individuals with PHIV, and there is a correlation between poor immunologic status and the risk of cardiac abnormalities. Noninvasive screening for cardiovascular disease (CVD), including echocardiograms and pulse wave velocity, can detect preclinical CVD. Recommending vitamin D3 supplementation, avoiding alcohol, and preventing hypertension may reduce premature CVD risk in this population.
- *Psychosocial and Behavioral Health:* behavioral health is an ongoing challenge for providers to consider in treating youth with PHIV. People with PHIV should be counseled on self-care, education, social capital, employment, and adherence to treatment to promote resilience while also treating intellectual and psychiatric diagnoses.
- *Immunologic Outcomes:* despite ART use, some PHIV experience continuous immune activation, which may have long-term health implications. Early ART initiation is encouraged to improve immunologic outcomes.

What changes in current practice are likely to improve outcomes?

- Based on this review, several changes in current practice are likely to improve outcomes for young adults living with PHIV:

- *Continued Access to ART:* ensuring continued access to free ART, especially in low- and middle-income countries, is crucial to removing barriers to treatment adherence.
- *Early Testing and Treatment:* collaborations between infectious disease and obstetric health care workers are needed to ensure that young women of reproductive age living with PHIV are virally suppressed and do not transmit HIV to their infants. Early testing and treatment during pregnancy are essential.
- *Multidisciplinary Approach:* a multidisciplinary approach is necessary to address the psychosocial, behavioral, and mental health challenges faced by individuals with PHIV, which includes addressing resilience, adherence to treatment, and overall well-being.
- *Regular Screening:* physicians who see individuals with PHIV should regularly screen for systemic long-term health outcomes, including cardiovascular health, immunologic outcomes, and ART resistance.
- *Research:* continued research is needed to better understand and address the challenges faced by individuals with PHIV, including psychosocial and behavioral issues, immune dysregulation, and drug resistance.

Recommendations

- Improving outcomes for young adults living with PHIV involves a comprehensive and multidisciplinary collaboration between clinicians and researchers that includes continued access to ART, early testing and treatment, and ongoing research to address the evolving challenges in this population.

DISCLOSURE

The authors have nothing to disclose.

REFERENCES

1. Yusuf H, Agwu A. Adolescents and young adults with early acquired HIV infection in the United States: unique challenges in treatment and secondary prevention. Expert Rev Anti Infect Ther 2021;19(4):457–71.
2. Preventing Perinatal Transmission of HIV. Available at: hivinfo.nih.gov/understanding-hiv/fact-sheets/preventing-perinatal-transmission-hiv#:~:text=Perinatal%20transmission%20of%20HIV%20is,to%2Dchild%20transmission%20of%20HIV. Accessed July 13, 2023.
3. AIDSinfo. 2022. Available at: aidsinfo.unaids.org/. Accessed July 13, 2023.
4. HIV statistics - global and regional trends. Unicef data. 2023. Available at: https://data.unicef.org/topic/hivaids/global-regional-trends/.
5. Cruz ML, Cardoso CA. Perinatally infected adolescents living with human immunodeficiency virus (perinatally human immunodeficiency virus). World J Virol 2015;4(3):277–84.
6. Tricco AC, Lillie E, Zarin W, et al. PRISMA extension for scoping reviews (PRISMA-ScR): checklist and explanation. Ann Intern Med 2018;169(7):467–73.
7. Williams PL, Abzug MJ, Jacobson DL, et al. International maternal pediatric and adolescent AIDS clinical trials P219219C study and the pediatric HIVAIDS cohort study. Pubertal onset in children with perinatal HIV infection in the era of combination antiretroviral treatment. AIDS 2013;27(12):1959–70.
8. Bellavia A, Williams PL, DiMeglio LA, et al. International maternal pediatric adolescent AIDS clinical trials (IMPAACT) P219/219C study, and the pediatric HIV/AIDS cohort study (PHACS). Delay in sexual maturation in perinatally HIV-infected youths is mediated by poor growth. AIDS 2017;31(9):1333–41.

9. Mwambenu B, Ramoloko V, Laubscher R, et al. Growth and the pubertal growth spurt in South African adolescents living with perinatally-acquired HIV infection. PLoS One 2022;17(1):e0262816.
10. Barlow-Mosha L, Eckard AR, McComsey GA, et al. Metabolic complications and treatment of perinatally HIV-infected children and adolescents. J Int AIDS Soc 2013;16(1):18600.
11. Gregson CL, Hartley A, Majonga E, et al. Older age at initiation of antiretroviral therapy predicts low bone mineral density in children with perinatally-infected HIV in Zimbabwe. Bone 2019;125:96–102.
12. Majaliwa ES, Mohn A, Chiarelli F. Growth and puberty in children with HIV infection. J Endocrinol Invest 2009 Jan;32(1):85–90.
13. Zash R, Holmes L, Diseko M, et al. Neural-tube defects and antiretroviral treatment regimens in Botswana. N Engl J Med 2019;381(9):827–40. https://doi.org/10.1056/NEJMoa1905230.
14. Kourtis AP, Zhu W, Lampe MA, et al. Dolutegravir and pregnancy outcomes including neural tube defects in the USA during 2008–20: a national cohort study. Lancet HIV 2023;10(9):e588–96.
15. Nichols SL. Central nervous system impact of perinatally acquired HIV in adolescents and adults: an update. Curr HIV AIDS Rep 2022;19(1):121–32.
16. Coutifaris P, Byrd D, Childs J, et al. Neurobehavioral outcomes in young adults with perinatally acquired HIV. AIDS 2020;34(14):2081–8.
17. Malee KM, Chernoff MC, Sirois PA, et al. Memory and executive functioning study of the pediatric HIV/AIDS cohort study. Impact of perinatally acquired HIV disease upon longitudinal changes in memory and executive functioning. J Acquir Immune Defic Syndr 2017;75(4):455–64.
18. Nichols SL, Chernoff MC, Malee KM, et al. Memory and executive functioning study of the pediatric HIV/AIDS cohort study. Executive functioning in children and adolescents with perinatal HIV infection and perinatal HIV exposure. J Pediatric Infect Dis Soc 2016;5(suppl 1):S15–23.
19. Crowell CS, Malee KM, Yogev R, et al. Neurologic disease in HIV-infected children and the impact of combination antiretroviral therapy. Rev Med Virol 2014;24(5):316–31.
20. Keesler MJ, Fisher SD, Lipshultz SE. Cardiac manifestations of HIV infection in infants and children. Ann N Y Acad Sci 2001;946:169–78.
21. Eckard AR, Raggi P, Ruff JH, et al. Arterial stiffness in HIV-infected youth and associations with HIV-related variables. Virulence 2017;8(7):1265–73.
22. Vallilo NG, Durigon GS, Lianza AC, et al. Echocardiographic follow-up of perinatally HIV-infected children and adolescents: results from a single-center retrospective cohort study in Brazil. Pediatr Infect Dis J 2020;39(6):526–32.
23. Ryscavage P, Macharia T, Trinidad LR, et al. Patterns of systemic hypertension among adults with perinatally acquired HIV. J Int Assoc Provid AIDS Care 2017;16(1):3–7.
24. Eckard AR, Raggi P, O'Riordan MA, et al. McComsey GA effects of vitamin D supplementation on carotid intima-media thickness in HIV-infected youth. Virulence 2018;9(1):294–305.
25. Koenig LJ, Nesheim S, Abramowitz S. Adolescents with perinatally acquired HIV: emerging behavioral and health needs for long-term survivors. Curr Opin Obstet Gynecol 2011;23(5):321–7.
26. Williams EF, Ferrer K, Lee MA, et al. Growing up with perinatal human immunodeficiency virus-A life not expected. J Clin Nurs 2017;26(23–24):4734–44.

27. Abrams EJ, Mellins CA, Bucek A, et al. Behavioral health and adult milestones in young adults with perinatal HIV infection or exposure. Pediatrics 2018;142(3): e20180938.
28. Wood SM, Shah SS, Steenhoff AP, et al. The impact of AIDS diagnoses on long-term neurocognitive and psychiatric outcomes of surviving adolescents with perinatally acquired HIV. AIDS 2009;23(14):1859–65.
29. Malee KM, Kerr S, Paul R, et al. PREDICT Resilience study. Emotional and behavioral resilience among children with perinatally acquired HIV in Thailand and Cambodia. AIDS 2019;33 Suppl 1(Suppl 1):S17–27.
30. Aurpibul L, Detsakunathiwatchara C, Khampun R, et al. Quality of life and HIV adherence self-efficacy in adolescents and young adults living with perinatal HIV in Chiang Mai, Thailand. AIDS Care 2023;35(3):406–10.
31. Vázquez-Pérez Á, Velo C, Escosa L, et al. Mental health in children, adolescents, and youths living with perinatally acquired HIV: at the crossroads of psychosocial determinants of health. Children 2023;10(2):405.
32. Zicari S, Sessa L, Cotugno N, et al. Immune activation, inflammation, and non-AIDS co-morbidities in HIV-infected patients under long-term ART. Viruses 2019;11(3):200.
33. Pollock KM, Pintilie H, Foster C, et al. Cross-sectional study of CD4: CD8 ratio recovery in young adults with perinatally acquired HIV-1 infection. Medicine (Baltim) 2018;97(8):e9798.
34. Boerma RS, Sigaloff KC, Akanmu AS, et al. Alarming increase in pretreatment HIV drug resistance in children living in sub-Saharan Africa: a systematic review and meta-analysis. J Antimicrob Chemother 2017;72(2):365–71.
35. HIV drug resistance report 2021. World Health Organization; 2021. Available at: https://www.who.int/publications/i/item/9789240038608. Accessed May 29, 2023.
36. Global action plan on HIV drug resistance 2017-2021. Pan American Health Organization/World Health Organization; 2017. Available at: https://www.paho.org/en/documents/global-action-plan-hiv-drug-resistance-2017-2021. Accessed May 29, 2023.
37. Regimens recommended for initial therapy of antiretroviral-naive children with HIV: NIH. Available at: https://clinicalinfo.hiv.gov/en/guidelines/pediatric-arv/regimens-recommended-initial-therapy-antiretroviral-naive-children?view=full. Accessed January 24, 2024.
38. Anderson K, Muloiwa R, Davies MA. Long-term outcomes in perinatally HIV-infected adolescents and young adults on antiretroviral therapy: a review of South African and global literature. Afr J AIDS Res 2020;19(1):1–12. https://doi.org/10.2989/16085906.2019.1676802.
39. Fokam J, Takou D, Njume D, et al. Alarming rates of virological failure and HIV-1 drug resistance amongst adolescents living with perinatal HIV in both urban and rural settings: evidence from the EDCTP READY-study in Cameroon. HIV Med 2021;22(7):567–80. https://doi.org/10.1111/hiv.13095.
40. Report on the global action plan on HIV drug resistance 2017-2021. World Health Organization; 2023. Available at: https://www.who.int/publications/i/item/9789240071087. Accessed May 29, 2023.
41. Update on the transition to dolutegravir-based antiretroviral therapy: report of a WHO meeting, 29–30 march 2022. World Health Organization; 2022. Available at: https://www.who.int/publications/i/item/9789240053335. Accessed May 29, 2023.

Neurocognitive Outcomes Following Perinatal Human Immunodeficiency Virus Infection

Sharon L. Nichols, PhD[a,*], Reuben N. Robbins, PhD[b], Shathani Rampa, MSc[c,d], Kathleen M. Malee, PhD[e]

KEYWORDS

• HIV • Perinatal • Cognitive • Neurodevelopment • AIDS • Infant • Child • Adolescent

KEY POINTS

- Perinatally acquired human immunodeficiency virus (HIV) infection increases risk for neurodevelopmental impairments, particularly following delays or gaps in antiretroviral therapy and HIV disease progression.
- Preventing HIV-related neurodevelopmental sequelae is best achieved by: preventing HIV infection in the infant with maternal and neonatal ART, prevention of viremia and disease progression in the child with PHIV with early and consistent ART and attention to regimen choice to avoid neurotoxicity. *Initiation of ART in early infancy with subsequent consistent viral suppression* is associated with greatest reduction in HIV-associated neurodevelopmental risk.
- Management of other risks to neurodevelopment common in HIV-affected children, and referral for appropriate interventions, is best accomplished through a multidisciplinary approach that includes timely neurodevelopmental evaluation, caregiver support, occupational, physical and speech therapy, mental health services, and school liaison, as needed and available.
- There exists a significant need for capacity building to support culturally appropriate neurodevelopmental assessment and intervention in low- and middle-income countries where the perinatal HIV burden is greatest.

[a] Department of Neurosciences, University of California, San Diego, 9500 Gilman Drive, #0935, La Jolla, CA 92093, USA; [b] Department of Psychiatry, Columbia University Vagelos College of Physicians and Surgeons, New York State Psychiatric Institute, 1051 Riverside Drive, Unit 15, New York, NY 10032, USA; [c] Department of Psychology, Queens College, The Graduate Center, CUNY, New York, NY, USA; [d] Department of Psychology, Queens College, E-324 Science Building, Flushing, NY 11367, USA; [e] Department of Psychiatry and Behavioral Science, Northwestern University Feinberg School of Medicine, 225 East Chicago Avenue, Box 155, Chicago, IL 60611, USA

* Corresponding author.

E-mail address: slnichols@health.ucsd.edu

Clin Perinatol 51 (2024) 865–879
https://doi.org/10.1016/j.clp.2024.08.004 **perinatology.theclinics.com**

INTRODUCTION

Since perinatal human immunodeficiency virus (PHIV) infection was first identified, the development of effective antiretroviral therapy (ART) and its use during pregnancy for women living with HIV has enabled prevention of its transmission and provided dramatic improvements in survival and quality of life for individuals who acquire HIV infection prenatally or perinatally. With the advent of better ART and greater access to it, children with perinatally acquired HIV (PHIV) can live well into adulthood. Today, there are 1.5 million children less than 15 years living with HIV, most with PHIV, and millions more adolescents and young adults (AYA) living with PHIV, mostly in sub-Saharan Africa.[1] While effective ART has all but ended PHIV in the United States—there were only 32 new cases of PHIV in 2019[2]—and greatly reduced transmission globally, there are still greater than 100,000 births globally every year and millions more infants with PHIV exposure without infection.[1] Those caring for an infant born with HIV today should plan for that child to live a long life with great opportunity, albeit with a highly stigmatised and chronic condition that demands lifelong ART adherence and places the child at heightened risk for neurodevelopmental (ND) problems, particularly in the presence of poor HIV management.

Among its many benefits, effective ART regimens have supported the development and functioning of the central and peripheral nervous systems, and the cognitive, behavioral, sensory and motor functions dependent upon them. Prompt identification of HIV infection and early ART initiation confer the most optimal ND protection.[3] Until HIV cure is achieved, ART must be continued lifelong. Assessment and continued monitoring of functioning, provision of appropriate interventions, and family and community support are also required for optimal outcomes (**Box 1**). Early, consistent ART is particularly critical given that progression of HIV disease can confer long lasting, potentially permanent, functional impacts. However, there are concerns that changes in brain functioning can develop and persist despite viral control.[4] Other concerns include increased risk for cognitive decline later in life, and interactions of HIV with social determinants of health, mental health or substance use problems.[5] Cognitive, behavioral and health equity issues (which can vary greatly across contexts and countries), along with treatment fatigue, can provoke challenges to ART adherence and further threaten brain health. It is important to acknowledge that ND risks and outcomes will differ among contexts depending on availability of resources, and political, cultural and social factors that impact HIV care. The greatest burden of PHIV is in low and middle-income countries (LMICs) where resources to support ND and its assessment may be scarce, and, within high-income countries, in minoritized and marginalized communities. Detection of changes in ND, provision of treatment or remediation, and supporting ART adherence are important aspects of clinical care for infants through young adults with HIV and must be considered within the context of mental health issues and available resources.

NEURODEVELOPMENTAL IMPACT OF PERINATAL HUMAN IMMUNODEFICIENCY VIRUS

Infancy and Early Childhood

Infants and young children living with *in utero* HIV exposure (CHEU) or HIV diagnosis (CHIV) at or following birth are uniquely different and more vulnerable than adults with HIV, with effects related to the presence and timing of direct HIV infection of brain perivascular macrophages and microglial cells, maternal-fetal immune interactions, efficacy and safety of antiviral therapy during pregnancy and early infancy, and severity of early HIV symptoms in the presence of HIV infection.[3,6,7] The neuropathogenesis of HIV acquired by children in utero, intrapartum, or postnatally differs from that

Box 1
Summary of recommendations for key neurodevelopmental issues in perinatal HIV

Minimizing risk via ART with sustained viral suppression in mothers with HIV and infants and children with PHIV

- Initiate preferred, safe ART in women with HIV ideally prior to conception, sustain maternal viral suppression, use prophylactic ART in newborn.
- Initiate ART in child upon HIV diagnosis, preferably as soon as possible after birth, using up-to-date guidelines.
- Prioritize consistent viral suppression; support access to care, medication, and treatment adherence.
- Consider neurotoxicity or CNS/psychiatric side effects when selecting ART regimens particularly for youth with impairments.

Early and regular neurodevelopmental assessment to detect and diagnose problems

- Assessment is ideally done by a specialist with expertise in HIV, considers other developmental risks and history of past HIV disease progression, and addresses cultural and linguistic context in using norms-based tests.
- Conduct early neurodevelopmental assessment for infants and young children to identify need for early intervention.
- For all ages, refer for assessment when cognitive, academic or functional concerns or deviation from typical developmental trajectory are observed. Consider prior HIV progression and ART regimens in evaluating medical history.
- See **Fig. 1** for domains of functioning to assess at different developmental stages, along with mental health, substance use, educational background, family and social/cultural resources, and other factors that contribute to risk or resilience.

Intervention recommendations to support neurodevelopment

- Interventions for younger children can include physical, speech/language and/or occupational therapies, enrichment of home environments, promoting/supporting parent-child interaction and play during infancy and other caregiver-based approaches.
- Support children and caregivers in collaborating with school staff and accessing physical, occupational, and/or speech therapies and early intervention/special education services in the presence of developmental or academic risk.
- Older adolescents and young adults may require assessment and assistance for career/vocational/educational planning and transition to independence, referrals for mental health/substance use treatment, and health care/medication adherence support.
- Both assessment and intervention should use best available resources and consider cultural and linguistic context. Capacity building and mentoring are important where resources are limited.

acquired in adults due to the immaturity of the blood brain barrier, greater susceptibility to chemokines, early immune cell vulnerability to environmental insults and HIV impact on neural progenitor cells.[8,9]

Neonatal prophylactic ART, and continuation (or transition to therapeutic ART in countries where the full ART regimen differs from the prophylactic) for infants with HIV infection, potentially limits the size of the HIV reservoir, reduces abnormal T-cell activation, and may support a polyfunctional HIV-1 specific T cell response.[10,11] However, such treatment is not universally available, particularly in sub-Saharan Africa; thus, outcomes in such areas may vary. In the absence of efficacious early ART, HIV may cause synaptodendritic injury which affects all brain systems, including fronto-striato-thalamo cortical circuits, and may result in reduced white matter (WM) volume and integrity and eventual neurocognitive challenges, including deficits in motor, language and other cognitive domains.[9] Neuroimaging studies have demonstrated underlying brain differences and abnormalities in WM development which may persist during childhood, even in the presence of early ART and viral suppression.[12] As well, PHIV and ART exposure among CHEU may influence WM microstructural integrity and early brain network development during the neonatal period and beyond, with potential impact upon single or multiple developmental outcomes that often vary according to the presence, timing and safety of specific exposures and other risk factors.[13–16]

Infants and young children with HIV and/or ART exposure during gestation, and especially CHIV, are at risk for ND challenges in motor, language, behavioral and cognitive functioning as they progress through childhood, although effects often vary among those in LMICs and high-income countries, where maternal HIV severity, ART exposures and access, infant feeding practices and access to appropriate support services differ.[14,17,18] In addition to risks associated with the effects of maternal immune activation and direct HIV/ART exposure during pregnancy, infants and young children may have heritable or prenatal and perinatal risks, including genetic predisposition to learning challenges or psychiatric disorders, prematurity, co-infections, and *in utero* exposure to teratogenic substances, such as nicotine, lead, alcohol and other substances.[16,19] Lower socioeconomic status, limited parental education, poor maternal and child nutrition, exposure to pollution, violence, early parental death, stress and intergenerational trauma, and limited access to societal support, including appropriate medical care and early education, each may alter neural and immune system development as well. These challenges, if present, may have unique, time-sensitive and reciprocal effects on health and developmental well-being during early development and beyond and may play a role in the development of ND deficits during childhood[20,21] (**Table 1**). Despite such risk, development of young children affected by HIV, whether CHIV or CHEU, is unique to the individual, environment and culture and may allow healthy adaptation and resilience across the lifespan in a positive, accommodating context[22] and, for CHIV, in the presence of effective and timely antiretroviral treatment and ongoing, responsive medical and developmental care.

Early, appropriate ART has potential to mitigate cerebral injury and ND risk among CHIV, although it may not fully protect against HIV-related damage.[5,9,11] ART initiated before the age of 3 months in South Africa supported greater immune reconstitution and achievement of early ND outcomes that were similar to CHEU, and HIV-unexposed and uninfected children (**Table 2** comparison groups), than in infants who deferred ART until immunologic progression.[23,24] ND impairment was significantly less likely among young children in Thailand with early ART initiation (22% with impairment), within 3 months of birth, compared to those with later ART initiation (44% with impairment).[25] CHIV with deferred ART in Thailand performed less adequately than CHIV with earlier ART.[26] Achievement of viral suppression by CHIV up to 5 years of age in the United States had significant but only clinically modest cognitive benefits.[27]

Developmental monitoring of children living with *in utero* HIV exposure and PHIV is crucial throughout early childhood, given the dynamic anatomic and physiologic brain changes and learning that normally occur during the early years of life. While CHEU are sometimes at risk for subtle impairment in expressive language and gross motor development by 2 years of age,[14] potentially related in part to specific antiretroviral exposures, CHIV may exhibit developmental challenges from mild to significant across single or multiple domains.[18,28] HIV encephalopathy and ensuing cognitive impairment were significant risks for CHIV prior to the advent of safe and effective ART,

Table 1
Neurodevelopment Risk and Protective Factors for Children with PHIV

Protective Factors	Risk Factors
• Maternal sustained virological suppression before, during, and after birth • Early HIV diagnosis • Early initiation of ART • Sustained virologic suppression • Active caregiver/familial/social support • Early identification of other comorbid conditions and infections	• Poor HIV management and ART nonadherence • ART neurotoxicity • HIV-related stigma • Chronic immune activation • Adverse socioeconomic conditions and stress/trauma and loss • Other prenatal and environmental exposures • Poor management of other health, mental health and learning comorbidities

yet rates and severity of developmental delay, if present, now tend to be variable, given differences in children's HIV and immune status, HIV subtypes, ART timing and efficacy, age, and nutrition. The use of ND assessments adapted for different cultural and linguistic contexts is important where possible; unfortunately, such tests may be unavailable in low- and middle-income countries where the burden of PHIV is greatest.

Early HIV diagnosis, appropriate, timely ART for CHIV with prevention of immune suppression, early identification of cognitive and brain integrity or abnormalities, and monitoring of antiretroviral safety, efficacy and adherence are necessary to reduce modifiable developmental and health risks among young children affected by HIV. Early access to targeted speech and language, occupational and physical therapies during early childhood is crucial as well, in the presence of developmental risk or delays. Finally, culturally sensitive, differentiated family care and early education for young CHIV and CHEU are essential to identify strengths and support cognitive development, resilience, and emotional well-being throughout childhood.[22,29,30]

Childhood

The effects of PHIV on neurodevelopment among school-age children are seen in multiple domains, including cognitive, social, academic, and adaptive functioning, as well as mental and behavioral health. Challenges in these domains can represent progression of the effects of PHIV during infancy and early childhood, although new delays and impairments can emerge in the presence of ongoing significant HIV disease and other ND insults. While no prototypical cognitive phenotype for CHIV has been fully defined, CHIV may exhibit deficits in verbal learning and memory, visuospatial functioning, executive functioning (eg, problem solving, inhibition, and abstract reasoning), and processing speed and, as a group, typically perform worse than age-matched HIV unexposed and uninfected peers in studies spanning several continents.[31–33] Among CHIV, those who have sustained HIV progression with CDC Class C (AIDS) diagnosis or, particularly, encephalopathy, typically have the lowest performance, while children who have had sustained virologic suppression have, in some studies, performed more similarly to CHEU,[4,34] emphasizing the importance of optimal HIV management. Executive functioning and other deficits observed among CHIV are often attributed to the early central nervous system (CNS) injuries associated with HIV-infection; however, differences in pathogenesis between children and adults, including the role of chronic immune activation and inflammation, are not yet fully understood.[35] Among CHIV, executive functioning deficits are associated with medication non-adherence and greater risk of HIV transmission.[35] Difficulties with reading,

Table 2
Comparison groups or data for evaluating neurodevelopment in children with perinatally acquired HIV: Advantages and disadvantages of different groups

Comparison Group	Best Use	Advantages	Disadvantages
Standardization normative group	• Clinical assessment of neurodevelopment and cognitive functioning	• Provides information about individual functioning relative to age and societal expectations.	• Normative data may not be available in many locations and countries • Available normative data may not accurately represent individuals across race/ethnicity, sex/gender, location/country, language, and other sociodemographic factors
Children with perinatal HIV exposure but without HIV infection	• Studies on the impact of PHIV on neurodevelopment • Establishing developmental expectations among similar individuals for clinical purposes	• Allows for isolation of HIV effects in research studies (eg, prenatal, maternal, and sociodemographic exposures most similar to PHIV individuals).	• Cannot distinguish between effects of HIV from those of prenatal and perinatal exposure to HIV and ART
Children without PHIV exposure or infection (unexposed uninfected)	• Studies on the impact of PHIV exposure and infection on neurodevelopment and neurocognition	• Can clarify effects of both HIV exposure and infection on neurodevelopment and neurocognition, *when well matched for maternal and sociodemographic factors*	• Matching children with PHIV and/or PHEU across key variables can be difficult
Individual baseline	• Clinical trials of medications and interventions • Follow-up clinical testing for ongoing monitoring of neurodevelopment and neurocognition	• Can determine individual change (decline or improvement) from previous testing while accounting for developmental, sociodemographic and exposure factors	• Individuals may benefit from practice effects and skew results

writing, and learning are observed and associated with poorer scores on tests of attention, sequential processing, planning and reasoning, simultaneous processing, and visual memory.[31] In general, deficits in learning/memory and processing speed can be detrimental to academic performance and, as academic and social demands increase, so too do cognitive demands for working memory and executive functioning.[31] Language development is also known to be affected by PHIV, with deficits often emerging in early childhood or when children transition from basic reading and literacy to more complex language usage, especially in the context of learning new information and socialization.[31]

Neuroimaging studies have elucidated patterns of CNS injury among CHIV, yet the evidence is inconclusive and further complicated by ongoing neuroplasticity during the early years of life.[36] Differences in cortical thickness and white matter hyperintensities have been reported, even among asymptomatic CHIV.[37] Notably, the structural abnormalities are consistent with worse performance in the cognitive domains commonly associated with those regions. Functional imaging studies found decreased activity in the brain regions associated with auditory, sensory, language, and motor networks, consistent with findings regarding cognitive deficits among children and adolescents with PHIV.[37]

Although early exposure to ART has reduced the likelihood of more severe cognitive impairments associated with PHIV, it has not eliminated them.[38,39] Other considerations of ART among CHIV are the effects of long-term ART on the developing brain and the increased risk of treatment failure and drug resistance, most notably seen during adolescence.[40,41] Poor ART adherence and inadequate retention in care among PHIV adolescents has been reported in multiple settings, leading to lower rates of viral suppression compared to other age groups[40,42] and risk of neurocognitive impact.

Factors predicting the ND trajectory of CHIV cannot be limited to neurologic injury and the impact of HIV and ART on the CNS. Living with a chronic illness and numerous familial, psychosocial and socioeconomic influences contribute to a complex interaction of risk and protective factors (see **Table 1**). Living with HIV may be associated with poverty, chronic parental illness, social isolation, and orphanhood.[43,44] Furthermore, regular medical check-ups and other health-related consequences of chronic HIV illness, such as cardiac, respiratory, and metabolic complications, lead to increased school absences, further separating CHIV from their peers.[45] HIV-related stigma continues to persist, and can manifest as bullying and exclusion, thus increasing the personal and social pressures placed on the still developing brains and emotions of children and adolescents with PHIV.[40] Mental health challenges have been consistently reported among children and adolescents with PHIV, at higher rates than the general public.[46] The most prevalent mental health challenges among children with PHIV, including attention-deficit/hyperactivity disorder, anxiety, depression, and substance use disorders, are, unfortunately, evident in middle and low income countries and communities where the HIV burden is highest and mental health care resources are lacking.[30,43,46]

Despite the myriad of risk factors for neurocognitive impairment, recent research describes the possibility of improved cognitive outcomes by addressing the environmental and psychological factors affecting children and adolescents with PHIV as well as their health care needs. Caregiver support in the form of caregiver training, provision of cash grants, and improving social support networks are associated with modest improvements in neurocognition among CHIV.[31,37,47] Evidence-based mental health interventions, such as Cognitive Behavioral Therapy (CBT), mindfulness training, development of self-regulation and healthy coping strategies, as well as psychiatric medication management, can manage the mental health and behavioral challenges of PHIV children and adolescents, although careful monitoring of drug interactions is required where psychopharmacological intervention is indicated.[37,46] Cognitive rehabilitation training is emerging as an option to support children and adolescents with PHIV to improve cognitive outcomes, with preference for computerized approaches due to the ease of standardization and administration.[48] A randomized controlled trial of a computerized cognitive rehabilitation training (CCRT) program in Uganda, targeting attention, working memory and visuospatial skills,[49] showed significantly better performance on tasks of learning and mental processing in the CCRT group, and these effects remained present 3 months post-intervention. A study examining the effects of a CCRT targeting working memory in South Africa also revealed improved verbal short term memory which translated to better performance on verbal tasks of executive functioning, attention, language, memory and learning on a cognitive battery.[48] While the CCRT findings are promising, resource and access considerations are important when making recommendations. Interventions that are contextually adapted, provide training for community members and local professionals, can be delivered by community members, and thus build capacity, are urgently needed.

Adolescence and Adulthood

Today, there are millions of adolescents and young adults (AYA) living with PHIV, mostly in sub-Saharan Africa.[1,50] In the United States there are just over 12,000 people living with PHIV, most of whom are AYA(2). These AYA are expected to grow well into adulthood, if optimally treated. ND delays that began early in life may persist into adolescence and young adulthood, with new issues emerging as people with PHIV grow older and encounter more complex demands on cognitive functioning. Furthermore, there is concern that poor virologic control throughout adolescence could lead to the development of new neurocognitive impairments in adulthood.[31]

Adolescence is a critical developmental period when all youth must adapt to more complex and demanding social interactions, environments, academic pressures, and individual responsibilities while also coping with significant physical, cognitive, emotional, and social change.[51] Adolescence involves identity development, increased risk taking, considering future prospects, navigating puberty and intimate relationships, greater understanding of the larger world, and developing self-direction and self-regulation.[37,40] Youth with PHIV must also contend with the life-long effects of viral infection, including cognitive and mental health problems, as well as the demands of lifelong ART adherence and living with a highly stigmatized disease. Mental health issues often emerge during this developmental stage,[52] and behavioral issues observed in childhood may persist in adolescence and develop into psychiatric problems. AYA with PHIV may struggle with navigating this developmental period which could affect their ART adherence, risk-taking behaviors, sexual debut, and negative coping skills.[31,43]

Longitudinal cohort studies of neurocognition in adolescence and young adulthood from the United States and LMICs indicate that those with PHIV often have lower cognition than age-matched HIV unexposed and uninfected (HUU) AYA, and similar, if not slightly lower cognition, than HEU AYA(4). A study from Thailand and Cambodia found that AYA (10–24 years) with PHIV had higher rates of impairment on tests of executive functioning than HEU and HUU AYA, as well as higher rates of internalizing and externalizing problems.[53] A longitudinal investigation in the United States with 9 to 18 year old PHIV and HEU youth found that PHIV with a Class C AIDS diagnosis performed significantly worse on tests of verbal and visual memory, prospective memory, and inhibitory control than PHIV youth without a Class C diagnosis, and PHIV youth without a Class C diagnosis performed more similarly to HEU, though trajectories over 2 years were similar across all groups.[34,54–56] Another US longitudinal study of neurocognition among AYA (15–29 years) with PHIV and HEU found that performance over time on tests of processing speed, working memory and executive functioning were fairly similar between the 2 groups,[57] with performance generally improving on tests of executive functioning and working memory. Only HEUs showed significant gains on processing speed as they aged. In a small US study that compared neurocognitive outcomes in YA (20–32 years) with PHIV and age matched adults with horizontally acquired HIV (HHIV) and older adults with HHIV (≥50–67 years), 85% of the YA with PHIV had neurocognitive impairment compared to 38% of their age matched HHIV counterparts. YA with PHIV in this small sample performed more similarly to the HHIV older adults.[57,58] Neuroimaging studies of PHIV have been limited in AYA with results indicating that white matter reductions found earlier can persist later on, though trajectories of white matter growth were similar to matched uninfected AYA.[34]

AYA with PHIV often exhibit high rates of mental health problems and suicidality. Mood, anxiety, and substance use disorders are the most common mental health problems among AYA with PHIV,[59–61] though lifetime prevalence of suicidal attempts has been estimated as high as 27%.[62] Psychiatric issues (ie, anxiety, mood, and behavior disorders), having been arrested in the past year, more negative life events, greater city stress, pregnancy, and greater HIV stigma increased odds of past suicide attempts.[62] In that same cohort of AYA with PHIV, about a third showed consistent and/or escalating psychiatric problems from ages 9 to 28; higher psychiatric burden was associated with greater likelihood of being viremic. Providers for adolescents with HIV should incorporate screening for suicidality into other mental health and psychiatric screenings, referring patients to age-appropriate services as needed.

All of these challenges can interfere with the achievement of AYA milestones, such as academics and employment, and key health behaviors such as ART adherence. Neurocognitive and mental health issues may exacerbate the normal impulsivity and risk-taking behavior observed in adolescence.[63] AYA with PHIV who are not virally suppressed and engage in sex without protection increase HIV transmission risk. Despite challenges, many AYA with PHIV have managed to thrive. Longer term outcomes are not yet known, as the population of people with PHIV is still mostly young (<30 years). We do know that among older adults (>50 years) with HHIV, signs of premature aging have been well documented, including higher rates of medical (eg, cardiovascular, renal), mental health (eg, depression, anxiety), and neurocognitive impairment compared to age-matched controls.[64–68] We do not yet know if older adults with PHIV will face a similar or worse landscape of HIV-related comorbidities. Treatment fatigue, which is common in all people with HIV, can lead to poor ART adherence and HIV-related health problems. AYA already struggle to maintain adequate ART adherence; we do not know yet what treatment fatigue will look like as these young people endure ART adherence requirements for many more decades. Long acting injectables may help ease treatment fatigue, but still require regular injections for the rest of one's life. Finally, as AYA with PHIV grow older and strive to reach their own goals and milestones, many will become parents. Little is known, yet, about the health of infants and children born to mothers with PHIV, though it will be essential for mothers to maintain virological suppression before, during and after birth.

ASSESSMENT

Detecting and differentiating the effects of HIV on neurodevelopment and making treatment recommendations requires expertise in PHIV and developmentally and culturally appropriate neuropsychological tests and assessment (see **Box 1**). Many

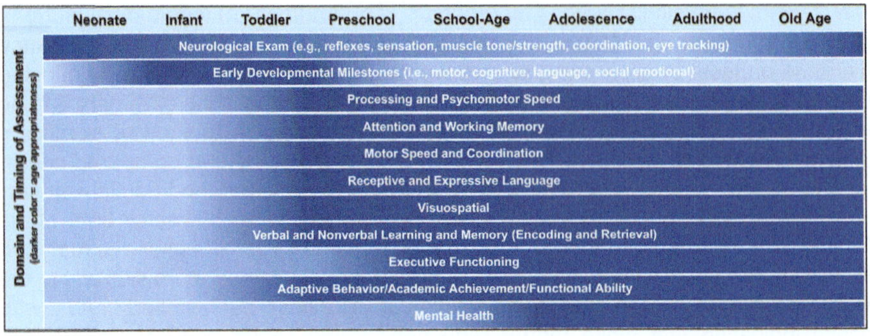

Fig. 1. Assessment of cognitive, neurologic, motor and behavioral domains across the lifespan.

LMICs have few, if any, such experts. Detection of ND, behavioral, and mental health problems early can help identify appropriate interventions (eg, occupational, physical or speech/language therapies, academic support, vocational planning, and behavioral health services) and caregiver support. Reports of changes in functioning, such as slowed processing or memory issues, are indications for assessment, as is significant HIV disease progression. Culturally and linguistically appropriate tests, as well as comparison groups, should be used, though many LMICs lack such tests (**Fig. 1**). See **Table 2** for comments regarding comparison groups for both clinical and research assessment. Assessment and intervention capacity building, particularly for portable and easily administered tests (eg, tablet-based) with local norms and professional and community development, is urgently needed in LMICs.[69,70]

SUMMARY

Prenatally or perinatally acquired HIV infection confers known risks for ND that may affect the person lifelong. Thus, it is important to consider protection of brain development and functioning from, or ideally before, conception. Prevention of HIV infection itself, through consistent viral suppression in the mother before or at least during pregnancy, is the first line of defense against ND risk. For the infant born with HIV, current guidelines call for prompt initiation of ART, with research showing better neurodevelopment with earlier treatment; similarly, later-diagnosed children should be provided ART according to guidelines at that time. Early ND assessment and regular, ongoing assessment to monitor neurodevelopment and cognitive abilities can identify cognitive, behavioral, and social problems as they arise and prompt referrals for appropriate interventions and therapies (see **Box 1**). As the child proceeds through development into adulthood, it is important to bear in mind the consistent literature showing long-term impacts of periods of significant immunosuppression, both for HIV acquired perinatally and later in life. Supporting caregivers as well as the child in accessing and adhering to ART regimens and maintaining viral suppression is critical, and continued support for HIV and health care management may be needed during adulthood, particularly for those with PHIV who have significant cognitive sequelae. Choice of ART should consider neurotoxicity and psychiatric side-effects or interactions. As outlined above, individuals with PHIV often live in contexts rife with other risks to neurodevelopment, particularly social and structural determinants of health such as poverty and food insecurity, poor access to health care, lower educational quality, and pollution; furthermore, they may have age-typical increases in mental health and substance use challenges that can impact their HIV care and potentially interact with HIV in the CNS. With increased emphasis on the whole-person context within which the brain develops, a multidisciplinary approach toward monitoring and intervening to support neurodevelopment, as well as capacity-building to do so in LMIC, should be recognized as critical goals for all those involved in clinical care and research involving those living with PHIV.

Best Practices

What is the current practice?

Current ART initiation guidelines support early initiation and include that treatment delay increases risk for neurodevelopmental problems. Still, resources for prompt identification and treatment of PHIV and developmental/neurocognitive evaluation when needed are not universally available.

*Best practice guidelines (for detailed recommendations, see **Box 1**)*

- Initiate approved ART for women living with HIV prior to pregnancy to support maternal health and reduce the risk of PHIV transmission.
- Initiate preferred ART in infants or children with HIV upon diagnosis, or according to current guidelines, to prevent and/or minimize health complications and ND sequelae.
- Support adherence and sustained virologic suppression in mothers before, during and post-pregnancy, and in the child throughout their life course.
- Evaluate neurodevelopment of infants and children with PHIV exposure or perinatally acquired HIV infection during infancy and childhood and continue lifespan monitoring.
- Identify and provide appropriate, targeted intervention services and therapies in the presence of developmental risk, delay, or impairment.
- Provide appropriate parental and family education to support both health care adherence and positive developmental outcomes for children affected by HIV.

DISCLOSURE

The authors have nothing to disclose.

REFERENCES

1. UNAIDS, Global HIV & AIDS statistics - fact sheet, 2022, Available at: https://www.unaids.org/en/resources/fact-sheet. Accessed December 3, 2023.
2. Centers for Disease Control and Prevention. HIV Surveillance Report, 2018 (Updated); vol. 31. Available at: http://www.cdc.gov/hiv/library/reports/hiv-surveillance.html. 2020. Accessed January 15, 2024.
3. Panel on Antiretroviral Therapy and Medical Management of Children Living with HIV, Guidelines for the use of antiretroviral agents in pediatric HIV infection, Available at: https://clinicalinfo.hiv.gov/en/guidelines/pediatric-arv, 2024. Accessed January 15, 2024.
4. Nichols SL. Central nervous system impact of perinatally acquired HIV in adolescents and adults: an update. Curr HIV AIDS Rep 2022;19(1):121–32.
5. Huff HV, Sportiello K, Bearden DR. Central nervous system complications of HIV in children. Curr HIV AIDS Rep 2024;21(2):40–51.
6. Panel on treatment of HIV during pregnancy and prevention of perinatal transmission. Recommendations for the use of antiretroviral drugs during pregnancy and interventions to reduce perinatal HIV transmission in the United States: Department

of Health and Human Services, Available at: https://clinicalinfo.hiv.gov/en/guidelines/pediatric-arv, 2024. Accessed Janary 15, 2024.
7. Ruck CF, Smolen KK. Effect of maternal HIV infection on infant development and outcomes. Front Virol 2022;2.
8. Crowell CS, Malee KM, Yogev R, et al. Neurologic disease in HIV-infected children and the impact of combination antiretroviral therapy. Rev Med Virol 2014; 24(5):316–31.
9. Blokhuis C, Kootstra NA, Caan MWA, et al. Neurodevelopmental delay in pediatric HIV/AIDS: current perspectives. Neurobehav HIV Med 2016;7:1–13.
10. Persaud D, Ray SC, Kajdas J, et al. Slow human immunodeficiency virus type 1 evolution in viral reservoirs in infants treated with effective antiretroviral therapy. AIDS Res Hum Retrovir 2007;23(3):381–90.
11. Garcia-Broncano P, Maddali S, Einkauf KB, et al. Early antiretroviral therapy in neonates with HIV-1 infection restricts viral reservoir size and induces a distinct innate immune profile. Sci Transl Med 2019;11(520).
12. Jankiewicz M, Holmes MJ, Taylor PA, et al. White matter abnormalities in children with HIV infection and exposure. Front Neuroanat 2017;11:88.
13. Tran LT, Roos A, Fouche JP, et al. White matter microstructural integrity and neurobehavioral outcome of HIV-exposed uninfected neonates. Medicine 2016; 95(4):e2577.
14. Wedderburn CJ, Weldon E, Bertran-Cobo C, et al. Early neurodevelopment of HIV-exposed uninfected children in the era of antiretroviral therapy: a systematic review and meta-analysis. Lancet Child Adolesc Health 2022;6(6):393–408.
15. Yao TJ, Malee K, Zhang J, et al. In utero antiretroviral exposure and risk of neurodevelopmental problems in HIV-exposed uninfected 5-year-old children. AIDS Patient Care STDS 2023;37(3):119–30.
16. Banik A, Kandilya D, Ramya S, et al. Maternal factors that induce epigenetic changes contribute to neurological disorders in offspring. Genes 2017;8(6).
17. Toledo G, Cote HCF, Adler C, et al. Neurological development of children who are HIV-exposed and uninfected. Dev Med Child Neurol 2021;63(10):1161–70.
18. Crowell CS, Malee K. Neurocognition in viral suppressed HIV-infected children. In: Pea Shapshak, editor. Global virology II - HIV and NeuroAIDS. New York, N.Y.: Springer; 2017. p. 257–82.
19. Spann MN, Monk C, Scheinost D, et al. Maternal immune activation during the third trimester is associated with neonatal functional connectivity of the salience network and fetal to toddler behavior. J Neurosci 2018;38(11):2877–86.
20. Marques AH, O'Connor TG, Roth C, et al. The influence of maternal prenatal and early childhood nutrition and maternal prenatal stress on offspring immune system development and neurodevelopmental disorders. Front Neurosci 2013; 7:120.
21. Buda A, Dean O, Adams HR, et al. Neighborhood-based socioeconomic determinants of cognitive impairment in zambian children with HIV: a quantitative geographic information systems approach. J Pediatric Infect Dis Soc 2021; 10(12):1071–9.
22. Osher D, Cantor P, Berg J, et al. Drivers of human development: how relationships and context shape learning and development. Appl Dev Sci 2018;24(1):6–36.
23. Payne H, Chan MK, Watters SA, et al. Early ART-initiation and longer ART duration reduces HIV-1 proviral DNA levels in children from the CHER trial. AIDS Res Ther 2021;18(1):63.
24. Laughton B, Cornell M, Grove D, et al. Early antiretroviral therapy improves neurodevelopmental outcomes in infants. AIDS 2012;26(13):1685–90.

25. Jantarabenjakul W, Chonchaiya W, Puthanakit T, et al. Low risk of neurodevelopmental impairment among perinatally acquired HIV-infected preschool children who received early antiretroviral treatment in Thailand. J Int AIDS Soc 2019;22(4):e25278.
26. Puthanakit T, Ananworanich J, Vonthanak S, et al. Cognitive function and neurodevelopmental outcomes in HIV-infected Children older than 1 year of age randomized to early versus deferred antiretroviral therapy: the PREDICT neurodevelopmental study. Pediatr Infect Dis J 2013;32(5):501–8.
27. Crowell CS, Huo Y, Tassiopoulos K, et al. Early viral suppression improves neurocognitive outcomes in HIV-infected children. AIDS 2015;29(3):295–304.
28. Smith R, Wilkins M. Perinatally acquired HIV infection: long-term neuropsychological consequences and challenges ahead. Child Neuropsychol 2015;21(2):234–68.
29. Lee S, Allison S, Brouwers P. Strengthening the evidence to improve health outcomes of children with perinatal HIV exposure. J Int AIDS Soc 2023;26(Suppl 4):e26160.
30. van Opstal SEM, Dogterom EJ, Wagener MN, et al. Neuropsychological and psychosocial functioning of children with perinatal HIV-Infection in The Netherlands. Viruses 2021;13(10).
31. Laughton B, Cornell M, Boivin M, et al. Neurodevelopment in perinatally HIV-infected children: a concern for adolescence. J Int AIDS Soc 2013;16(1):18603.
32. Phillips N, Amos T, Kuo C, et al. HIV-associated cognitive impairment in perinatally infected children: a meta-analysis. Pediatrics 2016;138(5).
33. Boivin MJ, Chernoff M, Fairlie L, et al. African multi-site 2-year neuropsychological study of school-age children perinatally infected, exposed, and unexposed to human immunodeficiency virus. Clin Infect Dis 2020;71(7):e105–14.
34. Nichols SL, Chernoff MC, Malee K, et al. Learning and memory in children and adolescents with perinatal HIV infection and perinatal HIV exposure. Pediatr Infect Dis J 2016;35(6):649–54.
35. Rowe K, Buivydaite R, Heinsohn T, et al. Executive function in HIV-affected children and adolescents: a systematic review and meta-analyses. AIDS Care 2021;33(7):833–57.
36. Van den Hof M, Ter Haar AM, Caan MWA, et al. Brain structure of perinatally HIV-infected patients on long-term treatment: a systematic review. Neurology Clinical practice 2019;9(5):433–42.
37. Bartlett AW, Williams PCM, Jantarabenjakul W, et al. State of the mind: growing up with HIV. Paediatr Drugs 2020;22(5):511–24.
38. Benki-Nugent S, Boivin MJ. Neurocognitive complications of pediatric HIV infections. Current topics in behavioral neurosciences 2019;50:147–74.
39. Benki-Nugent S, Tamasha N, Mueni A, et al. Early antiretroviral therapy reduces severity but does not eliminate neurodevelopmental compromise in children with HIV. J Acquir Immune Defic Syndr 2023;93(1):7–14.
40. Vreeman RC, Rakhmanina NY, Nyandiko WM, et al. Are we there yet? 40 years of successes and challenges for children and adolescents living with HIV. J Int AIDS Soc 2021;24(6):e25759.
41. Wilmshurst JM, Hammond CK, Donald K, et al. NeuroAIDS in children. Handb Clin Neurol 2018;152:99–116.
42. Foster C, Ayers S, Fidler S. Antiretroviral adherence for adolescents growing up with HIV: understanding real life, drug delivery and forgiveness. Ther Adv Infect Dis 2020;7. 2049936120920177.

43. Lowenthal ED, Bakeera-Kitaka S, Marukutira T, et al. Perinatally acquired HIV infection in adolescents from sub-Saharan Africa: a review of emerging challenges. Lancet Infect Dis 2014;14(7):627–39.
44. Lentoor AG. The association of home environment and caregiver factors with neurocognitive function in pre-school- and school-aged perinatally acquired HIV-positive children on cART in South Africa. Front Pediatr 2019;7:77.
45. Flynn PM, Abrams EJ. Growing up with perinatal HIV. AIDS 2019;33(4):597–603.
46. Dessauvagie AS, Jorns-Presentati A, Napp AK, et al. The prevalence of mental health problems in sub-Saharan adolescents living with HIV: a systematic review. Global mental health (Cambridge, England) 2020;7:e29.
47. Sherr L, Macedo A, Tomlinson M, et al. Could cash and good parenting affect child cognitive development? A cross-sectional study in South Africa and Malawi. BMC Pediatr 2017;17(1):123.
48. Fraser S, Cockcroft K. Working with memory: computerized, adaptive working memory training for adolescents living with HIV. Child Neuropsychol 2020; 26(5):612–34.
49. Boivin MJ, Nakasujja N, Sikorskii A, et al. A randomized controlled trial to evaluate if computerized cognitive rehabilitation improves neurocognition in ugandan children with HIV. AIDS Res Hum Retrovir 2016;32(8):743–55.
50. UNAIDS. UNAIDS data 2023, Available at: https://www.unaids.org/sites/default/files/media_asset/data-book-2023_en.pdf, Accessed December 18, 2023.
51. Dahl RE. Adolescent brain development: a period of vulnerabilities and opportunities. Keynote address. Ann N Y Acad Sci 2004;1021:1–22.
52. Nguyen N, Choi CJ, Robbins R, et al. Psychiatric trajectories across adolescence in perinatally HIV-exposed youth: the role of HIV infection and associations with viral load. AIDS 2020;34(8):1205–15.
53. Kerr SJ, Puthanakit T, Malee KM, et al. Increased risk of executive function and emotional behavioral problems among virologically well-controlled perinatally HIV-infected adolescents in Thailand and Cambodia. J Acquir Immune Defic Syndr 2019;82(3):297–304.
54. Malee KM, Chernoff MC, Sirois PA, et al. Impact of perinatally acquired HIV disease upon longitudinal changes in memory and executive functioning. J Acquir Immune Defic Syndr 2017;75(4):455–64.
55. Harris LL, Chernoff MC, Nichols SL, et al. Prospective memory in youth with perinatally-acquired HIV infection. Child Neuropsychol 2018;24(7):938–58.
56. Nichols SL, Brummel SS, Smith RA, et al. Executive functioning in children and adolescents with perinatal HIV infection. Pediatr Infect Dis J 2015;34(9):969–75.
57. Robbins RN, Zimmerman R, Korich R, et al. Longitudinal trajectories of neurocognitive test performance among individuals with perinatal HIV-infection and -exposure: adolescence through young adulthood. AIDS Care 2020;32(1):21–9.
58. Coutifaris P, Byrd D, Childs J, et al. Neurobehavioral outcomes in young adults with perinatally acquired HIV. AIDS 2020;34(14):2081–8.
59. Smith R, Huo Y, Tassiopoulos K, et al. Mental health diagnoses, symptoms, and service utilization in US youth with perinatal HIV infection or HIV exposure. AIDS Patient Care STDS 2019;33(1):1–13.
60. Abrams EJ, Mellins CA, Bucek A, et al. Behavioral health and adult milestones in young adults with perinatal HIV infection or exposure. Pediatrics 2018;142(3).
61. Mellins CA, Malee KM. Understanding the mental health of youth living with perinatal HIV infection: lessons learned and current challenges. J Int AIDS Soc 2013; 16(1):18593.

62. Kreniske P, Mellins CA, Dolezal C, et al. Predictors of attempted suicide among youth living with perinatal HIV infection and perinatal HIV-exposed uninfected counterparts. J Acquir Immune Defic Syndr 2021;88(4):348–55.
63. Nichols SL, Brummel S, Malee KM, et al. The role of behavioral and neurocognitive functioning in substance use among youth with perinatally acquired HIV infection and perinatal HIV exposure without infection. AIDS Behav 2021;25(9):2827–40.
64. Becker JT, Lopez OL, Dew MA, et al. Prevalence of cognitive disorders differs as a function of age in HIV virus infection. AIDS 2004;18(Suppl 1):S11–8.
65. Ettenhofer ML, Hinkin CH, Castellon SA, et al. Aging, neurocognition, and medication adherence in HIV infection. Am J Geriatr Psychiatr 2009;17(4):281–90.
66. Mateen FJ, Mills EJ. Aging and HIV-related cognitive loss. JAMA 2012;308(4):349–50.
67. Valcour V, Shikuma C, Shiramizu B, et al. Higher frequency of dementia in older HIV-1 individuals: the Hawaii Aging with HIV-1 Cohort. Neurology 2004;63(5):822–7.
68. Saloner R, Cysique LA. HIV-associated neurocognitive disorders: a global perspective. J Int Neuropsychol Soc 2017;23(9–10):860–9.
69. McHenry MS, Mukherjee D, Bhavnani S, et al. The current landscape and future of tablet-based cognitive assessments for children in low-resourced settings. PLOS Digit Health 2023;2(2):e0000196.
70. Robbins RN, Santoro AF, Ferraris C, et al. Adaptation and construct validity evaluation of a tablet-based, short neuropsychological test battery for use with adolescents and young adults living with HIV in Thailand. Neuropsychology 2022;36(8):695–708.

Care of the Child Perinatally Exposed to Human Immunodeficiency Virus

Catherine J. Wedderburn, MBChB, MA, MSc, DTM&H, MRCPCH[a,*], Grace M. Musiime, MBBCh, MSc, MMed, FC Paed (SA), DTM&H, Cert Neonatology[b], Megan S. McHenry, MD, MS, FAAP[c]

KEYWORDS

- Development • Morbidity • human immunodeficiency virus exposure • Pediatric • Integrated care

KEY POINTS

- Over 16 million children globally are perinatally exposed to human immunodeficiency virus (HIV), and the population who remains uninfected is growing.
- Children who are HIV-exposed but uninfected (CHEU) face unique health challenges and have higher risk of adverse neonatal outcomes, infectious morbidity, growth faltering, and poorer neurodevelopment compared to HIV-unexposed children.
- Etiologies of worse health and neurodevelopmental outcomes in CHEU are likely multifactorial, ranging from exposure to the virus itself or antiretroviral therapy to the complex psychosocial environment associated with living in an HIV-affected household.
- Interventions aimed at improving outcomes in CHEU should prioritize the optimization of perinatal HIV care, as well as creating a nurturing, safe environment for the mother-child dyad.
- A comprehensive package of care integrating general and HIV care from the antenatal period through early childhood is ideal for promoting optimal child outcomes.

INTRODUCTION

Over 39 million people are living with HIV globally, including 1.2 million pregnant women living with HIV.[1] The last 2 decades have brought great success in preventing perinatal HIV transmission, driven by the roll out of antiretroviral therapy (ART). This has led to a dramatic decline in new pediatric HIV infections from rates of 40% to

[a] Department of Paediatrics and Child Health and Neuroscience Institute, University of Cape Town, Cape Town, South Africa; [b] Department of Paediatrics, AIC Kijabe Hospital, Kiambu, Kenya; [c] Department of Pediatrics, Ryan White Center for Pediatric Infectious Disease and Global Health, Indiana University School of Medicine, 705 Riley Hospital Drive, Room 5900, Indianapolis, IN 46208, USA
* Corresponding author.
E-mail address: catherine.wedderburn@uct.ac.za
Twitter: @catwedderburn (C.J.W.); @MeganS_McHenry (M.S.M.)

Clin Perinatol 51 (2024) 881–894
https://doi.org/10.1016/j.clp.2024.08.011 perinatology.theclinics.com

less than 1%. As a result of this changing epidemiology, there is a rapidly increasing number of children born HIV-free following exposure in-utero.

Worldwide, over 16 million children under 15 years of age are estimated to be HIV-exposed and remain uninfected, with 50% of these children living in only 5 countries and 90% in sub-Saharan Africa (SSA).[1] The regional distribution of HIV reflects a generalized population-level epidemic in SSA where antenatal HIV rates remain high and, in some countries, over 20% of the child population are exposed to HIV, notably in South Africa, Botswana, and eSwatini.[2] In the current era of ART, most children with perinatal HIV exposure are additionally exposed to a minimum of 3 potent antiretroviral drugs throughout the perinatal period, along with the psychosocial factors associated with being born into a family affected by HIV.

There is substantial evidence that child HIV infection may affect health outcomes, even when ART is initiated early.[3] Separately, there is now an expanding evidence base on birth outcomes, morbidity, growth, and neurodevelopment of children who are HIV-exposed, uninfected (CHEU) compared to children who are HIV-unexposed, uninfected (CHUU) (**Fig. 1**).[4] This article will describe the literature on the health of CHEU and corresponding recommendations to optimize outcomes.

CLINICAL OUTCOMES

Prenatal/Neonatal Outcomes

The first 1000 days of a person's life, beginning at conception, are the most critical for growth and neurodevelopment, setting the foundation for future health.[5] The complex interaction of in-utero HIV and ART exposure during this vulnerable period,[5] increases the risk of adverse perinatal outcomes, such as stillbirth, preterm delivery, small-for-gestational age, and low birth weight.[6] However, the widespread scale-up of ART has resulted in a significant decline in the frequency of HIV-associated adverse pregnancy outcomes.[6–8] For example, in the pre-ART era, pregnant women with HIV were noted to have increased rates of stillbirth, but recently, only those *not* on ART showed increases in stillbirth.[6]

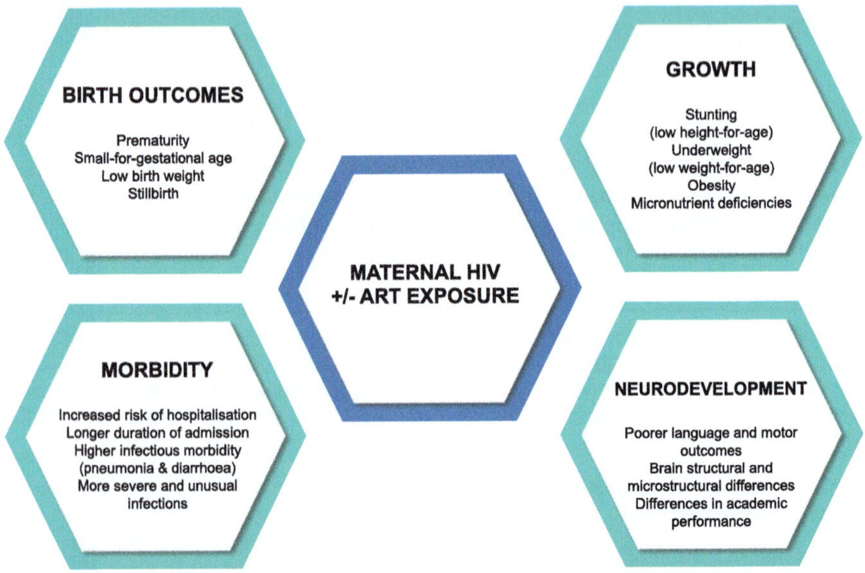

Fig. 1. Outcomes identified to be at risk in children with perinatal human immunodeficiency virus (HIV) exposure.

Despite these improved outcomes, in-utero ART exposure may influence fetal growth, and pre-conception ART has been associated with preterm delivery.[7,9] Exposure to protease inhibitors in particular has been associated with increased risk of small-for-gestational-age and preterm delivery, but evidence is conflicting.[10–12] Efavirenz was linked to central nervous system anomalies in early animal studies, but this was not shown in humans.[7] Dolutegravir was previously thought to be associated with neural tube defects;[13] however, this association attenuated as more individuals were studied. Furthermore, a large cohort study from the United States of America (USA) did not demonstrate increased risk of neural tube defects in infants with peri-conception or early-pregnancy exposure[14] and dolutegravir's safety profile is now well-documented.[10] Ongoing pharmacovigilance surveillance remains a critical component of perinatal HIV management.

The goal of postnatal care of CHEU is to prevent vertical HIV transmission and support infant well-being to optimize outcomes.[15] Morbidity may be influenced by several factors, including delivery in a facility and integration of evidence-based care practices for preterm, low birth weight newborns with HIV-specific interventions.[16] Infants born to mothers with an established HIV diagnosis without viral suppression and/or recent ART initiation, or who newly acquired HIV during pregnancy/breastfeeding are at high risk of perinatal HIV acquisition.[15] Breastfeeding confers multiple benefits for CHEU; however, even fully suppressive ART does not eliminate HIV transmission risk.[17] Care plans should be adapted to align with country-specific guidelines, as variations in the postnatal care of CHEU exist, specifically in high-income, low-burden settings regarding infant feeding and postnatal antiretroviral prophylaxis.

Morbidity and Mortality in Infancy

Overall, evidence suggests that CHEU have higher risk of mortality and morbidity compared to CHUU.[18–21] Similarly, multiple studies have reported increased early-life hospitalization in CHEU compared to CHUU in both low- and high-income countries,[22–25] along with longer duration of admission and more intensive care unit (ICU) admission.[23,26] The at-risk period for hospitalization appears to be the first year of life.[22,26] While all infants are most vulnerable in the earliest weeks of life, studies report comparable morbidity and mortality between neonatal CHEU and CHUU; however, when hospitalized, neonates with HIV exposure have greater ICU admission rates.[27] These outcomes may partly be attributable to adverse birth outcomes as CHEU are more likely to be very low birth weight and very preterm.[27] More data are needed to fully understand the other factors contributing to morbidity within this population, although associations with severe HIV disease in mothers and short ART duration, low breastfeeding, late vaccinations, and altered immunity have been reported.[22,26,28]

The excess morbidity in CHEU appears to be primarily driven by infections, notably pneumonia and diarrhea.[19,24,29–31] One study found that CHEU were 72% more likely to acquire severe or very severe pneumonia.[32] The etiology of pneumonia differed by age: respiratory syncytial virus (RSV) and tuberculosis dominated in the first year of life followed by tuberculosis and vaccine-serotype pneumococci in CHEU from ages 1 to 5 years, and non-b Haemophilus and RSV in CHUU. Furthermore, studies in Europe and SSA observed an increased risk of invasive and severe Group B streptococcal infection and pneumococcal infection in CHEU.[30,33–35] Prevalence of cytomegalovirus (CMV) has also been found to be higher in HIV-exposed neonates.[36]

The goal of reducing morbidity is focused on prevention and intervention strategies to target the confluence of HIV-related and universal factors contributing to worse outcomes within this population.[37] For example, elevated perinatal maternal HIV viral load and late initiation of ART in pregnancy have both been linked to morbidity and hospitalization.[22,25,38] Optimizing antenatal HIV care with early ART initiation is therefore recommended to benefit CHEU outcomes. Separately, existing evidence supports breastfeeding in preventing morbidity.[22,38–42] Socioeconomic and environmental factors, including the exposure to more infectious agents in HIV-affected households, emphasize the importance of timely vaccinations.[22,29]

Growth and Nutritional Outcomes

Globally, nearly half of all child deaths within the first 5 years of life are attributable to malnutrition,[43] specifically undernutrition. Beyond the neonatal period, CHEU frequently demonstrate higher rates of undernutrition, notably stunting (low height-for-age). By 6 weeks of age, CHEU have been found to have higher odds of stunting compared to their unexposed peers,[44,45] and by 12 to 18 months, these odds are estimated to be double that of CHUU. Some differences have also been noted in underweight status (low weight-for-age), while less consistent findings are seen for wasting status (low weight-for-height) and as children age.[46,47] Additionally, other factors found at higher rates within households affected by HIV, such as low maternal education, appear to be more strongly associated with worse growth outcomes compared to HIV/ART exposure alone.[48] Feeding choice is an important factor contributing to nutritional status. In some settings, breastfeeding may be performed at relatively low rates within CHEU even when it is highly encouraged, influenced by concerns for viral transmission, as well as a myriad of cultural and economic factors.[45,49] However, studies have found malnutrition to be independent of the differential breastfeeding durations between CHEU and CHUU.[40]

Micronutrient deficiencies are well-documented in children living with HIV (ie, vitamin A, zinc, iron); however, less is known about the impact of HIV exposure.[50] In some studies, young CHEU have shown higher rates of anemia, and trends toward higher rates of iron-deficiency anemia compared to CHUU.[51,52] This may be related to increased risk of maternal anemia and iron deficiency prior to and during pregnancy in women living with HIV.[53] More research is needed to understand associations and potential interventions.

While undernutrition is a primary concern within the regions of the world where HIV is most prevalent, overnutrition is an increasing concern in SSA with 16% of adolescent CHEU found to be obese in a South African study.[49] Within the US, adolescent CHEU had higher rates of obesity compared to unexposed peers,[54] and those US youth with obesity and HEU status had an increased risk of hypertension compared to their obese unexposed peers.[55] Action is needed to address both under- and over-nutrition within CHEU, including nutrition education and growth monitoring, with referral for further interventions if a child shows signs of faltering.

Neurodevelopmental Outcomes

A child's neurodevelopmental trajectory is influenced by a multitude of factors including biology, family, and the surrounding environment.[56] This early trajectory influences later school, economic, and health outcomes, with wide-ranging implications for the individual and society.[57] Several reviews and meta-analyses have indicated that CHEU are at risk for poorer neurodevelopmental outcomes compared to CHUU in the early years of life, although to a lesser extent than children living with HIV.[58,59] Language and motor domains appear to be the domains most negatively affected in CHEU compared to CHUU.[60] Nevertheless, there is heterogeneity across studies, and some have reported similar neurodevelopmental outcomes between CHEU and CHUU in both SSA[61] and USA.[62] Within this literature, addition of multiple, compounding risks increases the chances of poor neurodevelopmental outcomes, and children born into HIV-affected households may encounter more risk factors.[8,46,63,64]

Neuroimaging studies are important to gain insights into the rapidly developing brain. In the first few years of life, the brain doubles in size, and underlying neural pathways form the foundation of neurodevelopmental function.[65] The majority of neuroimaging studies among CHEU have examined white matter using diffusion tensor imaging, finding differences in white matter tracts compared to CHUU,[66] with some corresponding with neurologic outcomes.[67] Recent structural MRI studies examining young infants born to ART-treated mothers living with HIV have reported smaller basal ganglia nuclei in infant CHEU compared to CHUU. Brain volumes were associated with maternal CD4 cell count,[68] and one study found that earlier maternal ART initiation protected against differences.[69] Finally, differences in cortical brain structure have been found to mediate the poorer language outcomes in CHEU,[70] suggesting that HIV exposure may impact the developing brain with functional implications.

Optimizing early child brain development is important to ensure the best chance at reaching one's full potential. For children with neurodevelopmental delays, early interventions while the brain is most plastic are imperative to ameliorate outcomes.[71] Therefore, implementing monitoring of neurodevelopmental milestones with early referral, assessment, and intervention is advised. The neuroimaging findings indicate that changes relating to HIV exposure may happen in pregnancy and optimizing antenatal maternal HIV care is the key to addressing differences in neurodevelopment, alongside taking a holistic approach to address other environmental and caregiver-related factors.

Care of the School-Aged Child and Beyond

A growing population of individuals who are HEU is emerging, as more progress into adolescence and young adulthood. Few studies have examined this older population of individuals with perinatal HIV exposure. The limited existing research indicates poorer school performance across different academic subjects in CHEU in Botswana[72] and Zambia.[47,73] Questions remain regarding the persistence of morbidity and developmental differences seen in early childhood and whether these translate into worse academic, physical, and functional outcomes at older ages. Within many settings where HIV stigma is still prevalent, nondisclosure of maternal HIV status may render these youths unaware of their own HIV exposure status. Even when mothers disclose their status, many CHEU may be unwilling to engage in care that differentiates them from their HIV-unexposed peers. Little is known about the long-term effects of HIV and/or ART exposure within these youths, thus, research and care programs should focus on ensuring these individuals are also able to thrive over the long-term.

Current Evidence for Potential Mechanisms

Multiple interacting factors related to the in-utero and postnatal HIV environment, the health of the mother, the early life of the child, and the wider household may contribute to the clinical outcomes seen within CHEU (**Fig. 2**). A range of biologic factors influenced by maternal HIV disease severity have been associated with poorer child outcomes. Women living with HIV are at increased risk of co-infections and are more likely to be CMV viremic,[74] compared to mothers without HIV infection. Furthermore, reduced maternal antibody transfer through the placentas of women living with HIV have been reported,[75] increasing the likelihood for infectious morbidity within the first few months of life.[21,28] This is further compounded by reduced rates of breastfeeding, which limits post-partum maternal antibody transfer through breastmilk. ART may also play a role in the morbidity seen in CHEU, as older ART regimens are associated with mitochondrial toxicity, contributing to neuropathy and other metabolic and cardiac abnormalities.[76] Other inherent factors, such as inflammation, immune dysregulation, cellular immune defects, and chronic immune activation within young CHEU,[77,78]

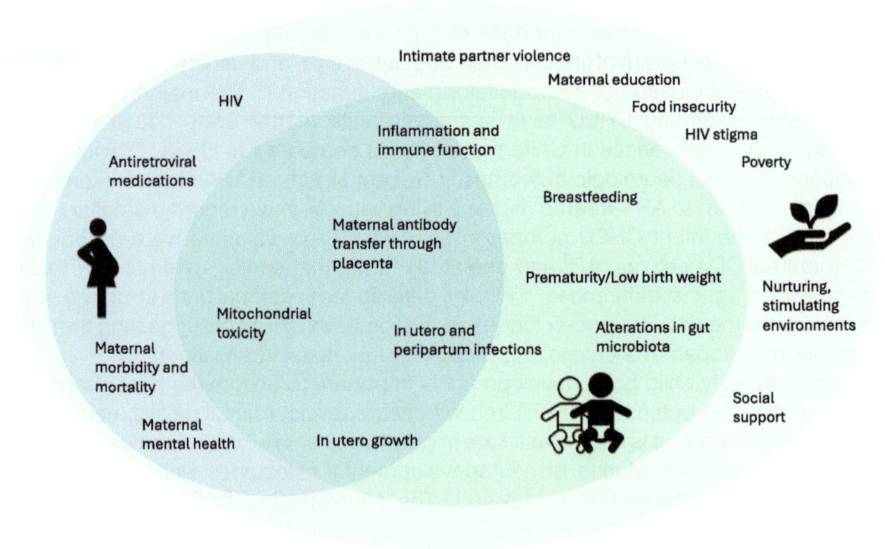

Fig. 2. Interacting factors that may impact outcomes of children with perinatal human immunodeficiency virus (HIV) exposure. Intersecting shapes represent factors related to the mother, the uterine environment, the child, and the wider household. (Data from Treatment Action Group clinical trials. https://www.treatmentactiongroup.org/cure/trials/.)

have been implicated in the worse health outcomes noted within this population. Early evidence also suggests HIV exposure may affect the microbiome with potential consequences, with limited data indicating over-diversification and over-maturity of the early life gut microbiome in CHEU.[79]

While these HIV-specific factors occur in children born to women with HIV (and to some extent, in pre-exposure prophylaxis-exposed children born to women without HIV), CHEU are also subject to other social and environmental exposures impacting their health. Certain risk factors, such as substance use, intimate partner violence, maternal mental health symptoms, food insecurity, and low child stimulation, have been found to be more closely linked to worse outcomes in CHEU compared to HIV/ART exposure alone.[8,46,63,64] Of note, these factors are more frequently experienced within HIV-affected households and contribute to the "syndemic" of co-occurring and mutually reinforcing exposures influencing worse health outcomes in CHEU.[63,80] Therefore, it is important to address family psychosocial risks and educate on risk factors for illness, including HIV exposure, particularly when accompanied by other risks for example, prematurity.[23,81]

Recommendations and Best Practices

A summary of the recommendations for care of CHEU can be found in **Fig. 3**.

Human immunodeficiency virus care for mothers

It is of the utmost importance to ensure that women are aware of their HIV status as early as possible, preferably prior to conception. ART should be initiated promptly with close monitoring of adherence to attain and maintain viral suppression. For breastfeeding mothers, the frequency of viral load monitoring should be increased in accordance with country-specific and the World Health Organization (WHO) guidelines. Mastitis, thrush, and bleeding or cracked nipples may increase vertical HIV transmission risk,[15,82] and thus should be screened for regularly and treated promptly. Additionally, interventions to prevent and treat anemia in pregnancy should be implemented.

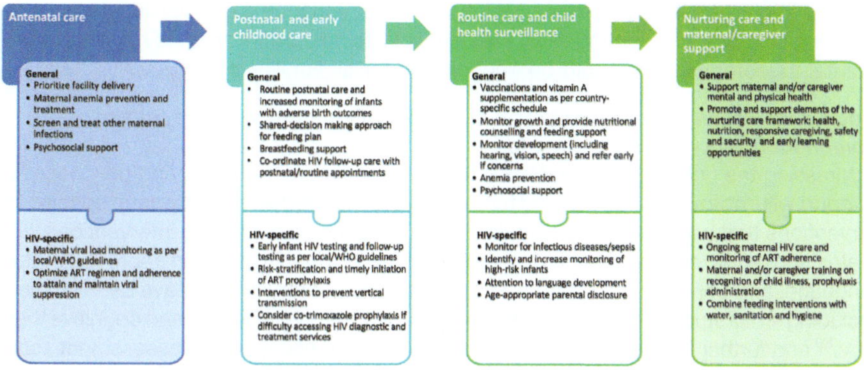

Fig. 3. Key components of care for children with perinatal human immunodeficiency virus (HIV) exposure.

Human immunodeficiency virus prevention and care for children

Early infant HIV testing and risk-stratification should be undertaken, and postnatal antiretroviral prophylaxis initiated promptly. Follow-up HIV testing should be performed, and ART initiated immediately in the event of a positive HIV diagnosis, as per country-specific and the WHO guidelines.[15] While co-trimoxazole prophylaxis is recommended for all children with confirmed HIV infection, it has not been shown to improve morbidity and mortality of CHEU, and is not routinely administered to HIV-exposed children in countries like the USA and South Africa who have adequate access to HIV diagnostic, treatment, and follow-up services.[83] In settings where there is suboptimal coverage or difficulty accessing HIV diagnostic and follow-up services, co-trimoxazole prophylaxis can be considered for HIV-exposed children, as delayed HIV diagnosis is associated with increased mortality.[84]

Recommendations for routine universal care

In alignment with the Nurturing Care Framework (https://nurturing-care.org/), promoting good health, adequate nutrition, responsive caregiving, safety and security, and opportunities for early learning is crucial to optimize child outcomes. To promote good health, families should be counseled on the importance of routine check-up and timely vaccinations, as per global guidelines.[85] There should be standard monitoring for growth, as well as sepsis and infectious diseases, and education given to caregivers on risk of infection alongside proactive prevention and intervention strategies.[29] In terms of nutrition and healthy growth, post-partum persons living in settings without safe access to formula should be encouraged to engage in early and exclusive breastfeeding until 6 months of age, with prolonged breastfeeding alongside appropriate complementary foods in alignment with WHO recommendations. In settings where formula is readily available, breastfeeding may be initiated with appropriate counseling and risk stratification. Wherever available, psychosocial support should be available for parents and caregivers to enable them to provide responsive caregiving.

Recommendations for early child neurodevelopment

Healthcare workers should be made aware of HIV exposure as a risk factor for poor child neurodevelopment. Routine monitoring of neurodevelopment, especially language and motor function, is important to ensure early identification of any delay, with prompt referral for assessment, support, and interventions where needed.[3] Screening tools should be appropriate for the context and ideally be incorporated into the health system, and, where needed, interventions should begin at the earliest chance to give the best outcomes.[86] Programs that enhance parent-child interactions, bonding, and teach parenting skills are beneficial to help optimize child neurodevelopmental trajectories and should be encouraged for all families of CHEUs.[87]

Additional interventions to optimize outcomes of children who are human immunodeficiency virus-exposed but uninfected

Addressing the unique needs of CHEU through healthcare, nutrition, and psychosocial support will improve outcomes, and further research is needed to understand specific interventions that will benefit this population. A combination of feeding interventions with water, sanitation, and hygiene (known as WASH) was found to result in improved motor, language, and behavioral scores in CHEU.[88] Few other interventions have been studied, including small studies including massage therapy, caregiver training, and cognitive therapy,[89] and further work is needed in this area. A risk stratification and assessment score may help identify CHEU at highest risk to allow for targeted interventions.

Recommendations for health system strengthening

Implementation of a comprehensive package of care, encompassing the mother-child dyad from the antenatal period through early childhood and integrating routine and HIV management, is the optimal strategy for delivering care.[15] Streamlining visits to include all aspects of care minimizes time and transport costs, and thereby improves access from the patient side. From the healthcare system perspective, this allows each visit to holistically assess the mother-child dyad, increasing efficiency and cost-effectiveness by addressing multiple health issues and lowering missed opportunities. This package of care may be different in high-burden versus low-burden HIV settings and vary depending on available resources.

SUMMARY

Up to 1 in every 4 children in some settings experience exposure to HIV and antiretroviral drugs in-utero. Evidence persists indicating that children born HIV-free to women with HIV on ART experience increased risk of infectious morbidity alongside worse birth, growth, and neurodevelopmental outcomes compared to unexposed children, across both high and low HIV-prevalence settings. To optimise outcomes of CHEU, a comprehensive integrated HIV and general care package targeted at preventing vertical transmission and supporting mother and child well-being should be provided.

Best Practices

Major Recommendations

- Implement a comprehensive holistic care package integrating both general and HIV care for mothers and children during the perinatal period through the early years. This includes coordination of follow-up care to minimize burden and missed visits
- Support optimization of maternal HIV care and ART adherence, as well as caregiver mental and physical health
- Take an individualized, unbiased evidence-based shared decision-making approach for feeding plans
- Promote and support elements of the nurturing care framework with a family-centric approach
- Implement growth monitoring, especially within the first few years of life
- Ensure early referral for nutritional consultation and supplementation if growth faltering is identified to reduce risk of long-term malnutrition sequelae

- Screen for neurodevelopment with implementation of evaluations and intervention if milestones are not reached.
- Identify CHEU who are at greatest risk of worse outcomes and focus interventions on this population.

Bibliographic Sources

Recommendations for the Use of Antiretroviral Drugs During Pregnancy and Interventions to Reduce Perinatal HIV Transmission in the United States

World Health Organization Policy Brief: Comprehensive Package of Care for Infants and Young Children Exposed to HIV. 2021.

Nurturing care framework: https://nurturing-care.org/

ACKNOWLEDGMENTS

The authors thank Dr Amy Slogrove for contributing support and information related to child outcomes.

FUNDING

Drs Wedderburn and Musiime have no disclosures for this work. During its development and writing, some of Dr McHenry's salary was supported by the National Institutes of Health (NIH) Grant #R01HD104552, titled: "Predicting neurodevelopmental risk in children born to mothers living with HIV in Kenya." This work's contents are solely the responsibility of the authors and do not necessarily represent the official views of the National Institutes of Health.

DISCLOSURE

The authors have nothing to disclose.

REFERENCES

1. UNAIDS. AIDSinfo. Available at: http://aidsinfo.unaids.org. Accessed April 3, 2024.
2. Slogrove AL, Powis KM, Johnson LF, et al. Estimates of the global population of children who are HIV-exposed and uninfected, 2000-18: a modelling study. Lancet Global Health 2020;8(1):e67–75.
3. Abubakar AA, Donald KA, Wilmshurst JM, Newton CR. Recent advances in the neurological and neurodevelopmental impact of HIV. 1st edition. London, UK: Mac Keith Press; 2023.
4. Prendergast AJ, Evans C. Children who are HIV-exposed and uninfected: evidence for action. AIDS 2023;37(2):205–15.
5. Jonathan CD, Panagiotis DB, Janice B, et al. The First Thousand Days: early, integrated and evidence-based approaches to improving child health: coming to a population near you? Arch Dis Child 2020;105(9):837.
6. Slogrove AL, Bovu A, de Beer S, et al. Maternal and birth outcomes in pregnant people with and without HIV in the Western Cape, South Africa. AIDS 2024;38(1):59–67.
7. Eke AC, Mirochnick M, Lockman S. Antiretroviral therapy and adverse pregnancy outcomes in people living with HIV. N Engl J Med 2023;388(4):344–56.
8. Wedi CO, Kirtley S, Hopewell S, et al. Perinatal outcomes associated with maternal HIV infection: a systematic review and meta-analysis. Lancet HIV 2016;3(1):e33–48.

9. Sexton H, Kumarendran M, Brandon Z, et al. Adverse perinatal outcomes associated with timing of initiation of antiretroviral therapy: systematic review and meta-analysis. HIV Med 2023;24(2):111–29.
10. Beck K, Cowdell I, Portwood C, et al. Comparative risk of adverse perinatal outcomes associated with classes of antiretroviral therapy in pregnant women living with HIV: systematic review and meta-analysis. Front Med 2024;11:1323813.
11. Cowdell I, Beck K, Portwood C, et al. Adverse perinatal outcomes associated with protease inhibitor-based antiretroviral therapy in pregnant women living with HIV: a systematic review and meta-analysis. EClinicalMedicine 2022;46:101368.
12. Saint-Lary L, Benevent J, Damase-Michel C, et al. Adverse perinatal outcomes associated with prenatal exposure to protease-inhibitor-based versus non-nucleoside reverse transcriptase inhibitor-based antiretroviral combinations in pregnant women with HIV infection: a systematic review and meta-analysis. BMC Pregnancy Childbirth 2023;23(1):80.
13. Zash R, Holmes L, Diseko M, et al. Neural-tube defects and antiretroviral treatment regimens in Botswana. N Engl J Med 2019;381(9):827–40.
14. Kourtis AP, Zhu W, Lampe MA, et al. Dolutegravir and pregnancy outcomes including neural tube defects in the USA during 2008–20: a national cohort study. Lancet HIV 2023;10(9)::e588–e596.
15. Policy Brief from the World Health Orgnaization. Comprehensive package of care for infants and young children exposed to HIV. 2021.
16. Hofmeyr GJ, Black RE, Rogozińska E, et al. Evidence-based antenatal interventions to reduce the incidence of small vulnerable newborns and their associated poor outcomes. Lancet 2023;401(10389):1733–44.
17. Prendergast AJ, Goga AE, Waitt C, et al. Transmission of CMV, HTLV-1, and HIV through breastmilk. Lancet Child Adolesc Health 2019;3(4):264–73.
18. Arikawa S, Rollins N, Newell ML, et al. Mortality risk and associated factors in HIV-exposed, uninfected children. Trop Med Int Health 2016;21(6):720–34.
19. Brennan AT, Bonawitz R, Gill CJ, et al. A meta-analysis assessing all-cause mortality in HIV-exposed uninfected compared with HIV-unexposed uninfected infants and children. AIDS 2016;30(15):2351–60.
20. Evans C, Chasekwa B, Ntozini R, et al. Mortality, human immunodeficiency virus (HIV) transmission, and growth in children exposed to HIV in rural Zimbabwe. Clin Infect Dis 2021;72(4):586–94.
21. Brennan AT, Bonawitz R, Gill CJ, et al. A meta-analysis assessing diarrhea and pneumonia in HIV-exposed uninfected compared with HIV-unexposed uninfected infants and children. J Acquir Immune Defic Syndr 2019;82(1):1–8.
22. le Roux SM, Abrams EJ, Donald KA, et al. Infectious morbidity of breastfed, HIV-exposed uninfected infants under conditions of universal antiretroviral therapy in South Africa: a prospective cohort study. Lancet Child Adolesc Health 2020;4(3):220–31.
23. Anderson K, Kalk E, Madlala HP, et al. Increased infectious-cause hospitalization among infants who are HIV-exposed uninfected compared with HIV-unexposed. AIDS 2021;35(14):2327–39.
24. Labuda SM, Huo Y, Kacanek D, et al. Rates of hospitalization and infection-related hospitalization among human immunodeficiency virus (HIV)-Exposed uninfected children compared to HIV-unexposed uninfected children in the United States, 2007-2016. Clin Infect Dis 2020;71(2):332–9.
25. Goetghebuer T, Smolen KK, Adler C, et al. Initiation of antiretroviral therapy before pregnancy reduces the risk of infection-related hospitalization in human immunodeficiency virus-exposed uninfected infants born in a high-income country. Clin Infect Dis 2019;68(7):1193–203.

26. Wedderburn CJ, Bondar J, Lake MT, et al. Risk and rates of hospitalisation in young children: a prospective study of a South African birth cohort. PLOS Global Public Health 2024;4(1):e0002754.
27. Anderson K, Kalk E, Madlala HP, et al. Preterm birth and severe morbidity in hospitalized neonates who are HIV exposed and uninfected compared with HIV unexposed. AIDS 2021;35(6):921–31.
28. Abu-Raya B, Kollmann TR, Marchant A, et al. The immune system of HIV-exposed uninfected infants. Front Immunol 2016;7:383.
29. Requejo J, Diaz T, Park L, et al. Assessing coverage of interventions for reproductive, maternal, newborn, child, and adolescent health and nutrition. BMJ 2020; 368:l6915.
30. von Mollendorf C, von Gottberg A, Tempia S, et al. Increased risk for and mortality from invasive pneumococcal disease in HIV-exposed but uninfected infants aged <1 year in South Africa, 2009-2013. Clin Infect Dis 2015;60(9):1346–56.
31. Slogrove AL, Esser MM, Cotton MF, et al. A prospective cohort study of common childhood infections in South African HIV-exposed uninfected and HIV-unexposed infants. Pediatr Infect Dis J 2017;36(2):e38–44.
32. Moore DP, Baillie VL, Mudau A, et al. The etiology of pneumonia in HIV-uninfected South African children: findings from the pneumonia etiology research for child health (PERCH) study. Pediatr Infect Dis J 2021;40(9s):S59–68.
33. Dauby N, Chamekh M, Melin P, et al. Increased risk of group B Streptococcus invasive infection in HIV-exposed but uninfected infants: a review of the evidence and possible mechanisms. Front Immunol 2016;7:505.
34. Manzanares Á, Prieto-Tato LM, Escosa-García L, et al. Increased risk of group B streptococcal sepsis and meningitis in HIV-exposed uninfected infants in a high-income country. Eur J Pediatr 2023;182(2):575–9.
35. Slogrove AL, Goetghebuer T, Cotton MF, et al. Pattern of infectious morbidity in HIV-exposed uninfected infants and children. Front Immunol 2016;7:164.
36. Pathirana J, Groome M, Dorfman J, et al. Prevalence of congenital cytomegalovirus infection and associated risk of in utero human immunodeficiency virus (HIV) acquisition in a high-HIV prevalence setting, South Africa. Clin Infect Dis 2019;69(10):1789–96.
37. Wedderburn CJ, Evans C, Yeung S, et al. Growth and neurodevelopment of HIV-exposed uninfected children: a conceptual framework. Current HIV/AIDS reports 2019;16(6):501–13.
38. Yeganeh N, Watts DH, Xu J, et al. Infectious morbidity, mortality and nutrition in HIV-exposed, uninfected, formula-fed infants: results from the HPTN 040/PACTG 1043 trial. Pediatr Infect Dis J 2018;37(12):1271–8.
39. Eckard AR, Kirk SE, Hagood NL. Contemporary issues in pregnancy (and offspring) in the current HIV era. Curr HIV AIDS Rep 2019;16(6):492–500.
40. Pillay L, Moodley D, Emel LM, et al. Growth patterns and clinical outcomes in association with breastfeeding duration in HIV exposed and unexposed infants: a cohort study in KwaZulu Natal, South Africa. BMC Pediatr 2021;21(1):183.
41. Ásbjörnsdóttir KH, Slyker JA, Maleche-Obimbo E, et al. Breastfeeding is associated with decreased risk of hospitalization among HIV-exposed, uninfected Kenyan infants. J Hum Lactation 2016;32(3):NP61–6.
42. Tchakoute CT, Sainani KL, Osawe S, et al. Breastfeeding mitigates the effects of maternal HIV on infant infectious morbidity in the Option B+ era. AIDS 2018; 32(16):2383–91.

43. World Health Organization, United Nations Children's Fund (UNICEF)' International Bank for Reconstruction and Development/The World Bank. Levels and trends in child malnutrition. 2023.
44. Mabaya L, Matarira HT, Tanyanyiwa DM, et al. Growth trajectories of HIV exposed and HIV unexposed infants. A prospective study in Gweru, Zimbabwe. Glob Pediatr Health 2021;8. 2333794x21990338.
45. Neary J, Langat A, Singa B, et al. Higher prevalence of stunting and poor growth outcomes in HIV-exposed uninfected than HIV-unexposed infants in Kenya. AIDS 2022;36(4):605–10.
46. McHenry MS, Oyungu E, Yang Z, et al. Neurodevelopmental outcomes of young children born to HIV-infected mothers: a pilot study. Front Pediatr 2021;9:697091.
47. Nicholson L, Chisenga M, Siame J, et al. Growth and health outcomes at school age in HIV-exposed, uninfected Zambian children: follow-up of two cohorts studied in infancy. BMC Pediatr 2015;15:66.
48. Cherkos AS, LaCourse SM, Kinuthia J, et al. Maternal breastfeeding and education impact infant growth and development more than in-utero HIV/antiretroviral therapy exposure in context of universal antiretroviral therapy. AIDS 2024;38(4): 537–46.
49. le Roux SM, Abrams EJ, Donald KA, et al. Growth trajectories of breastfed HIV-exposed uninfected and HIV-unexposed children under conditions of universal maternal antiretroviral therapy: a prospective study. Lancet Child Adolesc Health 2019;3(4):234–44.
50. Julia L, Finkelstein HA, Herman HS, et al. Micronutrients and HIV in pediatric populations. In: Mehta SFJ, editor. Nutrition and HIV: epidemiological evidence to public health. New York: CRC Press; 2018. p. 276–303.
51. Oyungu E, Roose AW, Ombitsa AR, et al. Anemia and iron-deficiency anemia in children born to mothers with HIV in Western Kenya. Glob Pediatr Health 2021;8: 2333794x21991035.
52. Moraleda C, de Deus N, Serna-Bolea C, et al. Impact of HIV exposure on health outcomes in HIV-negative infants born to HIV-positive mothers in Sub-Saharan Africa. J Acquir Immune Defic Syndr 2014;65(2):182–9.
53. Levine AM, Berhane K, Masri-Lavine L, et al. Prevalence and correlates of anemia in a large cohort of HIV-infected women: women's interagency HIV study. J Acquir Immune Defic Syndr 2001;26(1):28–35.
54. Fourman LT, Pan CS, Zheng I, et al. Association of in utero HIV exposure with obesity and reactive airway disease in HIV-negative adolescents and young adults. J Acquir Immune Defic Syndr 2020;83(2):126–34.
55. Jao J, Jacobson DL, Yu W, et al. A comparison of metabolic outcomes between obese HIV-exposed uninfected youth from the PHACS SMARTT study and HIV-unexposed youth from the NHANES study in the United States. J Acquir Immune Defic Syndr 2019;81(3):319–27.
56. Black MM, Walker SP, Fernald LCH, et al. Early childhood development coming of age: science through the life course. Lancet 2017;389(10064):77–90.
57. Grantham-McGregor S, Cheung YB, Cueto S, et al. Developmental potential in the first 5 years for children in developing countries. Lancet 2007;369(9555): 60–70.
58. Sherr L, Croome N, Parra Castaneda K, et al. A systematic review of psychological functioning of children exposed to HIV: using evidence to plan for tomorrow's HIV needs. AIDS Behav 2014;18(11):2059–74.

59. McHenry MS, McAteer CI, Oyungu E, et al. Neurodevelopment in young children born to HIV-infected mothers: a meta-analysis. Pediatrics 2018;141(2): e20172888.
60. Wedderburn CJ, Weldon E, Bertran-Cobo C, et al. Early neurodevelopment of HIV-exposed uninfected children in the era of antiretroviral therapy: a systematic review and meta-analysis. Lancet Child Adolesc Health 2022;6(6):393–408.
61. Boivin MJ, Maliwichi-Senganimalunje L, Ogwang LW, et al. Neurodevelopmental effects of ante-partum and post-partum antiretroviral exposure in HIV-exposed and uninfected children versus HIV-unexposed and uninfected children in Uganda and Malawi: a prospective cohort study. Lancet HIV 2019;6(8):e518–30.
62. Sirois PA, Huo Y, Williams PL, et al. Safety of perinatal exposure to antiretroviral medications: developmental outcomes in infants. Pediatr Infect Dis J 2013; 32(6):648–55.
63. le Roux SM, Abrams EJ, Zerbe A, et al. Children of a syndemic: co-occurring and mutually reinforcing adverse child health exposures in a prospective cohort of HIV-affected mother-infant dyads in Cape Town, South Africa. J Int AIDS Soc 2023;26 Suppl 4(Suppl 4):e26152.
64. Alimenti A, Forbes JC, Oberlander TF, et al. A prospective controlled study of neurodevelopment in HIV-uninfected children exposed to combination antiretroviral drugs in pregnancy. Pediatrics 2006;118(4):e1139–45.
65. Wedderburn CJ, Subramoney S, Yeung S, et al. Neuroimaging young children and associations with neurocognitive development in a South African birth cohort study. Neuroimage 2020;219:116846.
66. McHenry MS, Balogun KA, McDonald BC, et al. In utero exposure to HIV and/or antiretroviral therapy: a systematic review of preclinical and clinical evidence of cognitive outcomes. J Int AIDS Soc 2019;22(4):e25275.
67. Tran LT, Roos A, Fouche JP, et al. White matter microstructural integrity and neurobehavioral outcome of HIV-exposed uninfected neonates. Medicine (Baltim) 2016;95(4):e2577.
68. Wedderburn CJ, Groenewold NA, Roos A, et al. Early structural brain development in infants exposed to HIV and antiretroviral therapy in utero in a South African birth cohort. J Int AIDS Soc 2022;25(1):e25863.
69. Ibrahim A, Warton FL, Fry S, et al. Maternal ART throughout gestation prevents caudate volume reductions in neonates who are HIV exposed but uninfected. Front Neurosci 2023;17:1085589.
70. Wedderburn CJ, Yeung S, Subramoney S, et al. Association of in utero HIV exposure with child brain structure and language development: a South African birth cohort study. BMC Med 2024;22(1):129.
71. Cusick SE, Georgieff MK. The role of nutrition in brain development: the golden opportunity of the "first 1000 Days". J Pediatr 2016;175:16–21.
72. Powis KM, Lebanna L, Schenkel S, et al. Lower academic performance among children with perinatal HIV exposure in Botswana. J Int AIDS Soc 2023;26 Suppl 4(Suppl 4):e26165.
73. Nichols E, Ng DK, Hayat S, et al. Measurement differences in the assessment of functional limitations for cognitive impairment classification across geographic locations. Alzheimers Dement 2023;19(5):2218–25.
74. Slyker JA, Lohman-Payne BL, Rowland-Jones SL, et al. The detection of cytomegalovirus DNA in maternal plasma is associated with mortality in HIV-1-infected women and their infants. AIDS 2009;23(1):117–24.

75. Jones CE, Naidoo S, De Beer C, et al. Maternal HIV infection and antibody responses against vaccine-preventable diseases in uninfected infants. JAMA 2011;305(6):576–84.
76. Brinkman K, ter Hofstede HJ, Burger DM, et al. Adverse effects of reverse transcriptase inhibitors: mitochondrial toxicity as common pathway. AIDS 1998; 12(14):1735–44.
77. Smith C, Huo Y, Patel K, et al. Immunologic and virologic factors associated with hospitalization in human immunodeficiency virus-exposed, uninfected infants in the United States. Clin Infect Dis 2021;73(6):1089–96.
78. Dirajlal-Fargo S, Mussi-Pinhata MM, Weinberg A, et al. HIV-exposed-uninfected infants have increased inflammation and monocyte activation. AIDS 2019;33(5): 845–53.
79. Robertson RC, Edens TJ, Carr L, et al. The gut microbiome and early-life growth in a population with high prevalence of stunting. Nat Commun 2023;14(1):654.
80. Slogrove AL. It is a question of equity: time to talk about children who are HIV-exposed and "HIV-free". J Int AIDS Soc 2021;24(11):e25850.
81. Miller JE, Hammond GC, Strunk T, et al. Association of gestational age and growth measures at birth with infection-related admissions to hospital throughout childhood: a population-based, data-linkage study from Western Australia. Lancet Infect Dis 2016;16(8):952–61.
82. Centers for Disease Control and Prevention; HIV Medicine Association of the Infectious Diseases Society of America; Pediatric Infectious Diseases Society; HHS Panel on Treatment of HIV During Pregnancy and Prevention of Perinatal Transmission— A Working Group of the Office of AIDS Research Advisory Council (OARAC). Recommendations for the Use of Antiretroviral Drugs During Pregnancy and Interventions to Reduce Perinatal HIV Transmission in the United States. [Updated 2024 Jan 31]. In: ClinicalInfo.HIV.gov [Internet]. Rockville (MD): US Department of Health and Human Services; 2002. Available at: https://www.ncbi.nlm.nih.gov/books/NBK586310/.
83. Wedderburn CJ, Evans C, Slogrove AL, et al. Co-trimoxazole prophylaxis for children who are HIV-exposed and uninfected: a systematic review. J Int AIDS Soc 2023;26(6):e26079.
84. Mathur S, Smuk M, Evans C, et al. Estimating the impact of alternative programmatic cotrimoxazole strategies on mortality among children born to mothers with HIV: a modelling study. PLoS Med 2024;21(2):e1004334.
85. World Health Organisation, UNCEF, World Bank Group. Nurturing care for early childhood development: a framework for helping children survive and thrive to transform health and human potential. 2018.
86. Nelson CA, Gabard-Durnam LJ. Early adversity and critical periods: neurodevelopmental consequences of violating the expectable environment. Trends Neurosci 2020;43(3):133–43.
87. Daelmans B, Black MM, Lombardi J, et al. Effective interventions and strategies for improving early child development. BMJ 2015;351:h4029.
88. Chandna J, Ntozini R, Evans C, et al. Effects of improved complementary feeding and improved water, sanitation and hygiene on early child development among HIV-exposed children: substudy of a cluster randomised trial in rural Zimbabwe. BMJ Glob Health 2020;5(1):e001718.
89. McHenry MS, McAteer CI, Oyungu E, et al. Interventions for developmental delays in children born to HIV-infected mothers: a systematic review. AIDS Care 2019;31(3):275–82.

Research Toward a Cure for Perinatal HIV

Kristen Kelly, BS[a], Soumia Bekka, BS[a], Deborah Persaud, MD[b,c,*]

KEYWORDS

• Perinatal HIV-1 • ART-Free HIV-1 remission • HIV-1 cure

KEY POINTS

- Perinatal HIV-1 infection is unique, with distinct reservoir properties that enhance the potential for achieving antiretroviral therapy (ART)-free remission.
- Significant scientific advances have highlighted the importance of very early infant diagnosis and treatment of in utero HIV-1 infection to achieve ART-free remission and a potential cure.
- Efforts to achieve ART-free remission and a cure have the potential to expand the therapeutic armamentarium for perinatal HIV-1 infection. These include immunotherapeutics such as broadly neutralizing antibodies, therapeutic HIV-1 vaccines, and innate immune-enhancing agents aimed at attaining ART-free remission.

INTRODUCTION

Achieving antiretroviral therapy (ART)-free remission and ultimately curing HIV-1 is an aspirational goal for HIV-1 therapeutics, aiming to free individuals from a lifetime of ART and the associated stigma. This goal is rooted in the hope that newer antiviral therapies will emerge, enhancing both the health and quality of life for people living with HIV-1 (PLWH). Out of the 39 million PLWH, 2.58 million are children or adolescents under 19 years of age.[1] Children are particularly at risk for vertical transmission, which can occur prenatally in utero, peripartum during labor and delivery, or postnatally during breast/chest-feeding. All 3 modes of perinatal HIV-1 transmission are preventable if maternal infection is identified and treated. The overall risk of vertical transmission is estimated to be less than 1% when maternal viremia is controlled to clinically undetectable levels and postnatal prophylaxis is administered to the neonate.[2] Prevention of perinatal HIV-1 transmission should remain the mainstay of maternal and pediatric

[a] Department of Molecular Microbiology and Immunology, Johns Hopkins Bloomberg School of Public Health, Ross 1133, 720 Rutland Avenue, Baltimore, MD 21205, USA; [b] Department of Pediatrics, Division of Infectious Diseases, Johns Hopkins University School of Medicine, 1170, 720 Rutland Avenue, Baltimore, MD 21205, USA; [c] Department of Molecular Microbiology and Immunology, Johns Hopkins Bloomberg School of Public Health, Baltimore, MD 21205, USA
* Corresponding author. Department of Pediatrics, Division of Infectious Diseases, Johns Hopkins University School of Medicine, 1170, 720 Rutland Avenue, Baltimore, MD 21205.
E-mail address: dpers@jhmi.edu

Clin Perinatol 51 (2024) 895–910
https://doi.org/10.1016/j.clp.2024.08.006 perinatology.theclinics.com

HIV-1 care and global treatment programs. However, given the continued occurrence of transmissions in children, it is crucial to develop new treatment strategies that enable periods of ART-free remission, thereby improving quality of life and reducing drug toxicities, cost, and stigma for children living with perinatal HIV-1.[3]

HISTORY

Of the 2.58 million children aged 0 to 14 years living with HIV-1 (CLWH), an estimated 84,000 died in 2022, underscoring the high mortality associated with the perinatal HIV-1 infection.[4] Additionally, approximately 130,000 (90,000–120,000) new infections were reported.[4] Access to ART for children remains far below the 95% target goal set by the United Nations Joint Program on HIV/AIDS (UNAIDS) Project 95-95-95, with only 43% of CLWH receiving life-saving ART, leaving approximately 660,000 children without treatment.[4] These statistics highlight the critical need for cure strategies for this population.

While ART effectively controls HIV-1 replication, it is not curative. Currently, virtually all PLWH must adhere to a lifelong ART regimen to maintain clinically undetectable levels of plasma viremia and benefit from the survival advantages ART confers. In most PLWH, including children, viremic rebound occurs within 2 to 4 weeks of ART discontinuation due to the presence of the latent HIV-1 reservoir (LR).[5–8] The LR is established during acute infection, primarily through the infection of susceptible effector $CD4^+$ T cells that transition to memory $CD4^+$ T cells.[6,9] These memory $CD4^+$ T cells harbor integrated, intact HIV-1 proviruses, maintaining the LR of HIV-1 through clonal expansion and homeostatic proliferation.

Within resting memory $CD4^+$ T cells, HIV-1 proviruses express little-to-no viral genes.[10] In the absence of viral gene expression, neither ART nor immune-mediated clearance can target these infected cell populations.[10] However, some latent proviruses can be reactivated to produce infectious virus.[11] Without ART, virions produced from the LR can infect susceptible cells, reigniting viral replication and causing viremic rebound.[11] The goal of ART-free remission and cure therapies is to delay the period of viremic rebound off ART for years through LR reduction or by establishing immunity to control virus replication. A significant component of ART-free remission is the requirement for trial participants to stop their ART regimen to assess for remission or eventual cure (**Fig. 1**).

DEFINITIONS

Provirus: HIV-1 DNA integrated within a host chromosome.

Latent reservoir (LR): A population of cells capable of carrying intact, integrated infectious HIV-1 proviruses in a quiescent state that prevents proviral elimination.

Early ART: Initiating therapy within 2 to 3 months of life.

Very early ART: Initiating therapy within 48 hours to 7 days of life.

ART-free remission:* Here, we define ART-free remission for those living with perinatal HIV-1 as the maintenance of virologic control lasting a minimum of 48 weeks in the absence of ART or immnotherapeutics. To definitively confirm *lifelong ART-free remission*, those living with perinatal HIV-1 meeting the criteria of ART-free remission will require monitoring and follow ups for a minimum of 10 to 20 years.[12]

*Note: In the recently published HIV Language Guide, the use of "ART-free remission" is currently under reconsideration, and the term "ART-free virologic control" is suggested as an alternative. The guide defines remission as individuals who have experienced periods of virologic control but eventually rebounded. However, in the current context of the perinatal HIV-1, extended periods of aviremia off ART in

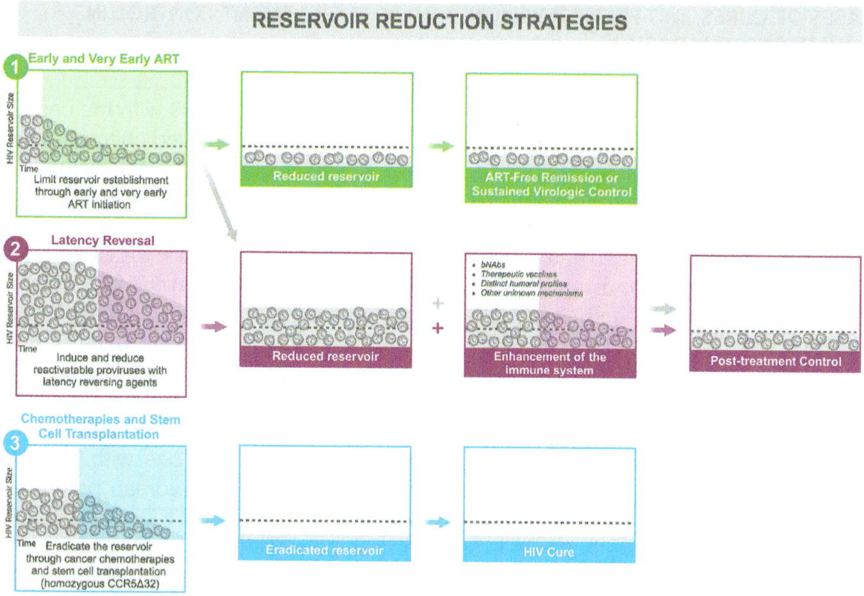

Fig. 1. General Approaches for ART-free Remission, Post-treatment Control and Cures. Each panel depicts the HIV reservoir size over time. Gray arrows indicate HIV reservoirs that are insufficiently reduced and require further intervention to achieve post-treatment control. Dotted lines represent an undefined reservoir threshold, which could enable ART-free remission, post-treatment control, or HIV cure.

neonates, children, and adolescents who received therapies aimed at remission is considered remission, regardless of whether viremic rebound occurs. For the purposes of this publication, we will use "ART-free remission".

Cure: For any person living with HIV-1 in whom HIV-1 reservoirs were completely eradicated, leading to a lifetime off ART without viremic rebound.

Elite controller (EC): A small subset of individuals who spontaneously control plasma viral loads to undetectable levels without ART due to natural production of HIV-1-specific CD4+ T cells generated from carrying specific human lymphocyte antigen (HLA) alleles.

Spontaneous cure: ECs who have maintained viremic control for decades off ART and have no detectable intact proviral reservoir.

Post-treatment control: Children, adolescents, or adults who achieve sustained control of viremia off ART following immunotherapeutic interventions such as broadly neutralizing antibodies (bNAbs), therapeutic HIV-1 vaccines, or latency reversal agents (LRAs). Alternatively, for the rare child, adolescent, or adult who following early ART are found to control HIV-1 viremia off ART and immunotherapeutics, have detectable HIV-1 proviruses, and have yet undefined HIV-1-specific immune responses.

Analytical treatment interruption (ATI): Planned ART discontinuation to assess efficacy of HIV-1 remission and cure interventions, where plasma viral loads are frequently monitored to detect viremic rebound and to describe the duration of aviremia off ART.

bNAbs: HIV-1-specific antibodies that neutralize diverse isolates of HIV-1 through targeting of the surface envelope (Env) glycoprotein.

LRAs: This class of drugs non-specifically target HIV-1 proviruses to increase their transcriptional activity and may lead to HIV-1 protein expression to enhance reservoir elimination.

CASES OF CURES, ART-FREE REMISSION, AND POSTTREATMENT CONTROL IN ADULTS AND CHILDREN

Cases of Cures

The proof-of-concept for HIV-1 cure was first demonstrated in 2009 with the case of Timothy Brown.[13] Brown, also known as the "Berlin patient," received chemotherapy and total body irradiation for relapsed acute myelogenous leukemia (AML), including 2 hematopoietic stem cell transplants from a donor with a homozygous base pair deletion in the gene encoding the main HIV-1 coreceptor C-C chemokine receptor type 5 (CCR5). Homozygosity for a naturally occurring 32 base pair deletion in the CCR5 gene (CCR5Δ32) leads to natural resistance to HIV-1 infection. Approximately 1% of individuals of Northern European descent are homozygous carriers of this mutation. Transplantation of CCR5Δ32 stem cells leads to immune reconstitution with $CD4^+$ T cells inherently resistant to HIV-1, rendering the transplant curative. Since then, 4 additional cases of HIV-1 cure mediated by hematopoietic stem cell transplantation with CCR5Δ32 homozygous cells have been reported in ALWH treated for underlying malignancies.[14–17] Three individuals were diagnosed with AML and one with Hodgkin lymphoma. Notably, one individual with AML, who was the first woman potentially cured of HIV-1, is of mixed race and underwent a unique haplo-cord transplantation.[16] These cases demonstrate that HIV-1 reservoirs can be sufficiently reduced to achieve cures but highlight the drastic measures needed for reservoir reduction and immune reconstitution with CCR5Δ32, HIV-1-resistant cells. No cases of HIV-1 cure from stem cell transplantation have been reported in children. A CCR5Δ32 cord blood transplant was used to treat acute lymphoblastic leukemia in a 12 year old adolescent living with perinatal HIV-1, but the adolescent succumbed to graft versus host disease 73 days later.[18] One clinical trial is currently investigating CCR5Δ32 cord blood transplantation as a treatment of hematological malignancies in infants, children, and adults living with HIV-1 (NCT04083170; **Table 1**).

Two women, the "San Francisco patient" reported in 2020 and the "Esperanza patient" reported in 2022, have exhibited "spontaneous cures" of HIV-1.[17,19–21] In these cases, the spontaneous cure was presumably achieved through immune-mediated mechanisms that led to the clearance of intact proviruses of HIV-1, leaving only defective proviruses incapable of fueling rebound. A case of perinatal HIV-1 clearance was first reported in 1995 in a 5 year old child diagnosed with HIV-1 infection through positive viral cultures from peripheral-blood mononuclear cells (PBMCs) and plasma at 19 and 51 days of life. Before initiating ART, the child became HIV-1 antibody negative and maintained seronegative status with subsequent negative viral cultures between 1 and 5 years of age. The mechanism of clearance was not determined, and no follow-up information on serostatus has been reported.[22]

ECs represent a unique population of PLWH who spontaneously and effectively suppress plasma viremia to undetectable levels (<50 copies/mL) without ART.[23] ECs are rare, occurring approximately 1% worldwide (from the CASCADE cohort of 25,692 HIV seroconverters), have small LRs with replication-competent proviruses, but they can prevent disease progression for many years without ART.[24] ECs have been found to harbor inherent anti-HIV-1 immunity, including enrichment of protective genes encoding class I HLA, enhanced cytotoxic T lymphocyte capacities, and distinct sites of proviral integration.[19,25,26] While viral rebound is prevented for many years in ECs, rebound can still occur due to the persistence of the LR.[27] Pediatric ECs are less common compared to ALWH. One study reported 11 cases of pediatric ECs, with 7 maintaining control of viremia for a median of over 6 years.[28] Other studies have documented long-term non-progressors and slow progressors to AIDS in pediatric populations.[29–32]

Table 1
Pediatric HIV cure-related studies

Study Name	Study ID	Study Phase	Study Intervention	Study Timeline	Country
Clinical Trials					
EIT: Early infant HIV treatment in Botswana	NCT02369406	Phase II/III	Treatment intensification/ Early treatment	Current Clinical Trial	Botswana
Cord blood transplantation: with OTS for the treatment of HIV + hematologic cancers	NCT04083170	Phase II	Stem cell transplantation	Current Clinical Trial	USA
HVRRICANE: HIVIS DNA + MVA-CMDR vaccines ± TLR4 agonist	NCT04301154	Phase I	Combination therapeutic immunization ± toll-like receptor agonist	Current Clinical Trial	South Africa
TATELO: VRC01LS + 10–1074 bNAbs in early treated children	NCT03707977	Phase I/II	Antibodies	Completed	Botswana
Antiretroviral regime for viral eradication in newborns	NCT02712801	Phase IV	Treatment intensification/ early treatment	Completed	China
LEOPARD: Latency and early neonatal provision of antiretroviral drugs clinical trial	NCT02431975	Phase IV	Treatment intensification/ early treatment	Completed	South Africa

(*continued on next page*)

Table 1 (*continued*)

Study Name	Study ID	Study Phase	Study Intervention	Study Timeline	Country
IMPAACT P1115: Very early intensive treatment of infants with HIV-1 to achieve HIV remission — *Version 1.0:* Very early intensive treatment within 48 h of birth; *Version 2.0:* Very early intensive treatment within 48 h of birth + RAL, ± VRC01 bNAb; *Version 3.0:* Very early intensive treatment within 48 h of birth + RAL, transition to DTG, ± VRC07–523LS bNAb	NCT02140255	Phase I/II	Very early treatment	Current Clinical trial	USA, Argentina, Brazil, Haiti, Kenya, Malawi, Puerto Rico, South Africa, Tanzania, Thailand, Uganda, Zambia, Zimbabwe
IMPAACT 2008: VRC01 bNAb in infants	NCT03208231	Phase I/II	Antibodies	Completed	Botswana, Brazil
IMPAACT 2039: Randomized study of an HIV vaccine regimen in combination with bNAbs in children living with HIV	No clinicaltrials.gov entry, listed on IMPAACT website	Phase I/II	Therapeutic vaccine +/_ bNAbs	In Development	To be determined
Observational Studies					
EARTH: Early antiretroviral treatment in HIV + children	NCT05784584	N/A	Treatment intensification/ Early treatment	Current Observational Study	Mali, Mozambique, South Africa
EPIICAL: Early-treated Perinatally HIV-infected Individuals: Improving Children's Actual Life with Novel Immunotherapeutic Strategies	No clinicaltrials.gov entry	N/A	Observational study	Completed	Italy, Mali, Mozambique, South Africa
PediacamNEG: Negative serology in children with HIV treated early with ART	NCT06302933	N/A	Treatment intensification/ Early treatment	Current Observational Study	Cameroon

AVIR: Characterization of HIV-1 reservoirs in adolescents with non-B HIV-1 on ART in Cameroon	NCT06363500	N/A	Treatment intensification/ Early treatment	Completed	Cameroon
CLEAC: Comparison of late vs early antiretroviral therapy in HIV-infected children	NCT02674867	N/A	Treatment intensification/ Early treatment	Completed	France
EPIC4: Early Pediatric Initiation: Canada Child cure Cohort Study	CTN S 281	N/A	Treatment intensification/ Early treatment	Completed	Canada
IMPAACT 2028: Long-term clinical, immunologic, and virologic profiles of children who received early treatment for HIV	NCT05154513	N/A	Treatment intensification/ Early treatment	Current Observational Study	USA
IMPAACT 2015: Evaluation of the HIV-1 reservoir in the CNS of perinatally-infected youth and young adults with cognitive impairment	NCT03416790	N/A	Observational study	Completed	USA, Puerto Rico
IMPAACT P1107: Cord blood transplantation with CCR5Δ32 donor cells in HIV-1 infected subjects who require bone marrow transplantation for any indication and its observed effects on HIV-1 persistence	NCT02140944	N/A	Cord blood transplantation CCR5Δ32	Completed	USA

Data from the Treatment Action Group (TAG) Research Toward a Cure Trials.

Post-treatment Control

Post-treatment control of HIV-1, where biomarkers of HIV-1 infection persist but aviremia or low-level viremia off ART occurs, was first reported in 2013 in a small subset of adults in the VISCONTI cohort who were treated during primary HIV-1 infection. In adult post-treatment controllers, HIV-1 DNA and/or HIV-1-specific antibodies are detected, suggesting that immune-mediated mechanisms are controlling the LR.[33] A long-term follow-up of post-treatment controllers from the VISCONTI cohort revealed distinct humoral responses associated with long-lasting viral suppression.[33] Post-treatment control in perinatal HIV-1 infection was subsequently identified in 2017 in a French Adolescent girl and in 2019 in a South African boy. Both were treated in early infancy, at 3 and 2 months of age, respectively, for 5.5 to 7 years and 40 weeks, and did not experience viremic rebound off ART for 12 and 8.5 years, respectively.[33,34] In-depth characterization of these cases provides key insights into potential immune mechanisms that may aid in controlling HIV-1 off ART.

An alternative approach to achieving post-treatment control through very early ART includes a treatment switch from daily ART to monthly intravenous infusions of bNAbs to maintain undetectable viral loads off ART. In the Tatelo Study (NCT03707977), the bNAbs VRC01-LS and 10-1074, which bind to the CD4 binding site and the V3 glycan supersite in the HIV-1 envelope glycoprotein respectively, were administered in later childhood to very early treated children who initiated ART in the first 7 days of life in the EIT study (see **Table 1**).[35] In this cohort, 56% of 25 children experienced viral rebound within 4 weeks of stopping ART. However, 11 of the 25 children maintained virologic suppression, with plasma viral load levels less than 400 HIV-1 RNA copies per mL, for the study period of 24 weeks off ART. These children were found to have low levels of HIV-1 DNA at ART initiation, indicating that combination bNAbs may sustain virologic suppression in the context of low proviral reservoirs with very early ART.[35]

ART-free Remission

In 2013, we reported on the well-documented case of ART-free remission in "the Mississippi baby."[36] Perinatal HIV-1 transmission was confirmed in utero through repeated detection of viremia within the first 19 days of life, which declined after the initiation of very early ART within 30 hours of birth. Undetectable levels of HIV-1 RNA, DNA, or HIV-1-specific antibodies at 23 months of age after stopping ART for 5 months. With close follow-up and monitoring, the child did not experience viremic rebound off ART for 12 months at the time of the first report, signifying HIV-1 remission.[37] After 27 months off ART, viremic rebound occurred despite the absence of detectable replication-competent HIV-1 in the LR during the ART discontinuation/ART-free remission period.[36,37] This case provided evidence for the very early formation and persistence of the LR in perinatal HIV-1 infection. While not curative, this case provided a proof-of-concept that very early ART in neonates can reduce the HIV-1 LR sufficiently to promote ART-free remission of 48 weeks or longer. Furthermore, it provided the scientific rationale to examine very early treatment of neonates with in utero HIV-1 as a strategy for ART-free remission and potential cure efforts in perinatal HIV-1.

The International Maternal Pediatric Adolescent AIDS Clinicals Trials (IMPAACT) Network P1115 clinical trial (NCT02140255; see **Table 1**) was subsequently developed and is ongoing.[38] This trial aims to achieve ART-free remission through very early ART, measuring the duration off ART without viremic rebound following the intervention. We recently reported our findings from IMPAACT P1115 on 4 cases of 48 weeks or more of ART-free remission in very early treated children enrolled in version 1.0 of the protocol.[39] Three other studies of very early ART of newborns have been conducted, although ATI has not been conducted to assess for remission (see **Table 1**).[40–42] One study in South Africa reported on 5 male individuals experiencing periods of 3 to 19 months of sustained control of viremia after self-discontinuing ART.[43] Altogether, these studies support the relationship between very early ART, reservoir reduction, and potential for ART-free remission (see **Fig. 1**).[44]

CURRENT STATE OF PEDIATRIC HIV-1 CURES AND RESEARCH GAPS

To date, there are 11 clinical trials and 9 observational studies across 21 countries focused on ART-free remission and cure strategies in children and adolescents (**Fig. 2**). Twelve studies focus on intensification and/or early/very early ART, 4 incorporate an immunotherapeutic intervention, 2 focus on stem cell transplantation, and 2 are observational (see **Table 1**).

An alternative approach to achieving ART-free remission is being studied in IMPAACT P1115 (version 2.0 and 3.0) and IMPAACT 2008 (NCT03208231; see **Table 1**). In these trials, very early ART initiation is combined with bNAbs in neonates with in utero HIV-1 infection or in infants initiating early ART when diagnosed at 2 to 3 months of age. This combination aims to improve virologic suppression rates and the clearance of infected cells. These studies will provide insights into the extent to which eliciting HIV-1-specific immune responses can promote ART-free remission in children.

Therapeutic HIV-1 Vaccines

Studies of HIV-1 vaccines show promise in eliciting HIV-1-specific immune responses, which can result in lower levels of viremia off ART. In the IMPAACT/PACTG 1059 study (NCT00107549), a therapeutic HIV-1 vaccine regimen using Ankara/fowlpox virus-based and MVA vaccines was administered to young adults with perinatal and non-perinatal infections. The regimen was found to be immunogenic and to

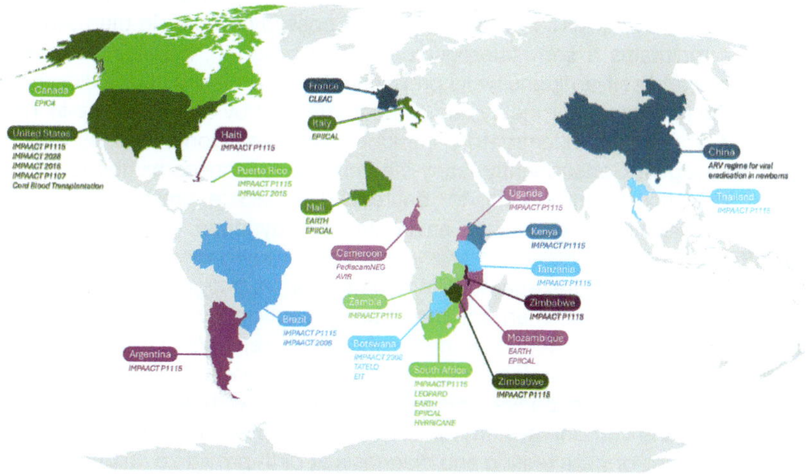

Fig. 2. The Global Distribution of Pediatric HIV Cure-Related Studies. World map showing all past and current clinical trials and observational studies on perinatal HIV-1. *Study location information is sourced from the Treatment Action Group (TAG).*

transiently decrease the size of the replication-competent LR.[45] Another study involving a multigene, multi-subtype A, B, C HIV-DNA (HIVIS) vaccine given to CLWH also showed a decrease in total HIV-1 DNA post-vaccination. A clinical trial of the HIVIS DNA vaccine, with or without a TLR-4 agonist, administered alongside a human papillomavirus vaccine to South African Adolescents treated from infancy was recently completed (NCT04301154; see **Table 1**). The main outcomes of this trial are immunogenicity and effects on LR size, but an ATI was not included, precluding analyses for ART-free remission. The IMPAACT Network (IMPAACT 2039; NCT TBD; see **Table 1**) is investigating another conserved element vaccine in combination with a triple bNAb regimen, aiming to achieve posttreatment control in very early and early treated children. These studies will provide valuable insights into the acceptability, safety, immunogenicity, and post-treatment control outcomes of these novel treatment approaches for children and adolescents with HIV-1, thereby advancing the field.

Latency Reversal

In the past 15 years, there have been many proof-of-concept clinical trials in PLWH examining latency reversal with histone deacetylase inhibitors such as vorinostat, romidepsin, panobinostat, or innate immune enhancing agents (TLR7 or TLR9 agonist) with hopes of reactivating the latent proviruses toward LR reduction and elimination[46,47] (see **Fig. 1**). LRAs administered as a single agent on ART have shown no meaningful change in the size of the LR or in delaying the time to viral rebound in adults treated during acute HIV-1 infection. This finding has driven the development of new combinatory strategies involving LRAs and immnotherapeutics, such as with bNAbs and therapeutic vaccines. Studies of HIV-1 vaccines show promise in eliciting HIV-1-specific immune responses to confer lower levels of viremia off ART. However, no studies on latency reversal have been conducted on perinatal HIV-1, highlighting a significant gap in research for this population.[47,48]

DISCUSSION

Perinatal HIV-1 infections possess distinctive immunologic features that offer potential pathways to achieving ART-free remission and possibly a cure. In utero, the developing fetus maintains a semi-tolerogenic immune program, balancing tolerance to both maternal and self-antigens while preparing for the transition to the external environment. The neonatal immune system is characterized by an imbalance in Th1/Th2 immunity, favoring anti-inflammatory immune responses dominated by Th2, Treg, and Th17 lineages. Consequently, early-life immune responses exhibit low levels of immune activation, contributing to decreased CCR5 expression observed in CLWH.[49] Furthermore, the immune environment is dynamic, evolving over the life course (**Fig. 3**).

Additionally, the neonatal adaptive immune system is antigenically inexperienced, creating an optimal environment for immunotherapeutic interventions. Children who initiate very early ART often lack detectable HIV-1-specific immune responses, indicating that very early virologic suppression may prevent the development of an HIV-1-specific memory response. This can be leveraged with early therapeutic vaccination to prime the immune system for better control or elimination of HIV-1.

Immediate point-of-care testing and diagnosis at birth provide a unique opportunity for very early or early ART initiation in infants with perinatal HIV-1. Early suppression of HIV-1 viremia with ART limits the establishment of the LR in terms of both size and complexity.[50,51] This contrasts with adult infections, where no difference in LR size

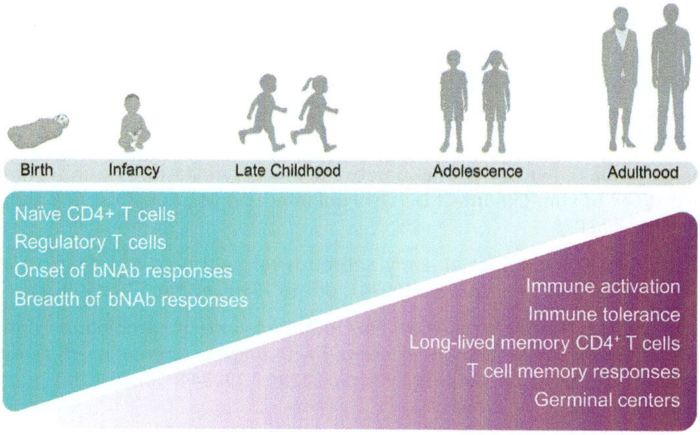

Fig. 3. Change in Immune Characteristics Throughout Childhood. Cell populations and immune processes change over time from infancy through childhood to adolescence.

is observed between those treated during acute versus chronic HIV-1 infection after 2 to 3 decades of continuous ART.[52] In fact, recent reports indicate that the LR can expand over 2 or more decades of ART in adults, with clonal expansion being a major contributor to LR persistence.[53] Regarding humoral responses, CLWH develop bNAbs earlier in infection, with greater breadth and potency compared to adults.[54,55] These unique aspects of perinatal HIV-1 infection suggest a higher likelihood of achieving ART-free remission and potential cure, warranting ongoing studies in this population.

SUMMARY

Despite significant advancements in the science of perinatal transmission prevention, the global epidemic of perinatal HIV-1 infection persists. The known timing of maternal HIV-1 exposure in most infants provides a unique opportunity to prevent perinatal HIV-1 infection through the initiation of very early and early ART, which can help limit HIV-1 reservoirs. Additionally, various immunotherapeutic approaches have been explored to enhance the chances of achieving ART-free remission, post-treatment control, or a cure for children living with HIV-1.

Best Practices

The current practice for ART-free remission and cure therapeutics

Considerable interest exists in treating perinatal HIV infection at very early stages of life to significantly reduce HIV reservoirs, aiming for a sustained low reservoir size throughout adolescence. This approach holds potential for achieving ART-free remission through immunotherapies.

Major Recommendations

Global attention to implementing very early and early infant diagnosis and treatment of perinatal HIV infection, combined with a focus on maintaining long-term viral suppression, represents the initial stride toward broadening the population of children and adolescents eligible for ART-free remission and curative therapies.

Bibliographic Source(s)

- Persaud D, Bryson Y, Nelson BS, et al. HIV-1 reservoir size after neonatal antiretroviral therapy and the potential to evaluate antiretroviral-therapy-free remission (IMPAACT P1115): a phase 1/2 proof-of-concept study. Lancet HIV. 2024;11(1):e20-e30. doi:10.1016/s2352 to 3018(23)00236-9
- Maswabi K, Ajibola G, Bennett K, et al. Safety and Efficacy of Starting Antiretroviral Therapy in the First Week of Life. Clin Infect Dis Off Publ Infect Dis Soc Am. 2020;72(3):388 to 393. doi:10.1093/cid/ciaa028
- Kuhn L, Strehlau R, Shiau S, et al. Early antiretroviral treatment of infants to attain HIV remission. EClinicalMedicine. 2020;18:100241. doi:10.1016/j.eclinm.2019.100241
- Millar JR, Bengu N, Fillis R, et al. HIGH-FREQUENCY failure of combination antiretroviral therapy in paediatric HIV infection is associated with unmet maternal needs causing maternal NON-ADHERENCE. EClinicalMedicine. 2020;22:100344. doi:10.1016/j.eclinm.2020.100344
- Sex-Specific Innate Immune Selection in Vertical HIV Transmission and cART-Free Aviraemia in Males–CROI Conference. Published March 7, 2024. Accessed June 3, 2024. https://www.croiconference.org/abstract/sex-specific-innate-immune-selection-in-vertical-hiv-transmission-and-cart-free-aviraemia-in-males/
- Khetan P, Liu Y, Dhummakupt A, Persaud D. Advances in Pediatric HIV-1 Cure Therapies and Reservoir Assays. Viruses. 2022;14(12):2608. doi:10.3390/v14122608

ACKNOWLEDGMENTS

This research was supported by the National Institutes of Health (R01A1150412), the PAVE collaboratory (UMIAI164566) Johns Hopkins Center for AIDS Research (P30 AI094189), and the Johns Hopkins Molecular and Cellular Basis of Infectious Diseases (MCBID) Program T32 (5T32AI007417-28).

DISCLOSURE

D. Persaud served on a Scientific Advisory Board Meeting for ViiV Healthcare.

REFERENCES

1. UNICEF. Global and regional trends. UNICEF DATA; 2023. Available at: https://data.unicef.org/topic/hivaids/global-regional-trends/. Accessed May 29, 2024.
2. Flynn PM, Taha TE, Cababasay M, et al. Prevention of HIV-1 transmission through breastfeeding: efficacy and safety of maternal antiretroviral therapy versus infant nevirapine prophylaxis for duration of breastfeeding in HIV-1-infected women with high CD4 cell count (IMPAACT PROMISE): a randomized, open label, clinical trial. J Acquir Immune Defic Syndr 2018;77(4):383–92. https://doi.org/10.1097/QAI.0000000000001612.
3. Dybul M, Attoye T, Baptiste S, et al. The case for an HIV cure and how to get there. Lancet HIV 2020;8(1):e51–8. https://doi.org/10.1016/S2352-3018(20)30232-0.
4. UNAIDS. UNAIDS 2023 report. UNAIDS - global report 2023. 2023. Available at: https://thepath.unaids.org/. Accessed May 29, 2024.
5. Davey RT, Bhat N, Yoder C, et al. HIV-1 and T cell dynamics after interruption of highly active antiretroviral therapy (HAART) in patients with a history of sustained viral suppression. Proc Natl Acad Sci USA 1999;96(26):15109–14. https://doi.org/10.1073/pnas.96.26.15109.

6. Pannus P, Rutsaert S, De Wit S, et al. Rapid viral rebound after analytical treatment interruption in patients with very small HIV reservoir and minimal on-going viral transcription. J Int AIDS Soc 2020;23(2):e25453. https://doi.org/10.1002/jia2.25453.
7. Paediatric European Network for Treatment of AIDS. Response to planned treatment interruptions in HIV infection varies across childhood. AIDS 2010;24(2):231. https://doi.org/10.1097/QAD.0b013e328333d343.
8. Borkowsky W, Yogev R, Muresan P, et al. Structured treatment interruptions (STI) in HIV-1 infected pediatric populations increases interferon gamma production and reduces viremia. Vaccine 2008;26(24):3086–9. https://doi.org/10.1016/j.vaccine.2007.12.017.
9. Chun TW, Finzi D, Margolick J, et al. In vivo fate of HIV-1-infected T cells: quantitative analysis of the transition to stable latency. Nat Med 1995;1(12):1284–90. https://doi.org/10.1038/nm1295-1284.
10. Fromentin R, Chomont N. HIV persistence in subsets of CD4+ T cells: 50 shades of reservoirs. Semin Immunol 2021;51:101438. https://doi.org/10.1016/j.smim.2020.101438.
11. Sengupta S, Siliciano RF. Targeting the latent reservoir for HIV-1. Immunity 2018;48(5):872–95. https://doi.org/10.1016/j.immuni.2018.04.030.
12. NIAID, HIV Language Guide, National Institute of Allergy and Infectious Diseases, 2024, No. 24-AI-740, https://www.niaid.nih.gov/sites/default/files/niaid-hiv-language-guide.pdf.
13. Gero H, Nowak D, Maximilian M, et al. Long-term control of HIV by CCR5 delta32/delta32 stem-cell transplantation. N Engl J Med 2009;360(7):692–8. https://doi.org/10.1056/NEJMoa0802905.
14. Gupta RK, Abdul-Jawad S, McCoy LE, et al. HIV-1 remission following CCR5Δ32/Δ32 haematopoietic stem-cell transplantation. Nature 2019;568(7751):244–8. https://doi.org/10.1038/s41586-019-1027-4.
15. Gupta RK, Peppa D, Hill AL, et al. Evidence for HIV-1 cure after CCR5Δ32/Δ32 allogeneic haemopoietic stem-cell transplantation 30 months post analytical treatment interruption: a case report. Lancet HIV 2020;7(5):e340–7. https://doi.org/10.1016/S2352-3018(20)30069-2.
16. Hsu J, Besien KV, Glesby MJ, et al. HIV-1 remission and possible cure in a woman after haplo-cord blood transplant. Cell 2023;186(6):1115–26.e8. https://doi.org/10.1016/j.cell.2023.02.030.
17. Jensen BEO, Knops E, Cords L, et al. In-depth virological and immunological characterization of HIV-1 cure after CCR5Δ32/Δ32 allogeneic hematopoietic stem cell transplantation. Nat Med 2023;29(3):583–7. https://doi.org/10.1038/s41591-023-02213-x.
18. Rothenberger M, Wagner JE, Haase A, et al. Transplantation of CCR5Δ32 homozygous umbilical cord blood in a child with acute lymphoblastic leukemia and perinatally acquired HIV infection. Open Forum Infect Dis 2018;5(5):ofy090. https://doi.org/10.1093/ofid/ofy090.
19. Jiang C, Lian X, Gao C, et al. Distinct viral reservoirs in individuals with spontaneous control of HIV-1. Nature 2020;585(7824):261–7. https://doi.org/10.1038/s41586-020-2651-8.
20. Turk G, Seiger K, Lian X, et al. A possible sterilizing cure of HIV-1 infection without stem cell transplantation. Ann Intern Med 2022;175(1):95–100. https://doi.org/10.7326/L21-0297.

21. Mendoza D, Johnson SA, Peterson BA, et al. Comprehensive analysis of unique cases with extraordinary control over HIV replication. Blood 2012;119(20): 4645–55. https://doi.org/10.1182/blood-2011-10-381996.
22. Bryson YJ, Pang S, Wei LS, et al. Clearance of HIV infection in a perinatally infected infant. N Engl J Med 1995;332(13):833–8. https://doi.org/10.1056/NEJM199503303321301.
23. Olson AD, Meyer L, Prins M, et al. An evaluation of HIV elite controller definitions within a large seroconverter cohort collaboration. PLoS One 2014;9(1):e86719. https://doi.org/10.1371/journal.pone.0086719.
24. Lambotte O, Boufassa F, Madec Y, et al. HIV controllers: a homogeneous group of HIV-1-infected patients with spontaneous control of viral replication. Clin Infect Dis 2005;41(7):1053–6. https://doi.org/10.1086/433188.
25. Gebara NY, El Kamari V, Rizk N. HIV-1 elite controllers: an immunovirological review and clinical perspectives. J Virus Erad 2019;5(3):163–6.
26. McLaren PJ, Carrington M. The impact of host genetic variation on infection with HIV-1. Nat Immunol 2015;16(6):577–83. https://doi.org/10.1038/ni.3147.
27. Borrell M, Fernández I, Etcheverrry F, et al. High rates of long-term progression in HIV-1-positive elite controllers. J Int AIDS Soc 2021;24(2):e25675. https://doi.org/10.1002/jia2.25675.
28. Vieira VA, Zuidewind P, Muenchhoff M, et al. Strong sex bias in elite control of paediatric HIV infection. AIDS Lond Engl 2019;33(1):67–75. https://doi.org/10.1097/QAD.0000000000002043.
29. De Maio FA, Rocco CA, Aulicino PC, et al. Unusual substitutions in HIV-1 vif from children infected perinatally without progression to AIDS for more than 8 years without therapy. J Med Virol 2012;84(12):1844–52. https://doi.org/10.1002/jmv.23261.
30. Chaudhuri RP, Neogi U, Rao SD, et al. Genetic factors associated with slow progression of HIV among perinatally-infected Indian children. Indian Pediatr 2014;51(10):801–3. https://doi.org/10.1007/s13312-014-0505-x.
31. Radhakrishna M, Durga K, Rao RK, et al. Factors associated with conversion of long-term non-progressors to progressors: a prospective study of HIV perinatally infected paediatric survivors. Indian J Med Res 2013;138(3):322–8.
32. Foster C, Kaye S, Smith C, et al. HIV-1 co-receptor tropism and disease progression in children and young adults with perinatally acquired HIV-1 infection. The HICCUP Study. J Virus Erad 2015;1(3):173–8.
33. Sáez-Cirión A, Bacchus C, Hocqueloux L, et al. Post-treatment HIV-1 controllers with a long-term virological remission after the interruption of early initiated antiretroviral therapy ANRS VISCONTI study. PLoS Pathog 2013;9(3):e1003211. https://doi.org/10.1371/journal.ppat.1003211.
34. Frange P, Faye A, Avettand-Fenoël V, et al. HIV-1 virological remission lasting more than 12 years after interruption of early antiretroviral therapy in a perinatally infected teenager enrolled in the French ANRS EPF-CO10 paediatric cohort: a case report. Lancet HIV 2016;3(1):e49–54. https://doi.org/10.1016/S2352-3018(15)00232-5.
35. Shapiro RL, Ajibola G, Maswabi K, et al. Broadly neutralizing antibody treatment maintained HIV suppression in children with favorable reservoir characteristics in Botswana. Sci Transl Med 2023;15(703):eadh0004. https://doi.org/10.1126/scitranslmed.adh0004.
36. Persaud D, Gay H, Ziemniak C, et al. Absence of detectable HIV-1 viremia after treatment cessation in an infant. N Engl J Med 2013;369(19):1828–35. https://doi.org/10.1056/NEJMoa1302976.

37. Luzuriaga K, Gay H, Ziemniak C, et al. Viremic relapse following prolonged antiretroviral-free HIV-1 remission in a perinatally infected child. N Engl J Med 2015;372(8):786–8. https://doi.org/10.1056/NEJMc1413931.
38. Persaud D, Bryson Y, Nelson BS, et al. HIV-1 reservoir size after neonatal antiretroviral therapy and the potential to evaluate antiretroviral-therapy-free remission (IMPAACT P1115): a phase 1/2 proof-of-concept study. Lancet HIV 2024;11(1): e20–30. https://doi.org/10.1016/S2352-3018(23)00236-9.
39. ART-free HIV-1 remission in very early treated children: results from IMPAACT P1115 - CROI conference. 2024. Available at: https://www.croiconference.org/abstract/art-free-hiv-1-remission-in-very-early-treated-children-results-from-impaact-p1115/. Accessed June 4, 2024.
40. Maswabi K, Ajibola G, Bennett K, et al. Safety and efficacy of starting antiretroviral therapy in the first week of life. Clin Infect Dis 2020;72(3):388–93. https://doi.org/10.1093/cid/ciaa028.
41. Kuhn L, Strehlau R, Shiau S, et al. Early antiretroviral treatment of infants to attain HIV remission. EClinicalMedicine 2020;18:100241. https://doi.org/10.1016/j.eclinm.2019.100241.
42. Millar JR, Bengu N, Fillis R, et al. HIGH-FREQUENCY failure of combination antiretroviral therapy in paediatric HIV infection is associated with unmet maternal needs causing maternal NON-ADHERENCE. EClinicalMedicine 2020;22:100344. https://doi.org/10.1016/j.eclinm.2020.100344.
43. Sex-specific innate immune selection in vertical HIV transmission and cART-free aviraemia in males - CROI conference. 2024. Available at: https://www.croiconference.org/abstract/sex-specific-innate-immune-selection-in-vertical-hiv-transmission-and-cart-free-aviraemia-in-males/. Accessed June 3, 2024.
44. Khetan P, Liu Y, Dhummakupt A, et al. Advances in pediatric HIV-1 cure therapies and reservoir Assays. Viruses 2022;14(12):2608. https://doi.org/10.3390/v14122608.
45. Persaud D, Luzuriaga K, Ziemniak C, et al. Effect of therapeutic HIV recombinant poxvirus vaccines on the size of the resting CD4+ T-cell latent HIV reservoir. AIDS Lond Engl 2011;25(18):2227–34. https://doi.org/10.1097/QAD.0b013e32834cdaba.
46. Kroon EDMB, Ananworanich J, Pagliuzza A, et al. A randomized trial of vorinostat with treatment interruption after initiating antiretroviral therapy during acute HIV-1 infection. J Virus Erad 2020;6(3):100004. https://doi.org/10.1016/j.jve.2020.100004.
47. Debrabander Q, Hensley KS, Psomas CK, et al. The efficacy and tolerability of latency-reversing agents in reactivating the HIV-1 reservoir in clinical studies: a systematic review. J Virus Erad 2023;9(3):100342. https://doi.org/10.1016/j.jve.2023.100342.
48. Research Toward a Cure Trials. Treatment action group. Available at: https://www.treatmentactiongroup.org/cure/trials/. Accessed June 3, 2024.
49. Bunders MJ, van der Loos CM, Klarenbeek PL, et al. Memory CD4(+)CCR5(+) T cells are abundantly present in the gut of newborn infants to facilitate mother-to-child transmission of HIV-1. Blood 2012;120(22):4383–90. https://doi.org/10.1182/blood-2012-06-437566.
50. Persaud D, Ray SC, Kajdas J, et al. Slow human immunodeficiency virus type 1 evolution in viral reservoirs in infants treated with effective antiretroviral therapy. AIDS Res Hum Retrovir 2007;23(3):381–90. https://doi.org/10.1089/aid.2006.0175.
51. Persaud D, Patel K, Karalius B, et al. Influence of age at virologic control on peripheral blood human immunodeficiency virus reservoir size and serostatus in

perinatally infected adolescents. JAMA Pediatr 2014;168(12):1138–46. https://doi.org/10.1001/jamapediatrics.2014.1560.
52. McMyn NF, Varriale J, Fray EJ, et al. The latent reservoir of inducible, infectious HIV-1 does not decrease despite decades of antiretroviral therapy. J Clin Invest 2023;133(17). https://doi.org/10.1172/JCI171554.
53. Crooks AM, Bateson R, Cope AB, et al. Precise quantitation of the latent HIV-1 reservoir: implications for eradication strategies. J Infect Dis 2015;212(9): 1361–5. https://doi.org/10.1093/infdis/jiv218.
54. Mishra N, Sharma S, Dobhal A, et al. Broadly neutralizing plasma antibodies effective against autologous circulating viruses in infants with multivariant HIV-1 infection. Nat Commun 2020;11:4409. https://doi.org/10.1038/s41467-020-18225-x.
55. Ditse Z, Muenchhoff M, Adland E, et al. HIV-1 subtype C-infected children with exceptional neutralization breadth exhibit polyclonal responses targeting known epitopes. J Virol 2018;92(17):e00878–918. https://doi.org/10.1128/JVI.00878-18.

Research on Perinatal Human Immunodeficiency Virus in Asia

Data on Treatment Outcomes and Emerging Co-Morbidities from the TREAT Asia Network

Tavitiya Sudjaritruk, MD, PhD[a,b,*], Aarti Kinikar, MD, MRCP[c],
Annette H. Sohn, MD, PhD[d]

KEYWORDS

• Pediatric • Adolescent • Youth • Young adult • Perinatal • HIV • Asia • Treatment

Continued

BACKGROUND

The Asia-Pacific region has half of the world's population and about one-sixth of people living with human immunodeficiency virus (HIV), with 6.5 million in 2022.[1] However,

Funding: The TREAT Asia Pediatric HIV Observational Database is an initiative of TREAT Asia, a program of amfAR, The Foundation for AIDS Research, with support from the US National Institutes of Health's National Institute of Allergy and Infectious Diseases, the *Eunice Kennedy Shriver* National Institute of Child Health and Human Development, United States, National Cancer Institute, United States, National Institute of Mental Health, United States, National Institute on Drug Abuse, the National Heart, Lung, and Blood Institute, United States, the National Institute on Alcohol Abuse and Alcoholism, United States, the National Institute of Diabetes and Digestive and Kidney Diseases, United States, and the Fogarty International Center, as part of the International Epidemiology Databases to Evaluate AIDS (IeDEA; U01AI069907). The Kirby Institute is funded by the Australian Government Department of Health and Ageing, and is affiliated with the Faculty of Medicine, UNSW Australia. A. H. Sohn is additionally supported by a grant from the Fogarty International Center and National Institute of Mental Health (D43TW011302). This work is solely the responsibility of the authors and does not necessarily represent the official views of any of the institutions mentioned earlier.

[a] Division of Infectious Diseases, Department of Pediatrics, Faculty of Medicine, Chiang Mai University, Chiang Mai, Thailand; [b] Clinical and Molecular Epidemiology of Emerging and Re-emerging Infectious Diseases Research Cluster, Faculty of Medicine, Chiang Mai University, Chiang Mai, Thailand; [c] Department of Pediatrics, BJ Government Medical College and Sassoon General Hospital, Pune, India; [d] TREAT Asia, amfAR - The Foundation for AIDS Research, Bangkok, Thailand

* Corresponding author. Division of Infectious Diseases, Department of Pediatrics, Faculty of Medicine, Chiang Mai University, 110 Intavaroros Road, Sriphum, Muang, Chiang Mai 50200, Thailand.

E-mail address: tavitiya.s@cmu.ac.th

Clin Perinatol 51 (2024) 911–923
https://doi.org/10.1016/j.clp.2024.08.008 **perinatology.theclinics.com**
0095-5108/24/

Continued

KEY POINTS

- As implementation of effective prevention strategies to reduce vertical transmission of human immunodeficiency virus (HIV) in the Asia-Pacific region has increased, the numbers of children and adolescents with newly perinatally acquired HIV (PHIV) have gradually declined.
- Maternal HIV treatment, early infant diagnosis, prompt antiretroviral treatment initiation, and comprehensive clinical and social support services for children and adolescents with PHIV are the core strategies for the region to progress toward ending the pediatric AIDS epidemic by 2030.
- As children age, they should be screened and treated appropriately for associated comorbidities and coinfections to improve long-term health outcomes and quality of life.

only about 130,000 are children younger than 15 years and 150,000 are adolescents 10 to 19 years of age, with 440,000 being young adults 15 to 24 years of age. Although a few countries have achieved high rates of prevention of vertical transmission, others have persistently low antiretroviral therapy (ART) coverage for pregnant women, high vertical transmission rates, and low early infant diagnostic testing (**Table 1**). As a result, the predominant features of the regional pediatric HIV epidemic have been its relatively small numbers of those with perinatally acquired HIV (PHIV) and the heterogeneity of risk across countries. Similar to other regions, older "lifetime survivors" of HIV have more complex clinical histories than their peers.[2]

When treatment of children with HIV at the national level in Asia started in the mid-2000s, there were small pockets of expertise in clinical management and research. This was largely in Thailand and India, where clinical trials were being conducted on preventing vertical transmission.[3,4] amfAR's TREAT Asia Pediatric HIV Initiative was started in 2007 to bring experts from across the region together into a network that could more efficiently study treatment outcomes through longitudinal, multisite cohort studies.[5] Through collaborations under the International Epidemiology Databases to Evaluate AIDS (IeDEA) global HIV research consortium, data also were leveraged to inform global pediatric estimates used for modeling and benchmarking treatment

Table 1
Vertical transmission metrics in selected Asian countries

Country	ART Coverage in Pregnancy (%)	Vertical Transmission (%)	Early Infant Diagnosis (%)
Malaysia	>98	2	>98
Thailand	97	2	94
Cambodia	89	10	86
Vietnam	77	13	27
India	64	20	n/a
Myanmar	43	24	12
Indonesia	18	30	8
Pakistan	12	41[a]	4[a]
Philippines	6	41	7

[a] UNAIDS 2019 data for transmission and 2020 data for infant diagnosis.[1]
Data from UNAIDS Estimates, 2023; with permission.

outcomes.[6] The TREAT Asia network remains the only regional source of epidemiology and clinical outcomes data for this population in the Asia region. Previous and ongoing studies described in this review have helped to characterize the health outcomes of children and adolescents with PHIV in Asia and identify gaps in care.

DISCUSSION

Epidemiology of Pediatric Human Immunodeficiency Virus in the Asia Region

The Joint United Nations Programme on HIV/AIDS (UNAIDS) estimates that about 84% of children younger than 15 years with HIV in the Asia-Pacific region have been diagnosed, but there are insufficient data to calculate regional ART coverage or HIV viral suppression rates.[1] Estimates are available on a national level for some countries and reflect the heterogeneity of the epidemic in pregnant women and access to diagnosis and treatment of infants and children. As of the end of 2022, the country in the region with the largest estimated number of children with HIV was India with 68,000, followed by Vietnam with 3800, Cambodia with 2000, Thailand with 1700, and the Philippines with less than 1000.[1] However, although 59% of children with HIV in Cambodia have been diagnosed and greater than 98% of those diagnosed were on ART, this compares to only 22% diagnosed and 78% of those on treatment in the Philippines.

Data from TREAT Asia network studies reflect the history of HIV care and treatment in the region. The pediatric cohort includes data from ~7700 children and adolescents with HIV who have been under care at up to 18 clinical centers in six countries: Cambodia, India, Indonesia, Malaysia, Thailand, and Vietnam (**Fig. 1**). About 90% of the cohort acquired HIV perinatally, and the median age at ART initiation went from 4.5 years for those enrolling between 2011 and 2013 to 6.7 years from 2017 to 2020, although the percentage of those with severe immunodeficiency went from 70% to 45%, with about one-third being severely underweight.[7] However, once ART was started, children in the cohort achieved immune recovery. Of those who ever started combination ART, the overall loss to follow-up rate in the cohort up to September 2023 was approximately 10%, and mortality was 7%. Analyses of causes of death showed that deaths were highest when diagnosis and treatment options were poorer (2008–2010: 19.8 per 1000 person-years) and decreased as the quality of pediatric care improved (2014–2017: 4.0 per 1000 person-years).[8]

Human Immunodeficiency Virus Treatment and Care

Antiretroviral treatment and outcomes

With effective ART and a strengthened HIV management and care in the Asian-Pacific region during the past decade, the authors' regional cohort data during 2014 to 2018 demonstrated that treatment failure, which included clinical, immunologic, and virologic failure, was approximately 7% in children and adolescents with PHIV (74% were on nonnucleoside reverse transcriptase inhibitor [NNRTI]-based regimens), corresponding to an overall rate of 3.8 per 100 person-years.

In addition, among individuals with treatment failure, 11% were switched to a new combined ART regimen within 6 months, which resulted in better immunologic and virologic outcomes compared with those retained on the original ART regimen.[9]

Approximately 13% of children in the authors' regional cohort experienced post-suppression virologic failure (a single viral load >1000 copies/mL) at a rate of 3.4 per 100 person-years after entering adolescence.[10] Being underweight, receiving second-line protease inhibitor (PI)-based regimens and prior virologic failure were associated with viremia.[10] Another study noted that 17% of virally suppressed

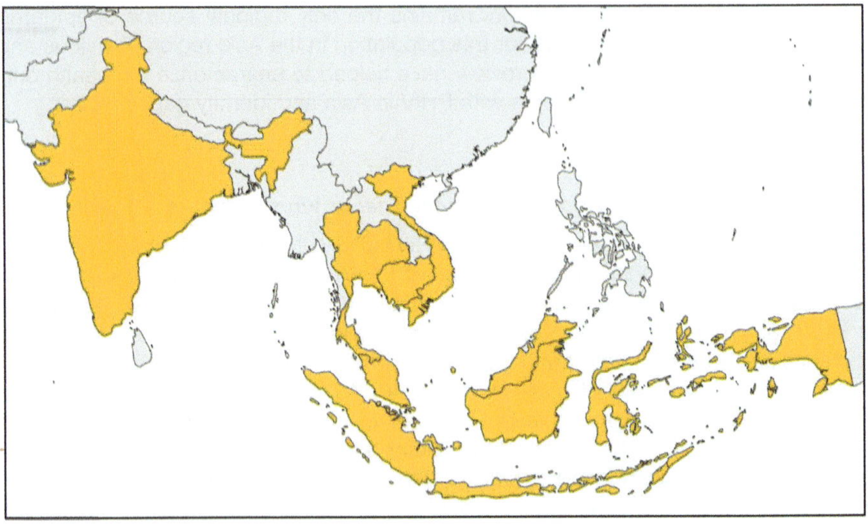

Fig. 1. Map of TREAT Asia pediatric network sites, 2007 to 2023. Site locations: *Cambodia:* National Center for HIV/AIDS, Dermatology and STD, Phnom Penh. *India:* BJ Medical College and Sassoon General Hospital, Pune; VHS-Infectious Diseases Medical Center, CART CRS, Chennai. *Indonesia:* Hospital Cipto Mangunkusumo, Jakarta; Prof. Dr. I.G.N.G. Ngoerah Hospital, Udayana University, Bali; Hasan Sadikin General Hospital, Bandung. *Malaysia* (closed in 2020): Hospital Likas, Kota Kinabalu; Hospital Raja Perempuan Zainab II, Kota Bharu; Penang Hospital, Penang; Women and Children's Hospital, Kuala Lumpur. *Thailand* (closed in 2020): Chiang Mai University and Research Institute for Health Sciences, Chiang Mai; Chiangrai Prachanukroh Hospital, Chiang Rai; Chulalongkorn University, Bangkok; Khon Kaen University, Khon Kaen; Siriraj Hospital, Mahidol University, Bangkok. *Vietnam:* Children's Hospital 1, Ho Chi Minh City; Children's Hospital 2, Ho Chi Minh City; National Hospital of Pediatrics, Hanoi.

children and adolescents with PHIV exhibited low-level viremia (viral load 50–1000 copies/mL) during study follow-up, of whom 37% had multiple low-level viremic episodes.[11] Importantly, children and adolescents with PHIV and low-level viremia had higher rates of virologic failure compared with those with sustained viral suppression (8.9 vs 3.3 per 100 person-years; $P<.001$).[11] These data emphasize the importance of careful monitoring during adolescence and earlier interventions to support adherence.

Treatment monitoring

Monitoring viral load helps ensure earlier identification of treatment failure than CD4 but has not been consistently available in low- to middle-income countries (LMICs).[12] A previous study among children and adolescents in the TREAT Asia cohort (97% on first-line NNRTI-based regimens) demonstrated that routine viral load monitoring (at least one viral load test after ≥24 weeks of ART and ≥1 time/year during the follow-up) was associated with a 46% increase in the relative risk of switching to second-line ART regimens after treatment failure.[13] Another study showed that rates of treatment failure (eg, viral failure, change of antiretroviral drug class, death) were not significantly different among virally suppressed children and adolescents with PHIV on first-line NNRTI regimens who had annual *versus* semi-annual viral load monitoring (5.4 vs 4.3 per 100 patient-years; $P = .27$).[14] In addition, among children and adolescents who were on second-line PI-based regimens (91% on boosted lopinavir) after failing first-line NNRTI-based regimens, 5% had viral loads higher than 1000 copies/mL at 1 year and 20% at 3 years after treatment switch.[15]

A study among virally suppressed children and adolescents on ART in the authors' network showed that the incidences of transient and confirmed immunodeficiency (eg, CD4 <200 cells/mm^3) and advanced clinical HIV disease during study follow-up were small: 0.73, 0.08, and 0.40 events per 100 patient-years, respectively.[16] Nevertheless, when there are concerns for adherence, at least intermittent CD4 testing may be useful to guide clinical management.

Adherence to antiretroviral therapy

Medication adherence is a critical determinant of ART success and long-term viral suppression. A prospective study among children and adolescents with HIV in Malaysia, Thailand, and Vietnam who were on ART for a median duration of 10 years found that the proportion of those with 95% or greater adherence declined from 69% to 60%, and the proportion of those with viral load higher than 1000 copies/mL increased from 14% to 17% between the study baseline and week 144 of follow-up.[17] Among those with poor adherence, common reasons they shared for not taking their medicines included boredom (30%–42%), inconvenience (29%–35%), and the number (22%–30%) and large size (18%–27%) of their pills.[17]

Non-AIDS Comorbidities

As a chronic illness, HIV infection *per se* and long-term use of ART are associated with a substantial burden of non-AIDS comorbidities among children and adolescents with PHIV while growing up into adulthood.

Adverse bone health

Children and adolescents with PHIV are at higher risk of adverse bone health.[18] A previous study reported a 16% prevalence of low bone mineral density (a lumbar spine bone mineral density Z-score <−2) among Thai children and adolescents with PHIV, as well as significantly lower bone mass compared with their age- and sex-matched HIV-negative peers.[19] Older age, female sex, low body mass index, low pre-ART CD4 count, and exposure to PI-based ART regimens were found to be associated with low bone mineral density.[19] In addition, vitamin D deficiency (25-hydroxyvitamin D <20 ng/mL) complicated with secondary hyperparathyroidism (intact parathyroid hormone >65 pg/mL) significantly contributed to increased bone turnover and reduced bone mass.[20]

Since experiencing low bone mineral density during adolescence may eventually contribute to early-onset osteoporosis and osteoporotic fracture during adulthood, several interventions have been investigated to prevent bone loss and optimize bone health, including improving nutrition, weight-bearing and muscle strengthening exercises, and pharmacologic interventions (eg, vitamin D and calcium supplementation, antiresorptive treatments).[18] In Thailand, where vitamin D–fortified foods are not generally available, a randomized, active-controlled, open-label trial was conducted among children and adolescents with PHIV and demonstrated that daily supplementation of vitamin D (high dose: 3200 IU/d or standard dose: 400 IU/d) and calcium (1200 mg/d) for 48 weeks significantly increased lumbar spine bone mineral density and reduced bone turnover markers.[21]

Liver disease

Before ART initiation, the prevalence of liver dysfunction (alanine aminotransferase [ALT] ≥3 times the upper limit of normal) among children with HIV in our cohort was

6%, of whom 0.1% were among those with hepatitis B virus coinfection; none had hepatitis C virus coinfection.[22] With effective ART, use of tenofovir disoproxil fumarate (TDF) and lamivudine to treat hepatitis B, and direct-acting antivirals to cure hepatitis C, the incidence of opportunistic liver infections has declined, whereas other forms of chronic liver disease, such as metabolic dysfunction–associated steatotic liver disease (MASLD) and hepatic fibrosis, are increasing in adults with HIV.[23] A multicenter cohort study among children and adolescents with PHIV in Thailand and Indonesia found that the prevalence of MASLD and significant hepatic fibrosis (transient elastography ≥7.4 kPa) were 8% and 9% at an initial evaluation, and 3% and 2% demonstrated evidence of persistent abnormalities at 1-year reassessments, respectively. Baseline ALT greater than 30 U/L and insulin resistance (homeostasis model assessment of insulin resistance >3.16) were found to be associated with persistent hepatic abnormalities.[24] Although non-AIDS liver comorbidities have not been prevalent in Asian children and adolescents with PHIV, noninvasive screening tests may be considered in at-risk individuals to identify those in need of early interventions to prevent liver damage.

Cardiovascular disease

There are increasing data around the associations between HIV infection, ART, and cardiovascular disease risks including in children and adolescents with PHIV. Importantly, cardiovascular events during childhood may increase the risk of premature cardiovascular disease in adulthood.[25] A cross-sectional study among Thai adolescents with PHIV without a previously identified cardiovascular condition found comparable myocardial function evaluated by echocardiogram (ejection fraction: 66% vs 66%; $P = .83$) and carotid intima media thickness evaluated by carotid ultrasonogram (constraint-induced movement therapy [cIMT]: 0.373 vs 0.371 mm; $P = .74$) to those of HIV-negative adolescents.[26] Receiving PI-containing regimens was associated with significantly increased cIMT among those with PHIV (0.364 vs 0.381 mm; $P = .009$).[26] Asymptomatic peripheral arterial disease is an indicator of systemic atherosclerosis and a well-known predictor of cardiovascular morbidity and death in adults.[27] This condition can be screened for by using an ankle brachial index—a simple, noninvasive, sensitive, and cost-effective tool.[28] In a cross-sectional study among Thai children and adolescents with PHIV, the prevalence of asymptomatic peripheral arterial disease (a resting ankle brachial index ≤0.9) were 11% in any extremity and 4% in both extremities.[29] Female sex and advanced HIV clinical stage before ART initiation were associated with a lower ankle brachial index among this population. Additional studies would help to guide the frequency of long-term follow-up with noninvasive assessments to evaluate cardiovascular disease risk in adults with PHIV.

Renal disease

Non–AIDS-related renal disease in children and adolescents with PHIV manifests in several ways, including acute kidney injury; glomerular, tubular, or interstitial disease; and ART-related kidney toxicity.[30] Among Thai children and adolescents with PHIV, the prevalence of glomerular dysfunction (persistent proteinuria or impaired estimated glomerular filtration rate) was 21% in those on TDF-containing regimens and 9% in those not taking TDF, which were significantly higher than age- and sex-matched HIV-negative individuals (1%).[31] In addition, the prevalence of proximal renal tubular dysfunction (phosphaturia, uricosuria, β2 microglobulinuria, or normoglycemic glucosuria) were 19% and 6% among those taking and not taking TDF, which also were significantly higher than age- and sex-matched HIV-negative individuals (1%).[32] As low-cost renal monitoring is widely available in the region, it is usually a standard component of HIV treatment monitoring for children and adolescents with PHIV.

Mental health

Mental health disorders, including psychiatric disorders, psychological distress, and emotional and behavioral problems, are a prevalent but neglected comorbidity among children and adolescents with PHIV in LMICs due to the lack of validated and culturally appropriate screening tools, limited awareness among health care providers, and an absence of adequate infrastructure and experienced providers to manage mental health disorders.[33] Chronic neuroinflammation, stress-induced neuroendocrine changes, and abnormal neurotransmitter signaling combined with side effects of antiretroviral medications, stigma and discrimination associated with HIV, and inadequate social support contribute to poor mental health among children and adolescents.[34,35] Importantly, mental health disorders can influence every step of the HIV care continuum, resulting in suboptimal adherence to ART, rapid disease progression, and increased morbidity and mortality.[35–37]

A previous prospective cohort study demonstrated that 21% of Thai children and adolescents with HIV had at least one mental health problem at the screening visit, which included depressive symptoms in 11%, anxiety symptoms in 7%, and lifetime suicidal ideation and/or attempted suicide in 11%.[38] Determinants of abnormal screening were younger age and living in urban areas. Notably, 61% of children and adolescents with an abnormal mental health screening had a mental health disorder confirmed by a psychiatrist at follow-up (eg, adjustment disorders, major depression, anxiety disorders).[38] A recent cross-sectional study among Thai children and adolescents with HIV (60% with PHIV) using a cross-culturally validated Thai version of the Columbia-Suicide Severity Rating Scale found that 29% reported lifetime suicidal ideation and 11% had previously attempted suicide.[39] As most children and adolescents with mental health disorders are not able to access specialized mental health services,[40] one key strategy is to integrate mental health screening and referral systems into primary HIV care. This strategy will likely be the only way to diagnose and treat mental health disorders among children and adolescents with HIV in LMICs in Asia.[41,42]

Coinfections

Although the scale-up of early diagnosis and ART initiation for children and adolescents with PHIV has reduced the incidence of opportunistic infections in many contexts in Asia, there are others where late diagnosis and associated poor clinical outcomes continue to occur (eg, Indonesia, Philippines). In addition, there remain HIV-associated coinfections that continue to present management challenges for adolescents with PHIV across LMICs, such as tuberculosis (TB) and hepatitis B.[43,44]

Tuberculosis

The WHO South-East Asia Region bears the highest burden of TB in the world. In 2022, an estimated 4.9 million people of all ages in this region had TB, of whom 628,000 (13%) were children and young adolescents age 0 to 14 years and 2% were among individuals living with HIV.[45] With the high TB incidence, children and adolescents with HIV remain at greater risk for TB even if they have stable CD4 counts and viral suppression.[43] The incidence of pulmonary TB within the first 2 years of ART initiation in the authors' regional cohort declined from 1.7 per 100 person-years between 2011 and 2013 to 1.3 between 2014 and 2016 and to 1.0 between 2017 and 2020 as HIV diagnostic testing coverage improved.[7] The elevated TB risk among children and adolescents with PHIV underscores the need to rapidly identify those at risk for TB as well as for widespread implementation of TB preventive treatment in this population.

Hepatitis B

The burden of chronic hepatitis B infection among Asian children and adolescents PHIV is not well described due to a lack of routine screening and surveillance. A cross-sectional study in the TREAT Asia network demonstrated a 5% prevalence of hepatitis B coinfection among children and adolescents with HIV.[46] Nevertheless, given the elevated risk of liver-related complications among those with HIV and hepatitis B virus coinfection, it is essential that infants with PHIV are vaccinated against hepatitis B (preferably starting with a birth dose) and older children have serologic screening for hepatitis B (eg, hepatitis B surface antigen, hepatitis B surface antibody [anti-HBs], hepatitis B core antibody) when vaccination status is unknown. Notably, vaccine-elicited immune responses could be suboptimal among those with history of severe immune deficiency after vaccination with a 3-dose primary series.[46] A previous study in the TREAT Asia network among children and adolescents with a history of completing the three-dose primary hepatitis B vaccination series during childhood showed that only 17% exhibited seroprotection against hepatitis B (anti-HBs >10 mIU/mL). Among those who were revaccinated after immune reconstitution, this frequency increased to 24% among those who had less than or equal to two additional doses and to 56% among those who had three doses.[46]

Transition to Adult Human Immunodeficiency Virus Care

In many Asian contexts, HIV care for children is initially provided in pediatric-specific clinics. Those who survive to young adulthood are then transitioned to adult HIV providers, sometimes in different health care facilities. Youth with PHIV who transitioned from pediatric sites in the TREAT Asia regional cohort through 2016 had been a median 5.5 years of age when they were diagnosed and 18 years at transition.[47] Although 85% were virally suppressed, 40% were on at least their second combination ART regimen. These findings led to a follow-up study of a cohort of 93 young adults (56% female) from Malaysia, Thailand, and Vietnam.[48] At 96 weeks of follow-up, they had been on ART for a median duration of 14 years, with 43% on second-line or subsequent regimens.[49] Self-reported ART adherence ranged from 97% to 100%, and viral suppression was 77%, which was higher than reports from some other cohorts and thought to be related in part to ongoing social support they were receiving from pediatric HIV clinics and peer groups. By this time, 65% were employed, 39% reported recent alcohol use, and 23% screened positive for moderate depression or reported suicidal ideation. In addition, 49% had been sexually active, and 53% of women and 36% of men intended to have children.

As young women with PHIV age, they have raised questions around their fertility and HIV risks to their infants. A TREAT Asia study is the only one reporting on these reproductive health outcomes in the region over time.[50] The authors analyzed data from 52 pregnancies in young women in Thailand and Vietnam that occurred between 2013 and 2018, representing an incidence in the cohort of 2.5 per 100 person-years (95% confidence interval: 1.9–3.3). Seventy-nine percent of the pregnancies they documented occurred among those between 15 and 19 years of age, and 51% were with an HIV-positive male partner. Overall, 90% resulted in live births and 10% in abortions (n = 4/5 elective). At delivery, 77% of mothers had HIV viral loads less than 400 copies/mL. Among the infants, 29% were low birth weight (<2500 gm), and one infant was diagnosed with HIV.

SUMMARY

As prevention of vertical transmission has improved in Asia, the numbers of infants with newly acquired HIV have decreased, whereas numbers of adolescents and young adults with PHIV have increased. In the TREAT Asia cohort, the median age of those in active follow-up is now almost 14 years, with less than 10% younger than 5 years. Network research has shown that those with PHIV are a unique population who experience the physical impacts of chronic coinfections and comorbidities, as well as the social and mental consequences of growing up with HIV over a lifetime. Translating these data into clinical practice across the region will help improve their ability to thrive as adults.

Best Practices

What is the current practice for managing pediatric HIV in the Asia region?

Coverage of pediatric diagnosis and treatment substantially varies across the region, with countries like Indonesia and the Philippines falling behind countries such as Malaysia and Thailand. In contexts where children with perinatally acquired HIV are in specialized pediatric HIV clinics, older adolescents are being transitioned to adult HIV care with inconsistent levels of preparation.

What changes in current practice are likely to improve outcomes?

Improvements in local public health infrastructure and investment are needed to address the heterogeneity of pediatric HIV prevention, testing, and treatment coverage between countries. On an individual level, adolescents and young adults with perinatally acquired HIV need access to comprehensive care that supports lifelong treatment adherence and addresses emerging comorbidities and sexual and reproductive health.

Major Recommendations

In Asia-Pacific countries that continue to struggle to achieve global targets for prevention of vertical transmission, efforts should focus on supporting care for pregnant women living with HIV and their infants, including early diagnosis. For older children, adolescents, and young adults with perinatally acquired HIV, greater attention is needed to prevent, screen, diagnose, and treat comorbidities (eg, mental health disorders). In addition, preparations for transition to adult HIV care should start in early adolescence to improve retention in care.

Bibliographic Sources

- UNAIDS. AIDSinfo. https://aidsinfo.unaids.org/
- World Health Organization. Consolidated guidelines on HIV prevention, testing, treatment, service delivery and monitoring: recommendations for a public health approach. Geneva: World Health Organization, 2021. Accessed February 7, 2024. https://www.who.int/publications/i/item/9789240031593
- Sohn AH, Singtoroj T, Chokephaibulkit K, et al. Long-Term Post-Transition Outcomes of Adolescents and Young Adults Living With Perinatally and Non-perinatally Acquired HIV in Southeast Asia. J Adolesc Health. Mar 2023;72(3):471-479. doi:10.1016/j.jadohealth.2022.10.021

ACKNOWLEDGMENTS

The authors thank Azar Kariminia for her assistance providing data from the TREAT Asia Pediatric HIV Observational Database.

DISCLOSURE

A. H. Sohn receives program funding to her institution from ViiV Healthcare, United States and United Kingdom. The other authors have nothing to disclose.

REFERENCES

1. UNAIDS. AIDSinfo. Available at: https://aidsinfo.unaids.org/. Accessed February 7, 2024.
2. The well project. Lifetime survivors of HIV. Available at: https://www.thewellproject.org/hiv-information/lifetime-survivors-hiv. Accessed February 7, 2024.
3. Shaffer N, Chuachoowong R, Mock PA, et al. Short-course zidovudine for perinatal HIV-1 transmission in Bangkok, Thailand: a randomised controlled trial. Bangkok collaborative perinatal HIV transmission study group. Lancet 1999; 353(9155):773–80.
4. Bedri A, Gudetta B, Isehak A, et al. Extended-dose nevirapine to 6 weeks of age for infants to prevent HIV transmission via breastfeeding in Ethiopia, India, and Uganda: an analysis of three randomised controlled trials. Lancet 2008; 372(9635):300–13.
5. Kariminia A, Chokephaibulkit K, Pang J, et al. Cohort profile: the TREAT Asia pediatric HIV observational database. Int J Epidemiol 2011;40(1):15–24.
6. Kassanjee R, Johnson LF, Zaniewski E, et al. Global HIV mortality trends among children on antiretroviral treatment corrected for under-reported deaths: an updated analysis of the International epidemiology Databases to Evaluate AIDS collaboration. J Int AIDS Soc 2021;24 Suppl 5(Suppl 5):e25780.
7. Sornillo JB, Ditangco R, Kinikar A, et al. The changing characteristics of a cohort of children and adolescents living with HIV at antiretroviral therapy initiation in Asia. PLoS One 2023;18(9):e0291523.
8. Sohn AH, Lumbiganon P, Kurniati N, et al. Determining standardized causes of death of infants, children, and adolescents living with HIV in Asia. AIDS 2020; 34(10):1527–37.
9. Bartlett AW, Sudjaritruk T, Mohamed TJ, et al. Identification, management, and outcomes of combination antiretroviral treatment failure in adolescents with perinatal human immunodeficiency virus infection in Asia. Clin Infect Dis 2021;73(7): e1919–26.
10. Sudjaritruk T, Aurpibul L, Ly PS, et al. Incidence of postsuppression virologic rebound in perinatally HIV-infected asian adolescents on stable combination antiretroviral therapy. J Adolesc Health 2017;61(1):91–8.
11. Sudjaritruk T, Teeraananchai S, Kariminia A, et al. Impact of low-level viraemia on virological failure among Asian children with perinatally acquired HIV on first-line combination antiretroviral treatment: a multicentre, retrospective cohort study. J Int AIDS Soc 2020;23(7):e25550.
12. Lecher S, Williams J, Fonjungo PN, et al. Progress with scale-up of HIV viral load monitoring - seven sub-saharan african countries, january 2015-june 2016. MMWR Morb Mortal Wkly Rep 2016;65(47):1332–5.
13. Jamal Mohamed T, Teeraananchai S, Kerr S, et al. Short communication: impact of viral load use on treatment switch in perinatally HIV-infected children in Asia. AIDS Res Hum Retrovir 2017;33(3):230–3.
14. Sudjaritruk T, Boettiger DC, Nguyen LV, et al. Impact of the frequency of plasma viral load monitoring on treatment outcomes among children with perinatally acquired HIV. J Int AIDS Soc 2019;22(6):e25312.
15. Prasitsuebsai W, Teeraananchai S, Singtoroj T, et al. Treatment outcomes and resistance patterns of children and adolescents on second-line antiretroviral therapy in Asia. J Acquir Immune Defic Syndr 2016;72(4):380–6.

16. Kosalaraksa P, Boettiger DC, Bunupuradah T, et al. Low risk of CD4 decline after immune recovery in human immunodeficiency virus-infected children with viral suppression. J Pediatric Infect Dis Soc 2017;6(2):173–7.
17. Ross JL, Teeraananchai S, Lumbiganon P, et al. A longitudinal study of behavioral risk, adherence, and virologic control in adolescents living with HIV in Asia. J Acquir Immune Defic Syndr 2019;81(2):e28–38.
18. Sudjaritruk T, Puthanakit T. Adverse bone health among children and adolescents growing up with HIV. J Virus Erad 2015;1(3):159–67.
19. Sudjaritruk T, Bunupuradah T, Aurpibul L, et al. Adverse bone health and abnormal bone turnover among perinatally HIV-infected Asian adolescents with virological suppression. HIV Med 2017;18(4):235–44.
20. Sudjaritruk T, Bunupuradah T, Aurpibul L, et al. Hypovitaminosis D and hyperparathyroidism: effects on bone turnover and bone mineral density among perinatally HIV-infected adolescents. AIDS 2016;30(7):1059–67.
21. Sudjaritruk T, Bunupuradah T, Aurpibul L, et al. Impact of vitamin D and calcium supplementation on bone mineral density and bone metabolism among Thai adolescents with perinatally acquired human immunodeficiency virus (HIV) infection: a randomized clinical trial. Clin Infect Dis 2021;73(9):1555–64.
22. Aurpibul L, Bunupuradah T, Sophan S, et al. Prevalence and incidence of liver dysfunction and assessment of biomarkers of liver disease in HIV-infected Asian children. Pediatr Infect Dis J 2015;34(6):e153–8.
23. Kalligeros M, Vassilopoulos A, Shehadeh F, et al. Prevalence and characteristics of nonalcoholic fatty liver disease and fibrosis in people living with HIV monoinfection: a systematic review and meta-analysis. Clin Gastroenterol Hepatol 2023;21(7):1708–22.
24. Sudjaritruk T, Bunupuradah T, Aurpibul L, et al. Nonalcoholic fatty liver disease and hepatic fibrosis among perinatally HIV-monoinfected Asian adolescents receiving antiretroviral therapy. PLoS One 2019;14(12):e0226375.
25. Idris NS, Grobbee DE, Burgner D, et al. Cardiovascular manifestations of HIV infection in children. Eur J Prev Cardiol 2015;22(11):1452–61.
26. Chanthong P, Lapphra K, Saihongthong S, et al. Echocardiography and carotid intima-media thickness among asymptomatic HIV-infected adolescents in Thailand. AIDS 2014;28(14):2071–9.
27. Doobay AV, Anand SS. Sensitivity and specificity of the ankle-brachial index to predict future cardiovascular outcomes: a systematic review. Arterioscler Thromb Vasc Biol 2005;25(7):1463–9.
28. Del Conde I, Benenati JF. Noninvasive testing in peripheral arterial disease. Interv Cardiol Clin 2014;3(4):469–78.
29. Sudjaritruk T, Aurpibul L, Anugulreungkit SCT, et al. Prevalence and associated factors of asymptomatic peripheral arterial disease among perinatally HIV-infected Thai adolescents. Paris, France: Presented at: the 9th international workshop on HIV pediatrics; 2017.
30. Bhimma R, Purswani MU, Kala U. Kidney disease in children and adolescents with perinatal HIV-1 infection. J Int AIDS Soc 2013;16(1):18596.
31. Sudjaritruk T, Kanjanavanit S, Aurpibul L, et al. Prevalence of glomerular dysfunction among perinatally HIV-infected Thai adolescents. Boston, United States of America: Presented at: the 25th conference on retroviruses and opportunistic infections; 2018.
32. Sudjaritruk T, Kanjanavanit S, Aurpibul L, et al. Prevalence and associated factors of proximal renal tubular dysfunction among perinatally HIV-infected Thai

adolescents. Amsterdam, The Netherlands: presented at: The 22nd International AIDS Conference; 2018.

33. Woollett N, Cluver L, Bandeira M, et al. Identifying risks for mental health problems in HIV positive adolescents accessing HIV treatment in Johannesburg. J Child Adolesc Ment Health 2017;29(1):11–26.
34. Lee SJ, Detels R, Rotheram-Borus MJ, et al. The effect of social support on mental and behavioral outcomes among adolescents with parents with HIV/AIDS. Am J Public Health 2007;97(10):1820–6.
35. Vreeman RC, McCoy BM, Lee S. Mental health challenges among adolescents living with HIV. J Int AIDS Soc 2017;20(Suppl 3):21497.
36. Kacanek D, Angelidou K, Williams PL, et al. Psychiatric symptoms and antiretroviral nonadherence in US youth with perinatal HIV: a longitudinal study. AIDS 2015;29(10):1227–37.
37. Lowenthal ED, Bakeera-Kitaka S, Marukutira T, et al. Perinatally acquired HIV infection in adolescents from sub-Saharan Africa: a review of emerging challenges. Lancet Infect Dis 2014;14(7):627–39.
38. Sudjaritruk T, Aurpibul L, Songtaweesin WN, et al. Integration of mental health services into HIV healthcare facilities among Thai adolescents and young adults living with HIV. J Int AIDS Soc 2021;24(2):e25668.
39. Sudjaritruk T, Mueangmo O, Saheng J, et al. Suicidal behaviors among Thai adolescents and young adults living with HIV. Brisbane, Australia: Presented at: the 12th IAS conference on HIV science; 2023.
40. Ngui EM, Khasakhala L, Ndetei D, et al. Mental disorders, health inequalities and ethics: a global perspective. Int Rev Psychiatry 2010;22(3):235–44.
41. Kaaya S, Eustache E, Lapidos-Salaiz I, et al. Grand challenges: improving HIV treatment outcomes by integrating interventions for co-morbid mental illness. PLoS Med 2013;10(5):e1001447.
42. Chuah FLH, Haldane VE, Cervero-Liceras F, et al. Interventions and approaches to integrating HIV and mental health services: a systematic review. Health Policy Plan 2017;32(suppl_4):iv27–47.
43. Kay AW, Rabie H, Maleche-Obimbo E, et al. HIV-associated tuberculosis in children and adolescents: evolving epidemiology, screening, prevention and management strategies. Pathogens 2021;11(1). https://doi.org/10.3390/pathogens11010033.
44. Kim HN. Chronic hepatitis B and HIV coinfection: a continuing challenge in the era of antiretroviral therapy. Curr Hepatol Rep 2020;19(4):345–53.
45. World Health Organization. Global tuberculosis report. 2023. Available at: https://www.who.int/teams/global-tuberculosis-programme/tb-reports/global-tuberculosis-report-2023. Accessed February 7, 2024.
46. Aurpibul L, Kariminia A, Vibol U, et al. Seroprevalence of hepatitis B among HIV-infected children and adolescents receiving antiretroviral therapy in the TREAT Asia pediatric HIV observational database. Pediatr Infect Dis J 2018;37(8):788–93.
47. Bartlett AW, Truong KH, Songtaweesin WN, et al. Characteristics, mortality and outcomes at transition for adolescents with perinatal HIV infection in Asia. AIDS 2018;32(12):1689–97.
48. Sohn AH, Chokephaibulkit K, Lumbiganon P, et al. Peritransition outcomes of southeast asian adolescents and young adults with HIV transferring from pediatric to adult care. J Adolesc Health 2020;66(1):92–9.

49. Sohn AH, Singtoroj T, Chokephaibulkit K, et al. Long-term post-transition outcomes of adolescents and young adults living with perinatally and non-perinatally acquired HIV in Southeast Asia. J Adolesc Health 2023;72(3):471–9.
50. Lumbiganon P, Kariminia A, Anugulruengkitt S, et al. Pregnancy and birth outcomes among young women living with perinatally acquired HIV in Thailand and Vietnam. AIDS Care 2023;35(6):818–23.

Penta Network: State-of-the-Art Research in Pediatric Human Immunodeficiency Virus

Pablo Rojo, PhD[a,*], Cinta Moraleda, PhD[b], Carlo Giaquinto, PhD[c]

KEYWORDS

• Perinatal HIV • Penta • HIV cure • Pediatric advanced HIV disease

KEY POINTS

- Commitment to Global Health: The Penta Network's research and partnerships aim to develop effective interventions and strategies not only to improve treatment and care for children living with human immunodeficiency virus (HIV) but also to enhance the overall management of pediatric infectious diseases worldwide.
- Innovative Treatment Research: The ODYSSEY trial demonstrated that dolutegravir-based antiretroviral therapy ART is superior to standard treatments in children and adolescents, leading to the inclusion of dolutegravir in pediatric HIV treatment guidelines and ensuring its availability in low- and middle-income countries.
- Focus on Cure and Remission: The Penta-led Early-treated Perinatally HIV-infected Individuals: Improving Children's Actual Life with Novel Immunotherapeutic Strategies consortium was established to influence early treatment strategies for HIV in children, focusing on reducing viral reservoirs and exploring potential pathways to remission through innovative approaches such as broadly neutralizing antibodies.
- Addressing Advanced HIV Disease: The Penta Network launched the EMPIRICAL trial to improve treatment outcomes for children with advanced HIV disease, particularly focusing on severe pneumonia, highlighting significant gaps in HIV diagnosis and the need for tailored treatment strategies in pediatric populations.

INTRODUCTION

The Penta Network emerged as a collaborative effort between European pediatric human immunodeficiency virus (HIV) centers in a time when there was no antiretroviral treatment (ART) available for children. Its primary focus was conducting independent clinical trials and observational studies to gather evidence to support the treatment of

[a] Department of Pediatrics, Pediatric Infectious Diseases Unit, Universidad Complutense, Avenida Puerta de Hierro, Madrid 28040, Spain; [b] Department of Pediatrics, Pediatric Infectious Diseases Unit, Hospital 12 de Octubre, Av. de Córdoba, s/n, Madrid, Spain; [c] Department of Pediatrics. University of Padova, Via Citolo da Perugia 126, Padova (PD) 35137, Italy
* Corresponding author.
E-mail address: projo01@ucm.es

Clin Perinatol 51 (2024) 925–933
https://doi.org/10.1016/j.clp.2024.08.013 perinatology.theclinics.com

children with HIV. After a few years, the Penta Network expanded its activities and clinical trials to countries with a significant number of children living with HIV (CLHIV) like Uganda, South Africa, Zimbabwe, Thailand, Argentina, and Brazil. More recently, Penta expanded its collaboration to areas affected by many years of social conflict like Mozambique and Mali, thereby supporting research and training where it is most needed. Later, recognizing the neglect of other childhood infections, the Penta Network broadened research endeavors (both clinical and basic) to encompass a wider range of pediatric infectious diseases. The Penta Network has become a worldwide organization with a vision to be at the forefront of clinical science that improves prevention, diagnosis, and treatment of infections in children.

Our aim in this article is to highlight the successes and also the ongoing trials and projects that the Penta Network is leading related to pediatric HIV. We have focused on 3 areas that we think the Penta Network has led state-of-the-art research and are or could be life-changing for CLHIV, research on pediatric ART treatment, and the contrasting topics of research on pediatric cure and remission and research on pediatric advanced HIV disease.

Pediatric Antiretroviral Treatment

Until a few years ago, we had very few good options of ART for children, especially for infants and young children and appropriate for low- and middle-income countries (LMICs). Nevirapine (NVP), efavirenz (EFV), and lopinavir/ritonavir (LPV/r) were the best main drugs available with strong data on good efficacy and safety results in children but had several drawbacks. NVP and EFV, both non-nucleoside reverse transcriptase inhibitors (NNRTIs), were initially highly effective but had a low genetic barrier for resistance, and their wide use in many sub-Saharan African countries increased the proportion of patients with resistant mutations to NNRTIs to over 10% by 2017.[1] LPV/r, a high genetic barrier protease inhibitor, is highly effective but needs to be given twice daily, and it was very problematic to produce a child-friendly formulation.

Dolutegravir (DTG), a second-generation HIV integrase strand-transfer inhibitor (INSTI), received the Food and Drug Administration (FDA) approval for adults in 2013. It offers advantages over first-generation INSTIs, including unboosted daily dosing, limited cross-resistance with raltegravir and elvitegravir, and a high barrier to resistance. Clinical trials have demonstrated its efficacy in both treatment-naïve and treatment-experienced adults.[2] DTG has outperformed other drugs, including protease inhibitors, in treatment-naïve patients and also in treatment-experienced adults.

For children, however, data on DTG and other licensed drugs and treatment strategies have been falling behind until recent years.

Penta Network research on pediatric antiretroviral therapy

Penta decided to design a trial, the ODYSSEY trial, also known as Penta 20, to compare the pharmacokinetics, efficacy, and safety of DTG-based ART with those of standard of care in children and adolescents who were starting first- or second-line ART in resource-limited and well-resourced settings.[3] The study took place in Germany, Spain, South Africa, Portugal, Thailand, Uganda, the United Kingdom, and Zimbabwe and enrolled 707 children. The trial showed that in children and adolescents with HIV-1 infection who were starting first- or second-line treatment, DTG-based ART was superior to the standard of care.[4] In a cohort of children weighing less than 14 kg, these results were also confirmed for the younger children and infants.[5] The odyssey trial included a strong pharmacokinetics component that allowed us to study different doses and formulations across all weight bands down to 3 kg, as well as the coadministration of DTG with rifampicin.[6] It showed as well that it was safe to use the DTG adult 50 mg formulation for children starting from 20 kg and that a child-friendly strawberry-flavored dispersible tablet had a great pharmacokinetic profile for children weighing between 3 and 20 kg.[7]

The evidence provided by the ODYSSEY trial was key to the approval of DTG in children by the FDA and the European Medicines Agency for its use in the United States and in Europe and the inclusion in the World Health Organization (WHO) ART Guidelines, but very important as well was the collaboration between many stakeholders to make the pediatric formulation available for LMICs. The Penta and the International Maternal Pediatric Adolescent AIDS Clinical Trials networks strongly collaborated with ViiV as the originator and owner of DTG, UNITAID, and Clinton health access initiative (CHAI) and several generic companies to engage in a quick transference of data, knowledge, and technical expertise to make pediatric DTG available around the world.

Penta is also running a trial in children and adolescents living with HIV with a new treatment strategy: The *D3 trial* (Penta 21). This study aims to find out whether treating children and young people living with HIV with 2 antiHIV medicines, DTG and lamivudine (3 TC), is safe and equally effective as the 3-medicine antiHIV treatments currently used in routine practice.[8] The trial that completed recruitment and is currently ongoing has included 370 children and young people from South Africa, Spain, Thailand, Uganda, and the United Kingdom. The focus is on optimizing treatment safety, adherence, and quality of life while maintaining virological suppression. Penta has supported the creation of a D3 youth trial board, where a group of young people living with HIV, actively participated in the trial in several activities. One of the main activities was that they collaborated with a designer to create a fun, engaging poster for their peers participating in the trial.

Another important trial sponsored by Penta is the ongoing SHIELD trial (Penta 22). The SHIELD trial focuses on evaluating the safety, pharmacokinetics, and antiviral activity of fostemsavir in children and adolescents living with HIV. These participants have developed resistance to 2 or more ART classes. Specifically, SHIELD investigates the use of fostemsavir in combination with optimized background ART. The trial aims to provide alternative treatment options for multi-drug-resistant pediatric patients who have limited therapeutic choices because of previous treatment failures and resistance mutations. The trial is recruiting children in South Africa and the United States of America and planning to open soon in Brazil.

Thanks to the great rollout of DTG, both in adult and pediatric formulations, around the world there has been a period of less resistant mutations to first-line or second-line ART all over the world, but new surveys are showing that although DTG has a high genetic barrier to resistance and great virological efficacy overall, recent real-world data show increasing emergence of resistance to DTG compared to what was seen in previous randomized clinical trials. The 2024 WHO brief report on HIV drug resistance shows that amongst the surveys reported, levels of DTG resistance ranged from 3.9% to 8.6%, with levels as high as 19.6% observed among highly treatment-experienced people who transitioned to a DTG-containing ART while having high HIV viral loads.[9] Children and adolescents are within the groups with higher levels of DTG resistance seen. Therefore, the SHIELD trial, aiming to enroll children with several resistance mutations and with few alternative options, is going to be very important to make fostemsavir approved and available for those children.

With the *UNIVERSAL project*, Penta has continued to focus on improving treatments and formulations for ART for CLHIV, especially focusing on LMIC. UNIVERSAL is a European–African project to evaluate and register 2 new antiretroviral formulations for infants and children newly diagnosed with HIV initiating ART and for children failing first-line therapy who need to switch to a new treatment regimen. These 2 new formulations contain approved drugs already used in adult and pediatric care in high-income settings: DTG combined with emtricitabine/tenofovir alafenamide and darunavir/ritonavir. The project will also monitor the long-term efficacy and safety of other pediatric ART formulations. This will help to fully address the main treatment gaps in the access of the best treatments to treat HIV in children living in sub-Saharan Africa, with a view to expand their availability also in South America and Asia.

Pediatric Human Immunodeficiency Virus Cure and Remission

Pediatric HIV cure and remission research have made significant strides in recent years, although challenges persist. Efforts to achieve a cure or sustained remission in CLHIV face unique obstacles compared with the adult population. The cornerstone of pediatric HIV management remains lifelong ART because of the persistence of latent viral reservoirs and the potential for viral rebound if treatment is interrupted.

Recent broadly neutralizing antibodies (bNAbs) treatment studies in adults indicate that bNAbs may be associated with a reduction in viral reservoirs, providing optimism that these agents may provide a pathway toward posttreatment control that rarely occurs with small-molecule ART.

Penta research on pediatric human immunodeficiency virus cure and remission

Penta led the creation of the *EPIICAL consortium* to work toward establishing new, scientific efforts on the early treatment of HIV to improve the lives of children and ultimately lead to the remission of HIV in children.[10] The main focus of the consortium was the development of a predictive platform to inform treatment strategies that would lead to HIV remission.[11]

EPIICAL succeeded in designing and conducting studies on pediatric HIV, which led to the development of different, well-established cohorts of CLHIV in Europe and Africa. The clinical cohorts were established with the intention to evaluate strategies to optimize the management of children with perinatal HIV. During the first phase of the project, the *Child and Adolescent Reservoir Measurements on early suppressive ART (CARMA) study* provided important information about the immunologic and virologic features of early-treated children and adolescents with long-term viral control. These data highlighted the impact of early-infant treatment on limiting the reservoir size after a decade of suppressive therapy.[12] Moreover, in this cohort it was demonstrated that the early initiation of ART preserves the functionality of the immune system.[13] The precious and informative data produced by the CARMA study inspired a new study, *CARMA Global*. CARMA Global has recruited children 7 years and older living with HIV from LMIC, who started ART in the first 3 months of life and remained in care while on ART.

In parallel, at this stage the consortium also established a large cohort of infants treated before 3 months of age in limited-resource settings to monitor the clinical, virologic, and immunologic features. These children were enrolled in *Early AntiRetroviral Treatment in children with HIV (EARTH) study* taking place in South Africa, Mozambique, and Mali, with the aim of providing data on the characteristics associated with the establishment of HIV reservoirs and identifying novel immunologic and virologic endpoints. Initial results from the EARTH study have shown that despite early ART, mortality remains high in infants living with HIV.[14]

EPIICAL succeeded in highlighting the strong possibility that early ART initiation plays a significant role in suppressing HIV. The high-quality data generated by the consortium are vital for improving the current understanding of HIV remission while paving the way to unravel the mechanisms behind viral remission. As there is currently no cure for HIV, we hope that the knowledge we generate will provide a clear picture of the evolution of HIV in early-treated children and that will guide a new therapeutic intervention. EPIICAL's success led to the development of the second phase of the project: Novel strategies to induce long-term viral remission in the EARTH study. One of the most promising tools is the use of bNAbs against HIV in CLHIV; therefore, the *ENABLE trial* has been developed to study the safety, pharmacokinetics, reduction in reservoir size, and increase in HIV-specific immune responses.[15]

Pediatric Advanced Human Immunodeficiency Virus Disease

Advanced HIV disease (AHD) in children poses a significant challenge to global public health. Despite advancements in ART and prevention strategies, children with AHD continue to experience high morbidity and mortality rates, especially in resource-limited settings. In 2022, children accounted for only 2% of all people living with HIV but represented 12% of all AIDS-related deaths.[16]

Any child younger than 5 years is considered to have AHD because younger children have an increased risk of disease progression and mortality regardless of clinical and immune conditions.[17] Many of these CLHIV present with AHD at diagnosis because of delayed testing. AHD is defined as WHO stage 3 or 4 or as a CD4 cell count below 200 cells/^{mm3} for children aged 5 years or older.

The major causes of morbidity and mortality related to AHD in children are different from adults and adolescents and include pneumonia (including *Pneumocystis jirovecii* pneumonia), tuberculosis, bloodstream infections, and diarrheal disease, all usually associated with severe acute malnutrition.[18] Therefore, AHD needs to be addressed in the context of the unique features of this population. In addition, for adolescents living with HIV, adult-type opportunistic infections also occur, including cryptococcal meningitis.[19]

The WHO recommends a specific package of care for people with AHD focused on screening, prevention, and rapid and adherent ART.[20] Evidence on managing AHD in children is however limited, particularly for those below 5 years old. No randomized controlled trials have investigated comprehensive intervention packages for this age group; as such, the WHO guidelines for children with AHD are primarily based on expert opinion.[21]

Thus, there are several gaps to address regarding children with AHD, such as issues in diagnosis, prevention, and treatment. Lack of available diagnostic tests or drug interactions are some examples. Opportunistic infections further exacerbate the health problems faced by CLHIV. The underdiagnosis or limited understanding of the further implications complicates the situation. Cytomegalovirus (CMV) coinfection contributes to the risk of death in people living with HIV, even during ART, and research on CMV dynamics to propose preventive approaches or treatments is needed for children.[22] Other diseases are not well studied, like histoplasmosis, which is often misdiagnosed as tuberculosis and neglected in African children.[23]

Penta research on pediatric advanced human immunodeficiency virus disease

The Penta Network is participating in the EMPIRICAL trial, focused on children with AHD. It is an ongoing clinical study focused on improving the treatment for severe pneumonia, which is the main cause of death in infants living with HIV. EMPIRICAL is a randomized controlled clinical trial taking place in 6 sub-Saharan African countries (Mozambique, Uganda, Zimbabwe, Zambia, Malawi, and Cote d'Ivoire) to assess the impact on mortality of empirical treatment against tuberculosis and/or CMV, in addition to current standard treatment for bacterial pathogens and *P jirovecii*, in infants hospitalized with severe HIV-associated pneumonia.[24]

The EMPIRICAL rationale is based on an autopsy study that showed that although bacteria were the most common underlying etiology (47%) among children with HIV who succumbed to respiratory tract infections, other important agents were tuberculosis (15%), CMV (9%), and *P jirovecii* (9%).[25] Empirical treatment with cotrimoxazole and steroids to treat *P jirovecii* pneumonia in infants with HIV and severe pneumonia is well established. However, even with appropriate treatment, in-hospital mortality of suspected *P jirovecii* pneumonia remains high.[26] Untreated CMV and tuberculosis are some of the proposed causes of this mortality.[27] However, CMV disease is neglected and there are no pragmatic CMV–pneumonia diagnostic criteria or treatment protocols, and tuberculosis continues to be underdiagnosed in children. EMPIRICAL results are expected in mid-2025. If the clinical trial confirms that the proposed empirical treatments decrease the mortality in CLHIV and severe pneumonia, it will have an important impact on public health, and it might change the AHD guidelines in children.

Although the EMPIRICAL trial has not finished, there are several learning points already noted. The mortality rate in the trial so far has been painfully high (44%) with a very impressive and high early mortality in the first days of hospitalization (57% of the total deaths). EMPIRICAL researchers have been surprised by an unbearable high postdischarge mortality (43% of the total deaths) even when those children have survived the first severe pneumonia and have started ART.[28] Urgent measures beyond EMPIRICAL are needed to counteract this loss of lives. Based on the EMPIRICAL trial data, the most common immediate cause of death during the first hospitalization was pneumonia, but sepsis was most prevalent among those dying post discharge.[29] In over 15% of cases, the cause of death could not be determined, particularly among children who died post discharge outside of a health care facility. Future analyses using minimally invasive autopsies will provide further insights into these findings.

Important gaps in HIV diagnosis in children with AHD have been identified. More than 70% of children admitted with severe pneumonia and AHD arrived at the hospital without an earlier HIV diagnosis during the EMPIRICAL trial implementation. Incident HIV in breastfeeding women is common, but early infant HIV diagnosis has not been fully implemented in all of the EMPIRICAL countries. Repeat HIV testing and counseling in the context of severe infant illness requiring hospitalization is a crucial first step to identify exposed infants, many of whom already have HIV. Point-of-care nucleic acid testing in hospitals is an important tool to supply deficiencies in the outpatient diagnosis where mother–baby pairs are frequently lost to follow-up or signs/symptoms that should prompt repeat virologic testing are missed.

An EMPIRICAL pharmacokinetic sub-study filled in an urgent need identified by the WHO showing that twice-daily dosing of DTG in infants receiving rifampicin resulted in adequate DTG exposure, supporting this treatment approach for infants with HIV–tuberculosis coinfection, which is a major achievement for CLHIV with AHD.[30] However, in infants with AHD and severe pneumonia, the tuberculosis treatment drug concentrations were low compared with the reference values for adults, supporting the need for studies on increased doses of first-line tuberculosis drugs in infants.[31]

Building on the lessons learned from EMPIRICAL, the Penta Network continues to promote research focused on AHD in children, and new research projects have been planned and launched in 2024. SUPPORT (Supporting the next generation of African researchers on preventing HIV pediatric mortality through a training network) is a

European Union–granted project that aims, through a full training program of young researchers, to develop a clinical study to better understand the causes of postdischarge mortality in CLHIV. Studies reporting postdischarge mortality showed that HIV infection, malnutrition status, and young age are the main predictors of postdischarge mortality, but information about the predictors of death specifically in the population of CLHIV is still missing.[32] Identification of the more vulnerable CLHIV among those with AHD appears to be essential to designing more targeted interventions to decrease mortality in this population.

SUPPORT is based on a multidisciplinary approach that involves clinicians, microbiologists, epidemiologists, statisticians, artificial intelligence experts, pharmacologists, and social science researchers, among others, to evaluate different diagnostic treatment tools that can have a real impact on mortality in children with AHD, taking into account the patient and his family, the community, and the environment. Some of the factors that will be evaluated include biomarkers of mortality, CMV viremia, colonization by multi-drug-resistant bacteria, prolonged respiratory virus infections, prolonged infections due to intestinal pathogens, and histoplasmosis, among others. These results will improve the management of children with AHD impacting clinical guidelines as well as morbidity and mortality.

The THRIVE project (Transforming advanced HIV disease caRe in LMICs through comprehensiVe and Equitable access), in which Penta joined the CHAI and African Community Advisory Board in a direct partnership with national governments and global partners, aims to dramatically reduce mortality among adults and CLHIV, by enabling global access to critical prevention, screening, and treatment commodities. This project centers local leadership and community-owned solutions to find and serve people living with AHD where they live. Penta is leading the pediatric aspect of THRIVE to generate replicable evidence on the implementation of the STOP AIDS guidance. Using mixed methods, the consortia will identify and overcome barriers to the implementation of the STOP AIDS package of care. It will allow the development of clear operational guidance for the STOP AIDS package of care to be disseminated to the Ministries of Health AHD programs, informing local guidance and supporting pediatric AHD strategy. THRIVE will develop this research in Mozambique focused on hospitalized children and in Uganda focused on the outpatient population. In consultation with health workers and communities, the design and implementation of innovative community-facility service delivery models will be implemented in health centers and the community in a rural area in Zimbabwe.

Effective implementation of existing and new interventions is crucial for combating AHD in children. The Penta Network focuses on implementation science to understand the best strategies for scaling up interventions, addressing barriers, and ensuring sustainable impact. In conclusion, the Penta Network has spearheaded crucial clinical trials and observational studies in recent years on pediatric HIV, including pediatric ART, HIV cure and remission, and pediatric AHD. The Penta Network is dedicated to furthering research in these areas and other pediatric infectious diseases that affect children around the world.

DISCLOSURE

The authors have nothing to disclose.

FUNDING

P. Rojo Participated in research projects funded by ViiV, also participated in Gilead and ViiV advisory boards.

REFERENCES

1. World Health Organization. HIV drug resistance report. Geneva: WHO; World Health Organization; 2017. Available at: www.who.int/hiv/pub/drugresistance/hivdr-report-2017/en.
2. Nickel K, Halfpenny NJA, Snedecor SJ, et al. Comparative efficacy, safety and durability of dolutegravir relative to common core agents in treatment-naïve patients infected with HIV-1: an update on a systematic review and network meta-analysis. BMC Infect Dis 2021;21:222.
3. Moore CL, Turkova A, Mujuru H, et al. ODYSSEY clinical trial design: a randomised global study to evaluate the efficacy and safety of dolutegravir-based antiretroviral therapy in HIV-positive children, with nested pharmacokinetic substudies to evaluate pragmatic WHO-weight-band based dolutegravir dosing. BMC Infect Dis 2021;21:5.
4. Turkova A, White E, Mujuru H, et al. Dolutegravir as first- or second-line treatment for HIV-1 infection in children. N Engl J Med 2021;385:2531–43.
5. Amuge P, Lugemwa A, Wynne B, et al. Once-daily dolutegravir-based antiretroviral therapy in infants and children living with HIV from age 4 weeks: results from the below 14 kg cohort in the randomised ODYSSEY trial. Lancet HIV 2022;9(9): E638–48.
6. Turkova A, Waalewijn H, Chan MK, et al. Dolutegravir twice-daily dosing in children with HIV-associated tuberculosis: a pharmacokinetic and safety study within the open-label, multicentre, randomised, non-inferiority ODYSSEY trial. Lancet HIV 2022;9(9):e627–37.
7. Waalewijn H, Chan MK, Bollen PD, et al. Dolutegravir dosing for children with HIV weighing less than 20 kg: pharmacokinetic and safety substudies nested in the open-label, multicentre, randomised, non-inferiority ODYSSEY trial. Lancet HIV 2022;9(9):e341–52.
8. Turkova A, Chan MC, Kityo C, et al. D3/Penta 21 clinical trial design: a randomised non-inferiority trial with nested drug licensing substudy to assess dolutegravir and lamivudine fixed dose formulations for the maintenance of virological suppression in children with HIV-1 infection, aged 2 to 15 years. Contemp Clin Trials 2024;142:107540.
9. HIV drug resistance: brief report 2024. Geneva: World Health Organization; 2024.
10. Palma P, Foster C, Rojo P, et al. The EPIICAL project: an emerging global collaboration to investigate immunotherapeutic strategies in HIV-infected children. J Virus Erad 2015;1(3):134–9.
11. Klein N, Palma P, Luzuriaga K, et al. Early antiretroviral therapy in children perinatally infected with HIV: a unique opportunity to implement immunotherapeutic approaches to prolong viral remission. Lancet Infect Dis 2015;15(9):1108–14.
12. Tagarro A, Chan M, Zangari P, et al. Early and highly suppressive antiretroviral therapy are main factors associated with low viral reservoir in european perinatally HIV-infected children. J Acquir Immune Defic Syndr 2018;79:269–76.
13. Rinaldi S, Pallikkuth S, Cameron M, et al. Impact of early antiretroviral therapy initiation on HIV-specific CD4 and CD8 T cell function in perinatally infected children. J Immunol 2020;204:540–9.
14. Tagarro A, Dominguez-Rodriguez S, Cotton M, et al. High mortality following early initiation of antiretroviral therapy in infants living with HIV from three African countries. eClinicalMedicine 2024;73:102648.
15. Ajibola G, Masheto G, Shapiro R, et al. Antibody interventions in HIV: broadly neutralizing mAbs in children. Curr Opin HIV AIDS 2023;18:217–24.

16. UNICEF Global and Regional HIV trends, 2023. Available at: https://data.unicef.org/topic/hivaids/global-regional-trends/. (Accessed 13 September 2024).
17. Guidelines for managing advanced HIV disease and rapid initiation of antiretroviral therapy. Geneva: World Health Organization; 2017. Available at: https://www.who.int/hiv/pub/guidelines/advanced-HIV-disease/en. Accessed July 10, 2024.
18. Ford N, Shubber Z, Meintjes G, et al. Causes of hospital admission among people living with HIV worldwide: a systematic review and meta-analysis. Lancet HIV 2015;2:e438–44.
19. Slogrove AL, Sohn AH. The global epidemiology of adolescents living with HIV: time for more granular data to improve adolescent health outcomes. Curr Opin HIV AIDS 2018;13:170–8.
20. Guidelines for managing advanced HIV disease and rapid initiation of antiretroviral therapy. World Health Organization; 2017. ISBN 978-92-4-155006-2 ©.
21. Package of care for children and adolescents with advanced HIV disease: stop AIDS. Technical brief WHO; 2020.
22. Slyker JA. Cytomegalovirus and paediatric HIV infection. J Virus Erad 2016;2:208–14.
23. Ekeng BE, Edem K, Akintan P, et al. Histoplasmosis in African children: clinical features, diagnosis and treatment. Ther Adv Infect Dis 2022;9. 204993612110685.
24. Rojo P, Moraleda C, Tagarro A, et al. Empirical treatment against cytomegalovirus and tuberculosis in HIV-infected infants with severe pneumonia: study protocol for a multicenter, open-label randomized controlled clinical trial. Trials 2022;23(1):531.
25. Bates M, Shibemba A, Mudenda V, et al. Burden of respiratory tract infections at post mortem in Zambian children. BMC Med 2016;14:99.
26. Newberry L, O'Hare B, Kennedy N, et al. Early use of corticosteroids in infants with a clinical diagnosis of Pneumocystis jiroveci pneumonia in Malawi: a double-blind, randomised clinical trial. Paediatr Int Child Health 2017;37:121–8.
27. Goussard P, Kling S, Gie RP, et al. CMV pneumonia in HIV-infected ventilated infants. Pediatr Pulmonol 2010;45:650–5.
28. Passanduca A, Buck WB, Tagarro A. High mortality in African infants hospitalized with severe pneumonia and advanced HIV disease. CROI 2023. abstract 810.
29. Madrid L, Buck WB, Musiime V. Causes of death among infants living with HIV and hospitalized with severe pneumonia in sub-Saharan African countries: preliminary results from the EMPIRICAL trial. Internat Ped Workshop 2024. Oral Abstract 8.
30. Jacobs TG, Mumbiro V, Cassia U, et al. Twice-daily dosing of dolutegravir in infants on rifampicin treatment: a pharmacokinetic substudy of the EMPIRICAL trial. Clin Infect Dis 2024 Mar 20;78(3):702–10.
31. Chabala C, Jacobs TG, Moraleda C, et al. First-line antituberculosis drug concentrations in infants with HIV and a history of recent admission with severe pneumonia. J Pediatric Infect Dis Soc. 2023 Nov 30;12(11):581–5.
32. Childhood Acute Illness and Nutrition (CHAIN) Network. Childhood mortality during and after acute illness in Africa and south Asia: a prospective cohort study. Lancet Global Health 2022;10(5):e673–84.

Maternal–Child Human Immunodeficiency Virus Clinical Trials Networks across the Ages

Sharon Nachman, MD

KEYWORDS

- Maternal HIV • Pediatric HIV • Clinical trial network

KEY POINTS

- The Pediatric AIDS Clinical Trial Group (PACTG) network grew out of combining a pediatric-focused research agenda along with that of the HIV Network (HIVNET).
- Studies developed and resulted from the PACTG and International Maternal Pediatric Adolescent AIDS Clinical Trials (IMPAACT) significantly contributed to guidelines for the care of HIV-infected infants, children, adolescents, and pregnant and postpartum people.
- The current structure of the IMPAACT network includes a strong community presence and leverages collaboration among academic, industry, and NIH. This multifaceted approach has resulted in 11 new therapeutics licensed over the past decade.

BACKGROUND

The history of the maternal–child human immunodeficiency virus (HIV) networks is multifaceted and developed from the division of the original AIDS Clinical Trial Network funded in 1986 to its current format known as the International Maternal Pediatric Adolescent AIDS Clinical Trials (IMPAACT). Its current mission is to improve health outcomes for infants, children, and adolescents as well as pregnant and postpartum people who are impacted by or living with HIV by evaluating novel treatments and interventions for HIV and its complications for tuberculosis (TB) and other related complications. This study reviews the history of the network and focuses on some of the key publications that have led to changes in guidelines and medical care over the years of development.

1981 TO 1986

The written history of the HIV epidemic started in 1981. In the June 5, 1981 Morbidity and Mortality Weekly Report (MMWR), the US Centers for Disease Control (CDC)

Pediatric Infectious Disease, Department of Pediatrics, Renaissance School of Medicine, State University of New York at Stony Brook, 101 Nicholls Road, Stony Brook, NY 11794-8111, USA
E-mail address: Sharon.nachman@stonybrookmedicine.edu

Clin Perinatol 51 (2024) 935–949
https://doi.org/10.1016/j.clp.2024.08.009 **perinatology.theclinics.com**

published a report on cases of a rare lung infection *Pneumocystis carinii* pneumonia (PCP), in 5 young, previously healthy, gay men in Los Angeles. These young men also had other unusual infections. By the time of publication, 2 had already died and the rest soon followed. Within the next few days and weeks, cases of other unusual opportunistic infections (OIs) were being reported around the United States. By year's end, there were a cumulative total of 337 reported cases of individuals with severe immune deficiency in the United States; 321 adults/adolescents and 16 children under the age of 13 years. Of those cases, 130 were already dead by December 31, 1981. By January 1983, the first cases were being reported in women and, by March of that year, the CDC reported in the MMWR that most cases of acquired immune deficiency syndrome (AIDS) have been identified in gay men with multiple sexual partners, people who inject drugs, Haitians, and people with hemophilia. The report suggested that AIDS may be caused by an infectious agent that is transmitted sexually or through exposure to blood or blood products and included recommendations for preventing transmission. During that same year, the World Health Organization (WHO) held its first meeting to assess the global AIDS situation and began its first international surveillance. However, it was not until 1985 that the first commercial diagnostic tests for HIV were available, and these were only testing for antibodies to the virus. Antibody testing cannot be used for identifying infants with HIV, as maternal antibodies cross the placenta and give a false result for infant testing. Over the next several years, public opinion was swayed by both the numbers of HIV-related deaths and the high profile of some who identified as HIV infected. These included Ryan White, a teenager who contracted HIV through a blood transfusion and was refused entry to his middle school, speaking out in public on the need for AIDS education.

1986 TO 1990

In 1986, the original AIDS Treatment and Evaluation Units in the United States were established by the National Institutes of Health. In 1987, the AIDS Clinical Trials Group (ACTG) was established by the National Institute of Allergy and Infectious Diseases (NIAID). It was in this year that the AIDS Coalition to Unleash Power (ACT UP) was founded. This organization was referenced as the most effective health activist group in history by *Time Magazine*. The CDC issued first-time recommendations regarding the practice of universal precautions in dealing with all patients. Also, during this year, the CDC released its first AIDS-related public service announcements. This clinical trial group did not focus on maternal infant health, but rather on adult clinical trials.

In 1987, the US Food and Drug Administration (FDA) approved zidovudine or azidothymidine (AZT) as the first antiretroviral (ARV) drug for the treatment of HIV. The American Medical Association declared in that same year that doctors have an ethical obligation to care for people with AIDS, as well as for those who have been infected with the virus but were considered asymptomatic. There were still no therapies for pregnant women or children, and pediatric formulations of any therapies were lacking. In essence, children aged over 18 months could be identified as HIV infected, but that diagnosis would be a death sentence. Children aged under 18 months would rarely be identified as HIV infected due to lack of available specific testing.

It was during the late 1980s that NIAID began funding several different HIV/AIDS research collaborations or networks focused initially on treatment and then largely on preparation for testing of vaccines. The first of these networks was focused on clinical trials and surveillance studies at US domestic sites only. Subsequent, concurrently funded networks with somewhat different funding periods and mandates included sites in other countries where HIV/AIDS was spreading rapidly and ravaging broader populations. A full overview of this timeline is presented in **Fig. 1**.

In 1988, the US Health Resources and Services Administration (HRSA) awarded $4.4 million in grants to 11 states and Puerto Rico for the first pediatric AIDS service demonstration projects. The projects were expected to demonstrate effective ways to reduce mother-to-child HIV transmission; develop coordinated, community-based, and family-centered services for infants and children living with HIV; and develop programs to reduce the spread of HIV to vulnerable populations of young people. With the death of Ryan White in 1990, this program would be renamed in his memory and is currently known as the HRSA Ryan White/AIDS Program (Ryan White Care Act). With the massive sit-in by ACT UP at the FDA during that year, shutting the agency down for an entire day, the FDA announced new regulations for speeding up federal drug approval processes for HIV-related treatments. These FDA changes helped move new therapeutics into care; however, they have not significantly increased the speed to licensure of these new therapies for pediatric and pregnant populations.

The next few years brought new guidelines into place for preventing PCP, hepatitis B, and infections in health care workers. It was not until 1990 that AZT was first approved for children.

1990 TO 1997

In 1991, the NIH-funded ACTG was divided into 2 groups: the Adult ACTG and the Pediatric ACTG (PACTG). This would allow, for the first time, a network to focus solely on populations that were almost always excluded from clinical trials; infants, children, adolescents, and pregnant and postpartum individuals, and they would now be the key focus of HIV-related clinical research. The Red Ribbon Project was developed to create a visual symbol to demonstrate compassion for people living with AIDS and their caregivers. The Red Ribbon became the international symbol of AIDS awareness,

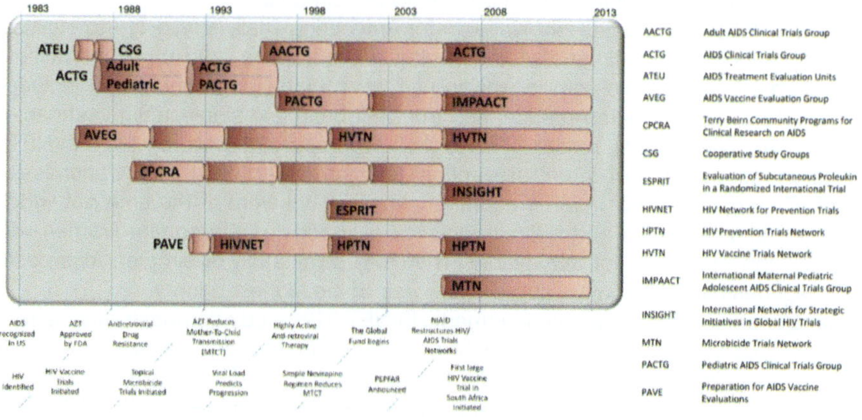

Timeline of NIAID's HIV/AIDS clinical trials networks by U.S. Government fiscal years (October 1 – September 30). Horizontal bars depict networks (or pre-network programs). Connections between bars represent time points where a program/network was competitively renewed.

Fig. 1. Evolution of the NIAID HIV/AIDS clinical trials networks. [a]Networks continuing beyond 2013 https://health-policy-systems.biomedcentral.com/articles/10.1186/1478-4505-7-12. (*From:* Kagan, J.M., Kane, M., Quinlan, K.M. et al. Developing a conceptual framework for an evaluation system for the NIAID HIV/AIDS clinical trials networks. *Health Res Policy Sys* 7, 12 (2009). https://doi.org/10.1186/1478-4505-7-12.)

and wearing that ribbon was a visual symbol for families that we, as providers, were there to care for them. The Red Ribbon project was a force for increasing awareness that children were dying of HIV, and care providers were often seen wearing these ribbons. This helped families see that they were not alone in their struggles.

Ideas for clinical trials were limited by lack of availability of therapeutics to be used in children. Some of PACTG's first studies included the use of intravenous immunoglobulin to prevent OIs, while others investigated the safety and pharmacokinetics (PK) of oral and intravenous (IV) AZT in children with HIV. In 1993, a critical study led by Ed Conner and Rhoda Sperling, called PACTG 076,[1] evaluated whether a combination of oral AZT given to pregnant women during pregnancy, IV AZT during delivery and oral AZT given to infants for 6 weeks, compared to placebo could prevent the transmission of HIV from mother to infant. Findings from this study changed the world's view of HIV, demonstrating that AZT when given as described in the study reduced perinatal transmission of HIV from 25% to 8%; a 67% reduction. These results prompted the US Public Health Service to recommend that pregnant women with HIV be given AZT to reduce the risk of perinatal transmission. They also changed the world view on pediatric and obstetric trials, showing that pregnant women could and would participate in clinical research and that, despite exposure to HIV in utero, transmission to the neonate can be prevented.

With the understanding that a study to understand progression of HIV disease was also needed, the PACTG developed a Pediatric Late Outcomes Protocol in 1993, otherwise known as PACTG 219, then PACTG 219C as it progressed across the years. This omnibus study included both HIV-infected and HIV-exposed uninfected (HEU) children and would form the basis for the cohort followed in the National Institute of Child Health and Development (NICHD)-funded US Pediatric HIV/AIDS Cohort Study (PHACS) network (https://onlinelibrary.wiley.com/doi/pdf/10.1002/%28SICI%291096-9926%28200005%2961%3A5%3C395%3A%3AAID-TERA15%3E3.0.CO%3B2-H). With over 50 publications to its credit and hundreds of citations, PHACS elucidated the long-term consequences of being born HEU in the United States as well as the long-term sequela of living with perinatally acquired HIV.

In 1993, NIAID funded the HIV Network for Prevention Trials (HIVNET)—to evaluate HIV prevention interventions (vaccines, microbicides, ARVs, and other modalities), with both a US domestic component and an international component that included sites in Asia, Africa, South America, and the Caribbean and significant investment in developing international research capacity. An important part of the HIVNET's research agenda focused on prevention of maternal-to-child HIV transmission (PMTCT) in mid-to-lower income countries where ARVs were at the time not widely available and the costs and difficult logistics of reaching all pregnant women with PMTCT services were not achievable. Therefore, evaluation of simpler, less costly ARV regimens and alternative approaches was of the highest priority.

A major achievement was the landmark HIVNET 012[2] study demonstrating in 1999 that a single oral dose of nevirapine to the mother during labor and a single oral dose to the infant within 48 hours of birth reduced the rate of vertical transmission by nearly half (47%) at 14 to 16 weeks postpartum compared to a short regimen of AZT; later results published in 2003 showed persistent benefits in the nevirapine (NVP) arm through 18 months. Other early HIVNET perinatal studies evaluated alternative, non-ARV interventions such as antibiotics to prevent chorioamnionitis-associated perinatal HIV (HIVNET 024)[3] and different concentrations of chlorhexidine for peripartum vaginal and infant washes (HIVNET 025).[4] Some perinatal studies developed during HIVNET were implemented in the subsequent network funding cycle when the US domestic and international components of HIVNET were combined under the first iteration of the HIV Prevention Trials Network (HPTN) and focused on testing interventions that could safely and effectively protect infants from HIV while breastfeeding (BF), as discouraging BF in low and middle income countries (LMIC) to protect against HIV would place infants at greater risk of poor growth and increased morbidity and mortality. These included the first pediatric HIV vaccine trial in Africa (HPTN 027),[5] which evaluated the safety and immunogenicity of ALVAC-HIV vCP1521 in infants born to women with HIV-1 in Uganda. HPTN 046[6] assessed the efficacy and safety of extending daily NVP among HIV-exposed breastfed infants from 6 weeks to 6 months compared to placebo to prevent postnatal infection in 4 African countries and demonstrated significantly reduced transmission at 6 months in the extended NVP arm compared to the placebo arm. The PMTCT landscape was rapidly evolving during the late 1990s and early 2000s, with contributions of a number of network and non-network studies that evaluated different ARV regimens—for example, different/improved drug combinations, initiated earlier in pregnancy, continued longer postpartum and/or given to BF infants throughout the period of exposure, as well as regimens for infants of mothers who delivered before starting treatment.

Along with the change supporting development of a separate pediatric clinical trial network came ideas about how to look broadly at HIV and related infections and comorbidities. The 1996 request for applications (RFA) for PACTG from the Division of AIDS of NIAID solicited applications interested in participating in a cooperative group to plan, direct, and conduct Phase I, II, and III clinical trials in the United States. These clinical trials would have to address high-priority research questions on the treatment and prevention of HIV disease and its sequelae. The focus would be on (1) treatment of primary HIV disease; (2) interventions designed to prevent perinatal transmission of HIV; and (3) prophylaxis and treatment of OIs. Modalities of intervention might include but were not limited to (1) drugs or combinations, (2) active and/or passive immune-based therapies, (3) immunomodulators, and (4) gene transfer techniques. For the first time in 1998, there would be one single RFA for clinical trial networks, with another RFA for Clinical Trial Units (CTUs). The funders also described the importance of performance evaluation, designation of new "reserve" funds, and a role for external advisory bodies to assist in meeting such challenges.

1998 TO 2006

In 1998, the CDC issued its first national treatment guidelines for the use of ARV therapies in adults and adolescents with HIV. Guidelines for children did not yet exist. HIV viral load testing was first being rolled out in the United States but was unaffordable and not widely available in international settings. In 1999, WHO acknowledged that HIV/AIDS had become the fourth biggest killer worldwide and the number one killer in Africa. In 2000, the US Congress reauthorized the Ryan White Care Act for the second time. For the first time, generic drugs were in development and drug manufacturers agreed to lower the prices of their newly developed ARV therapies. In 2002, the Global Fund to Fight AIDS, Tuberculosis and Malaria was established, and in its first year, $600 million in grant funding was approved. Worldwide, 10 million young people aged 15 to 24 years and over 3 million children under the age of 15 years were now living with HIV. In 2003, President George W Bush established the Presidents Emergency Plan for AIDS Relief (PEPFAR).

In 1998, the CDC published its first Public Health Service Task Force Recommendations for the Use of Antiretroviral Drugs in Pregnant Women Infected with HIV-1 for Maternal Health and for Reducing Perinatal HIV-1 Transmission in the United States.[7] These recommendations included both combination ARV regimens and the

PACTG 076 AZT regimen for PMTCT. In 2002, the US Department of Health and Human Services issued Guidelines for the Use of Antiretroviral Agents in Pediatric HIV Infection, its first recommendations on the topic. The FDA approved efavirenz for the treatment of HIV/AIDS in children and adults. This approval resulted, in part, from the findings of a study[8] conducted by the PACTG, supported by NICHD and NIAID. It was not until 2002 that the FDA granted approval for nevirapine for pediatric patients, 2 years after approving its use for adults.

In the years between 1998 and 2006, both new diagnostics for HIV, including HIV polymerase chain reaction (PCR) testing, and breakthroughs in PCR testing for TB were jump-started. At the same time, improved pediatric ARV formulations were being developed. PACTG studies expanded and included not only new therapies for HIV treatment in children, but also studies of responses to vaccines and newly developed combination therapies to lower maternal HIV transmission to less than 6%. During this era, the PACTG demonstrated that therapies from 2 classes of ARVs were needed to suppress viral load below the limit of detection and that the addition of nevirapine to AZT lowered vertical transmission rates to under 2%. Other key/critical studies during this cycle of the PACTG included trials of protease inhibitors (nelfinavir, ritonavir, saquinavir, and indinavir) in children,[9–12] studies of immunogenicity of routine vaccines in youth with HIV: pneumococcal conjugate in infants;[13] varicella, tetanus, acellular pertussis, meningococcal, and hepatitis A vaccines in children;[14–19] and best therapies to prevent OIs and when to stop them.[20] All of these studies contributed to CDC and WHO guidelines for care of infants, children, and adolescents living with HIV worldwide. In 2005, the FDA approved the use of emtricitabine (FTC) for treatment of HIV in children—2 years after it was approved in adults using data from PACTG and IMPAACT studies.[8]

2007 TO 2013

In preparation for response to the RFA for the next NIAID HIV/AIDS clinical trials network funding cycle to begin in 2006, investigators from the PACTG joined with investigators from the international pediatric component of the HPTN (previously under HIVNET) to propose a new, combined US domestic and international network focused specifically on infants, children, adolescents, and pregnant/postpartum people, which was to be named the International IMPAACT network and had a broader research agenda. This RFA would result in funding for 6 restructured HIV/AIDS clinical trials networks: IMPAACT, ACTG, and HPTN, as well as the HIV Vaccine Trials Network, *the* International Network for Strategic Initiatives in Global HIV Trials and the Microbicide Trials Network. Together, these networks supported studies at 73 CTU located around the world.

In 2007, WHO and UNAIDS issued guidance recommending provider-initiated HIV testing. In 2008, President Bush signed legislation reauthorizing PEPFAR for an additional 5 years, critical to changing the direction of the HIV epidemic worldwide. These actions brought more patients into the network's clinical trial sites with the resulting challenge of developing timely clinical trials to address their needs.

Studies during those years focused on not only HIV and related issues, but also on TB and complications from OIs.[21] During the first iteration of the IMPAACT network, the 2009 H1N1 influenza pandemic occurred. IMPAACT's unique ability to pivot when challenged with a pandemic demonstrated its scientific leadership, excellence in study design and participant enrollment capacity, and ability to move therapeutics rapidly along a licensure pathway. The network not only swiftly and comprehensively developed a study protocol for evaluation of a novel flu vaccine in a short time

(2 months) but also enrolled over 130 pregnant individuals with HIV in the successive 2 months, allowing for critical information regarding novel flu vaccines to be useful during the pandemic.[22]

In 2010, the IMPAACT network implemented the Promoting Maternal and Infant Survival Everywhere (PROMISE) studies, a constellation of trials designed to address in an integrated and comprehensive manner remaining critical questions facing pregnant and postpartum women with HIV and their infants. These included determining the optimal intervention for the prevention of antepartum and intrapartum HIV transmission, the optimal intervention for prevention of postpartum transmission in BF infants, and the optimal intervention for the preservation of maternal health after delivery.

PMTCT ends (either at delivery or cessation of BF). Combined, these multiple-component studies enrolled over 5000 participants between June 2010 and October 2014. Data from these studies showed that antenatal 3 drug antiretroviral therapy resulted in significantly lower rates of early HIV transmission than a simpler course of ART but a higher risk of adverse maternal and neonatal outcomes[23] and that continued ART postpartum was safe among women enrolled during pregnancy with high pre-ART CD4 + T-cell counts and was associated with a halving of the rate of WHO clinical staging grade 2 mildly symptomatic or stage 3 moderately symptomatic conditions such as unexplained weight loss, unexplained diarrhea, severe bacterial infections, and mucocutaneous conditions.[24]

Expanding to address other unmet needs including evaluating new ARV treatments for use in infants, children, and adolescents, the network also developed critical TB studies. In 2011, the network published results from the IMPAACT P1041[25] demonstrating that primary isoniazid (INH) prophylaxis, which was the recommended standard of care in populations with HIV at that time, did not improve TB disease-free survival among children with HIV or TB infection-free survival among HIV-uninfected children immunized with Bacillus Calmetter-Guerin vaccine (BCG) vaccine. This study and those downstream from it examined not only the utility of INH prophylaxis in HIV infected and exposed infants but also the degree of ARV uptake and development of ARV resistance in this population (at the age of 3 months to 4 years)[26] and helped set the stage for WHO consensus statements on evaluation of TB in children.

In 2010, the network reported that death rates of children with HIV had decreased more than 9 fold since the use of Highly Active Antiretroviral Therapy in the mid-1990s.[27] Despite this improvement, these findings showed that the rate of death among young people with HIV was still 30 times higher than among young people who do not have HIV, underscoring the idea that better drugs along with other measures are needed to lower deaths rates among children with HIV. Not surprisingly, many therapies were still not approved for children. It was only in 2010 that the FDA approved tenofovir for use in treating children infected with HIV ages 12 to 18 years; the decision came 9 years after it was approved for adults.

Building on prior work in adults, ARVs moved into being part of routine care for children. Toxicities and PK were key barriers to their use along with the need for sustainable pediatric formulations. Testing for resistance was not available at international sites and expensive at US domestic sites if not part of a clinical trial. Viral load testing became the norm, and both viral load and CD4 testing were routine markers of adherence and treatment failure.

In 2010, the first available integrase inhibitor raltegravir (RAL) was evaluated in children.[28] This IMPAACT study was performed not only for evaluation of safety and virologic control but also enabled licensure of the first of these therapies in children at both United States and international sites. Included in the study were critical arms and analyses regarding PK modeling from aged 18 years down to 4 weeks and inclusion of novel pediatric formulations. By working directly with pharmaceutical partners and developing teams with "boots on the ground" members and community representatives, the network set the stage for development of future studies that would hasten the approval and licensure of novel therapeutic agents in pediatric populations.

While the first sets of Guidelines for the Prevention and Treatment of OIs in HIV-Exposed and HIV-Infected Children were published in 2002[29] and 2004, they were combined for the first time into one comprehensive set in 2009.[30] That document and subsequent updates in 2013[31] set the standard for comprehensiveness, including sections on each OI, epidemiology, clinical presentation, diagnosis, treatment, as well as sections on discontinuation of primary and secondary prophylaxis. Data from PACTG and IMPAACT studies were incorporated across these documents, and authorship included many researchers involved in PACTG and IMPAACT studies.

2013 TO 2024

In 2013, 210,000 children younger than 15 years were newly infected with HIV worldwide and 190,000 died of AIDS. It was in this setting that the NIAID HIV/AIDS clinical trials network RFA was again refined; this iteration solicited applications for CTUs to implement the clinical research plans of one or more of the HIV/AIDS Clinical Trials Networks. Each CTU could have one or more clinical research site and should be optimally configured to conduct clinical research by recruiting, screening, enrolling, and following research participants from the populations most affected and/or endangered by the HIV/AIDS epidemic. This flexibility and the enormous investment in developing research capacity in the previous funding cycles positioned the networks well not only for dealing with HIV, but also, as demonstrated in 2020, developing and rolling out clinical trials for other emerging epidemics, specifically the novel coronavirus pandemic. This infrastructure was again leveraged in 2023, when the MPOX epidemic started, allowing for sites affiliated with any of the HIV networks to also enroll in these critical studies.

In 2014, WHO set the "90-90-90" targets, aiming to diagnose 90% of all people HIV positive, provide ART for 90% of those diagnosed, and achieve viral suppression for 90% of those treated, by 2020. During this era, focus was placed on getting new therapeutics licensed for children and pregnant people and expanding what we understood about the safety and PKs of licensed therapies in pregnant women. In July of the same year, the AIDS 2014 conference in Melbourne Australia drew nearly 14,000 delegates from over 200 nations. One key message of the conference was that a one-size-fits-all approach may not be suitable for all settings, especially given the diversity of the epidemic's geographic hotspots and key populations. Interventions and policies will require target-based strategies and greater support of key populations, especially in countries where discriminatory policies and legislation are hindering prevention and treatment efforts. In 2016, the US CDC reported that only 1 in 5 sexually active high school students had been tested for HIV. An estimated 50% of young Americans who were living with HIV did not know they were infected. While there was recognition that more would be needed to achieve WHO's 90/90/90 goals, focus would now need to turn to newer and better ARVs for both pre-exposure prophylaxis as well as treatment, and importantly, what would be the network's clinical trials for bringing these therapies to populations served by the IMPAACT network.

The report of a child who was HIV infected yet had undetectable circulating virus while off ARVs for over 2 years, also known as the Mississippi baby in 2013[32] brought another critical change to our thinking. Can analytical treatment interruption (ATI) be used with confidence in children and if so for whom and when can it be safely used? It also underscored the idea that better laboratory diagnostics must focus on HIV reservoirs in newly infected infants and that there may be surrogate markers that could be used to understand the types of individuals who might have the ability to undergo ATI. IMPAACT 2015 assessed cell-free HIV-RNA and cell-associated HIV pol/gag-DNA in paired cerebral spinal fluid (CSF) and blood and found persistent HIV-DNA in CSF in youth aged 13 to 27 years despite between 8 and 25 years of ARVs and being virally suppressed for more than the past 12 months, raising the concern that despite sustained viral load in plasma below the limit of detection, the central nervous system (CNS) continues to be a reservoir for virus and may need different therapeutics to eradicate virus.[33]

Key milestones for the IMPAACT network in the past decade alone included over 37 studies enrolling their first participants, over 14,000 participants followed on studies, with over 57% being children. There were over 300 publications during these years, many of which were referenced in national and international guidelines, adding to the large volume of over 1500 publications prior by the network. This was all due to enrollments from 52 sites in 12 countries. The current table of organization allows for input from our National Institutes Health (NIH) funders (NIAID, NICHD, and National INstitute Mental Health [NIMH]), as well as the community and our core scientific groups. Recognizing changes in the HIV pandemic, the network has realigned its scientific committees. **Fig. 2** shows the current focus of the network's 4 scientific committees. The current portfolio of studies under investigation by the network includes therapeutics, ART-free remission/cure, TB, and mental health studies (**Fig. 3**). A full reporting of studies and publications is available on the open access network Web site: www.impaactnetwork.org.

Licensure of new drugs has now been accelerated. With 11 drugs or formulations under direct IMPAACT study, understanding optimal dosing of these therapeutics in our key populations has changed both US and WHO guidelines as well as their country-specific standard of care use (**Fig. 4**). These include the safety and PK of both oral and injectable integrase inhibitors as well as fixed-dose combination therapies for young children and treatment of hepatitis C during pregnancy.

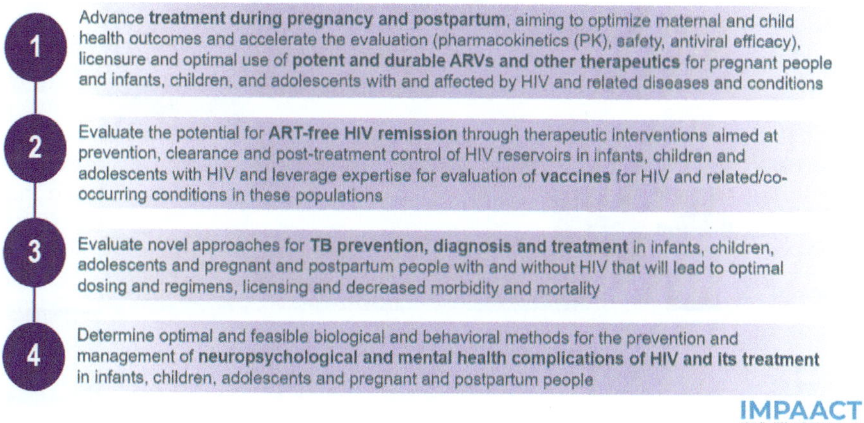

1
Advance treatment during pregnancy and postpartum, aiming to optimize maternal and child health outcomes and accelerate the evaluation (pharmacokinetics (PK), safety, antiviral efficacy), licensure and optimal use of potent and durable ARVs and other therapeutics for pregnant people and infants, children, and adolescents with and affected by HIV and related diseases and conditions
2
Evaluate the potential for ART-free HIV remission through therapeutic interventions aimed at prevention, clearance and post-treatment control of HIV reservoirs in infants, children and adolescents with HIV and leverage expertise for evaluation of vaccines for HIV and related/co-occurring conditions in these populations
3
Evaluate novel approaches for TB prevention, diagnosis and treatment in infants, children, adolescents and pregnant and postpartum people with and without HIV that will lead to optimal dosing and regimens, licensing and decreased morbidity and mortality
4
Determine optimal and feasible biological and behavioral methods for the prevention and management of neuropsychological and mental health complications of HIV and its treatment in infants, children, adolescents and pregnant and postpartum people
IMPAACT

Fig. 2. Scientific aims.

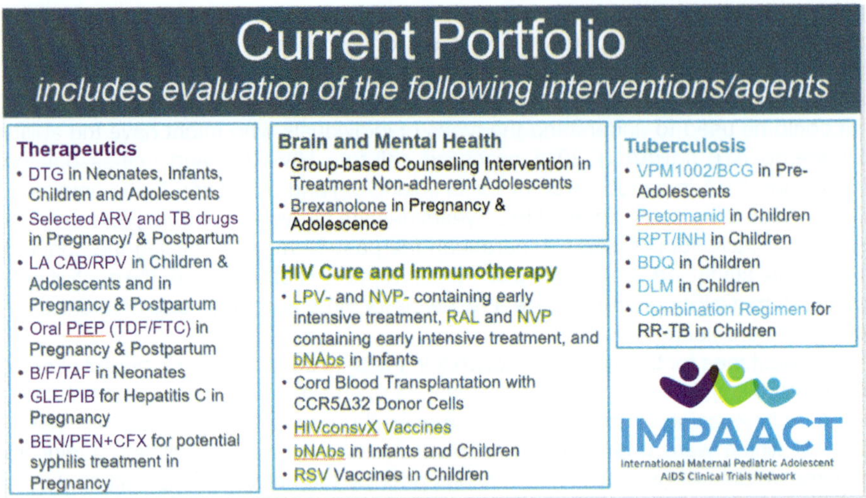

Fig. 3. Current site portfolio. B/F/TAF, Biktarvy; BDQ, bedaquiline; BEN/Pen, benzathine penicillin; bNABs, broadly neutralizing antibodies; CFX, ceftriaxone; DLM, delamanid; INH, isoniazid; RPT, rifapentine; RSV, respiratory syncytial virus.

The IMPAACT P1115 study focuses on very early identification of neonates with HIV and starting them on ARVs and broadly neutralizing antibodies (bNAbs) by 48 hours of life (mirroring the Mississippi baby approach) that might allow them to undergo an ATI at 4 years of life. Data presented in Denver at CROI 2024[34] demonstrated that this approach and recapitulation of the Mississippi baby was possible. Results of this ongoing study showed that, among those few infants who had sustained undetectable

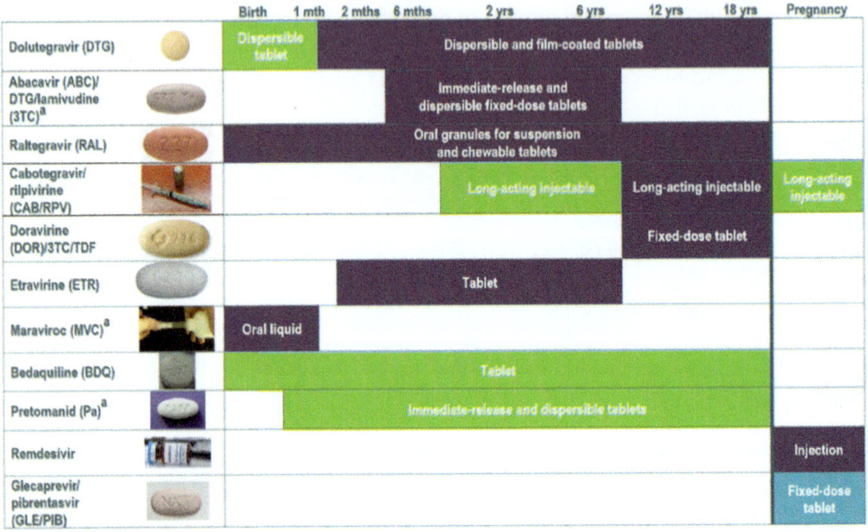

Fig. 4. Therapeutics licensed though IMPAACT clinical trials. [a]Approved in children using weight-based dosing.

virus after 4 years of treatment, ATI could be sustained for more than 48 weeks. Data such as this, and studies exploring the safety and PK of bNAbs in young infants, may help develop a path forward for getting to a "cure." IMPAACT 2017, evaluating long-acting injectable ARVs, has led to licensure in youth aged over 12 years, and we anticipate that IMPAACT 2036 in children aged 2 to 12 years will enable licensure of these therapeutics for that age group soon as well. Moving these therapies to children across the ages will also help achieve WHO's current last "95," getting 95% of those identified as having HIV and on ARVs to be undetectable.

A review of the network would be remiss if it does not discuss the importance of community engagement. A key strength of the network is the incorporation of community input at every level and in every aspect of our work. The network's top-down as well as bottom-up approach to community engagement means that each site must have its own local community advisory board (CAB), with each site also having representation on the broader network-level CAB. Community representation on both network management and scientific leadership committees, on each of the scientific committees and on each protocol team while the study is being developed and implemented, is invaluable and essential for ensuring the relevance and appropriateness of our research.

Strategic collaboration is also key to the network's success. The overall goal is to enhance and accelerate drug/intervention evaluation and accessibility for our populations of interest. Collaboration with other groups (eg, pharmaceutical partners, guidelines organizations, other research entities, and networks) provides opportunities for input and early influence on global research priorities for our populations of interest (eg, participating in guidelines committees and jointly convening workshops on targeted topics of mutual interest), ensures early access to novel study agents for evaluation in our key populations, broadens our scientific and public health footprint, and strengthens our research approach (eg, collaboration and co-enrollment with other trials networks). It also affords downstream influence and impact on guidelines, uptake, and care.

In 2020, WHO moved its prior 90-90-90 targets to now achieve 95-95-95, with the aim of diagnosing 95% of all individuals with HIV positive, providing ART for 95% of those diagnosed and achieving viral suppression for 95% of those treated by 2030. Globally, an estimated 38 million people were living with HIV in 2020; of these, 1.8 million were children aged under 15 years. We anticipate that data from IMPAACT studies will effectively help reach the WHO 95/95/95 goals, with the currently funded network focusing on novel and durable treatment and prevention interventions for HIV and associated conditions, ART-free HIV remission, TB, and complications of HIV, including mental health. Continuing the strong community partnership and involvement in all aspects of our research and strengthening and expanding collaborations with commercial or noncommercial product developers will facilitate evaluation and licensure of new ARVs and other agents in our key pediatric populations. The IMPAACT network is well positioned to continue its contributions to controlling and eliminating HIV and associated conditions in infants, children, adolescents, and pregnant and postpartum people worldwide. Investments made over the last 3 decades by the NIH in the infrastructure and research capacity of their HIV clinical networks have been integral to the resulting scientific advancements that have dramatically transformed the HIV landscape and improved lives in affected populations—including those of key interest to the IMPAACT network—across the globe.

SUMMARY

The current structure of the NIH funded maternal child HIV network, IMPAACT, has a robust portfolio of studies, is making progress in getting new therapeutics licensed for its populations, and is contributing to worldwide guidelines in the care of HIV-infected populations worldwide.

Best Practices

What is the current practice for treatment of infants, children adolescents, and pregnant people with HIV?

Standardization of treatment regimens is based on data from clinical trials supporting licensure of therapeutics across these populations. Clinical trials in these populations must continue as they have unique immunologic, hormonal, and physiologic differences from adult populations that impact PK, dosing, and safety of these products.

Best practice/guideline/care path objective(s)

Best practice treatment guidelines exist for identifying HIV in neonates, planning appropriate ARV treatment regimens across different pediatric populations and pregnant people with HIV. They are often informed from data collected from clinical trials developed and funded by governmental (NIH and other)-sponsored clinical trials. However, best practice guidelines for inclusion of children across the ages and for inclusion of pregnant and postpartum people do not exist.

What changes in current practice are likely to improve outcomes?

Timely evaluation of new ARVs including assessing both safety and PK will lead to improved outcomes and help lead to licensure of these products in both pediatric and onstetrics (OB) populations.

Pearls/pitfalls at the point-of-care

Care of populations with HIV will need to continue to include careful history and physical examination, assessment for CD4, POC viral load, presence of coinfections, and among those with detectable virus, assessment of resistance to current ARVs. Newer therapeutics will lead to better outcomes, and changes in length and quality of life for these populations.

Major recommendations

There continues to be a need for specific research in infants, children, adolescents, and pregnant/postpartum people. These key populations have unique biologic, social, and behavioral characteristics distinct from those in adults and nonpregnant people affecting their response to interventions to prevent, treat, or eradicate HIV and its coinfections and complications.

Bibliographic source(s):

Lantos JD. The "inclusion benefit" in clinical trials. J Pediatr. 1999 Feb;134(2):130–1. https://doi.org/10.1016/s0022-3476(9970400-2). PMID: 9931513.

Abrams EJ, Calmy A, Fairlie L, Mahaka IC, Chimula L, Flynn PM, Kinuthia J, Myer L, Khoo SH, Musoke P, Zwerski S, Zech JM, Lockman S, Siberry GK. Approaches to accelerating the study of new antiretrovirals in pregnancy. J Int AIDS Soc. 2022 Jul;25 Suppl 2(Suppl 2):e25916. https://doi.org/10.1002/jia2.25916. PMID: 35851757; PMCID: PMC9294864.

Illamola SM, Bucci-Rechtweg C, Costantine MM, Tsilou E, Sherwin CM, Zajicek A. Inclusion of pregnant and breastfeeding women in research—efforts and initiatives. Br J Clin Pharmacol. 2018 Feb;84(2):215-222. https://doi.org/10.1111/bcp.13438. Epub 2017 Oct 22. PMID: 28925019; PMCID: PMC5777434.

Nachman S, Ahmed A, Amanullah F, Becerra MC, Botgros R, Brigden G, Browning R, Gardiner E, Hafner R, Hesseling A, How C, Jean-Philippe P, Lessem E, Makhene M, Mbelle N, Marais B, McIlleron H, McNeeley DF, Mendel C, Murray S, Navarro E, Anyalechi EG, Porcalla AR, Powell C, Powell M, Rigaud M, Rouzier V, Samson P, Schaaf HS, Shah S, Starke

J, Swaminathan S, Wobudeya E, Worrell C. towards early inclusion of children in tuberculosis drugs trials: a consensus statement. Lancet Infect Dis. 2015 Jun;15(6):711–20. https://doi.org/10.1016/S1473-3099(1500007-9). Epub 2015 May 6. PMID: 25957923; PMCID: PMC4471052.

DISCLOSURE

Dr S. Nachman has nothing to disclose.

FUNDING

Overall support for the International Maternal Pediatric Adolescent AIDS Clinical Trials Network (IMPAACT) was provided by the National Institute of Allergy and Infectious Diseases (NIAID) with co-funding from the Eunice Kennedy Shriver National Institute of Child Health and Human Development (NICHD) and the National Institute of Mental Health (NIMH), all components of the National Institutes of Health (NIH), under Award Numbers UM1AI068632-15 (IMPAACT LOC), UM1AI068616-15 (IMPAACT SDMC) and UM1AI106716-15 (IMPAACT LC), and by NICHD contract number HHSN275201800001I. The content is solely the responsibility of the authors and does not necessarily represent the official views of the NIH.

REFERENCES

1. Connor EM, Sperling RS, Gelber R, et al. Reduction of maternal-infant transmission of human immunodeficiency virus type 1 with zidovudine Treatment.Pediatric AIDS clinical trials group protocol 076 study group. N Engl J Med 1994;331:1173–80.
2. Guay LA, Musoke P, Fleming T, et al. Intrapartum and neonatal single-dose nevirapine compared with zidovudine for prevention of mother-to-child transmission of HIV-1 in Kampala, Uganda: HIVNET 012 randomised trial. Lancet 1999;354(9181):795–802.
3. Taha TE, Brown ER, Hoffman IF, et al. A phase III clinical trial of antibiotics to reduce chorioamnionitis-related perinatal HIV-1 transmission. AIDS 2006;20(9):1313–21.
4. Wilson CM, Gray G, Read JS, et al. Tolerance and safety of different concentrations of chlorhexidine for peripartum vaginal and infant washes: HIVNET 025. J Acquir Immune Defic Syndr 2004;35(2):138–43.
5. Kaleebu P, Njai HF, Wang L, et al. HPTN 027 protocol team. Immunogenicity of ALVAC-HIV vCP1521 in infants of HIV-1-infected women in Uganda (HPTN 027): the first pediatric HIV vaccine trial in Africa. J Acquir Immune Defic Syndr 2014;65(3):268–77.
6. Coovadia HM, Brown ER, Fowler MG, et al. HPTN 046 protocol team. Efficacy and safety of an extended nevirapine regimen in infant children of breastfeeding mothers with HIV-1 infection for prevention of postnatal HIV-1 transmission (HPTN 046): a randomised, double-blind, placebo-controlled trial. Lancet 2012;379(9812):221–8.
7. Public health service Task force recommendations for the use of antiretroviral drugs in pregnant women infected with HIV-1 for maternal health and for reducing perinatal HIV-1 transmission in the United States. January 30, 1998/47(RR-2);1-30, Available at: https://www.cdc.gov/mmwr/preview/mmwrhtml/00053202.htm. Accessed April 12, 2024.

8. McKinney RE, Rodman J, Hu C, et al. Long-term safety and efficacy of a once-daily regimen of emtricitabine, didanosine, and efavirenz in HIV-infected, therapy-naive children and adolescents: pediatric AIDS clinical trials group protocol P1021. Pediatrics 2007;120(2):e416–23.
9. Nachman S, Stanley K, Yogev R, et al. A randomized trial of one or two nucleoside analogues plus ritonavir versus dual nucleoside analogue therapy in stable antiretroviral-experienced HIV-infected children. JAMA 2000;283(4):492–8.
10. Wiznia AA, Stanley K, Krogstad P, et al. Combination nucleoside analogue reverse transcriptase inhibitor(s) plus nevirapine, nelfinavir or ritonavir in stable antiretroviral therapy-experienced HIV-infected children. Week 24 Results of randomized controlled trial-PACTG 377. Pediatric AIDS Clinical Trials Group 377 Study Team. AIDS Res Hum Retrovir 2000;16(12):1113–21.
11. Pelton SI, Stanley K, Yogev R, et al. PACTG 338 Study Team. Switch from ritonavir to indinavir combination therapy for HIV-infected children. Clin Infect Dis 2005;40: 1181–7.
12. Floren LC, Wiznia A, Hayashi S, et al. Pediatric AIDS Clinical Trials Group 377 Team. Nelfinavir pharmacokinetics in stable HIV-positive children: PACTG 377. Pediatrics 2003;112(3):e220–7.
13. Nachman S, Kim S, King J, et al. for the PACTG 292 TeamSafety and immunogenicity of a heptavalent pneumococcal conjugate vaccine in HIV type-1 infected infecction. Pediatrics 2003;112(1):66–73.
14. Weinberg A, Gona P, Nachman SA, et al. PACTG 1008 Team. Antibody responses to hepatitis A vaccine among HIV-infected children with evidence of immunologic reconstitution on antiretroviral therapy. J Infect Dis 2006;193(2):302–11.
15. Abzug MJ, Pelton SI, Song LY, et al. Pediatric AIDS Clinical Trials Group P1024 Protocol Team. Immunogenicity, safety, and predictors of response after a pneumococcal conjugate and pneumococcal polysaccharide vaccine series in human immunodeficiency virus-infected children receiving highly active antiretroviral therapy. Pediatr Infect Dis J 2006;25(10):920–9.
16. Song LY, Fenton T, Nachman SA, et al. International Maternal Pediatric Adolescent AIDS Clinical Trials Group P1024 Protocol Team. Pertussis booster vaccination in HIV-infected children receiving highly active antiretroviral therapy. Pediatrics 2007;120(5):e1190–202.
17. Abzug MJ, Warshaw M, Rosenblatt HM, et al. International Maternal Pediatric Adolescent AIDS Clinical Trials Group P1024 and P1061s Protocol Teams. Immunogenicity and immunologic memory after hepatitis B virus booster vaccination in HIV-infected children receiving highly active antiretroviral therapy. J Infect Dis 2009;200(6):935–46.
18. Levin MJ, Gershon AA, Weinberg A, et al. Pediatric AIDS Clinical Trials Group 265 Team. Administration of live varicella vaccine to HIV-infected children with current or past significant depression of CD4(+) T cells. J Infect Dis 2006;194(2):247–55.
19. Siberry GK, Williams P, Lujan-Zilbermann J, et al. IMPAACT P1065 Protocol Team. Phase I/II, open-label trial of safety and immunogenicity of meningococcal (groups A, C, Y, and W-135) polysaccharide diphtheria toxoid conjugate vaccine in human immunodeficiency virus-infected adolescents. Pediatr Infect Dis J 2010; 29:391–6.
20. Nachman S, Gona P, Dankner W, et al. The rate of serious bacterial infections among HIV-infected children with immune reconstitution who have discontinued opportunistic infection prophylaxis. Pediatrics 2005;115(4):e488–94.
21. Gona P, Van Dyke RB, Williams PL, et al. Incidence of opportunistic and other infections in HIV-infected children in the HAART-era. JAMA 2006;296(3):292–300.

22. Abzug MJ, Nachman SA, Muresan P, et al. International Maternal Pediatric Adolescent AIDS Clinical Trials Group P1086 Protocol team. Safety and immunogenicity of 2009 pH1N1 vaccination in HIV-infected pregnant women. Clin Infect Dis 2013;56(10):1488–97.
23. Fowler MG, Qin M, Fiscus SA, et al. IMPAACT 1077BF/1077FF PROMISE Study Team. Benefits and risks of antiretroviral therapy for perinatal HIV prevention. N Engl J Med 2016;375(18):1726–37.
24. Currier JS, Britto P, Hoffman RM, et al. 1077HS PROMISE Team. Randomized trial of stopping or continuing ART among postpartum women with pre-ART CD4 $\geq$ 400 cells/mm3. PLoS One 2017;12(5):e0176009.
25. Madhi SA, Nachman S, Violari A, et al. P1041 Study Team: primary isoniazid prophylaxis against tuberculosis in HIV-exposed children. N Engl J Med 2011; 365(1):21–31.
26. Hesseling AC, Kim S, Madhi S, et al. IMPAACT 1041 Team. High Prevalence of drug resistance amongst HIV-exposed and –infected children in a tuberculosis prevention trial. Int J Tuberc Lung Dis 2012;16(2):192–5.
27. Brady MT, Oleske JM, Williams PL, et al. Pediatric AIDS Clinical Trials Group219/219C Team. Declines in mortality rates and changes in causes of death in HIV-1-infected children during the HAART era. J Acquir Immune Defic Syndr 2010; 53(1):86–94.
28. Nachman S, Zheng N, Acosta EP, et al. Pharmacokinetics, safety, and 48-week efficacy of oral raltegravir in HIV-1-infected children aged 2 through 18 years. Clin Infect Dis 2014;58(3):413–22.
29. CDC. Guidelines for preventing opportunistic infections among HIV-infected persons - 2002. Recommendations of the U.S. Public health service and the infectious diseases society of America. MMWR (Morb Mortal Wkly Rep) 2002;51(RR-08): 1–52. Available at: http://www.cdc.gov/mmwr/preview/mmwrhtml/rr5108a1.htm.
30. Mofenson LM, Brady MT, Danner SP, et al. Centers for Disease Control and Prevention; National Institutes of Health; HIV Medicine Association of the Infectious Diseases Society of America; Pediatric Infectious Diseases Society; American Academy of Pediatrics. Guidelines for the prevention and treatment of opportunistic infections among HIV-exposed and HIV-infected children: recommendations from CDC, the national Institutes of health, the HIV medicine association of the infectious diseases society of America, the pediatric infectious diseases society, and the American academy of pediatrics. MMWR Recomm Rep (Morb Mortal Wkly Rep) 2009;58(RR-11):1–166.
31. Siberry GK, Abzug MJ, Nachman S, et al. Panel on Opportunistic Infections in HIV-Exposed and HIV-Infected Children. Guidelines for the prevention and treatment of opportunistic infections in HIV-exposed and HIV-infected children: recommendations from the national Institutes of health, Centers for disease control and prevention, the HIV medicine association of the infectious diseases society of America, the pediatric infectious diseases society, and the American academy of pediatrics. Pediatr Infect Dis J 2013;2(4):293–308.
32. Persaud D, Gay H, Ziemniak C, et al. Absence of detectable HIV-1 viremia after treatment cessation in an infant. N Engl J Med 2013;369:1828–35.
33. Wagner TA, Tierney C, Huang S, et al. IMPAACT2015 Protocol Team. Prevalence of detectable HIV-DNA and -RNA in cerebrospinal fluid of youth with perinatal HIV and impaired cognition on antiretroviral therapy. AIDS 2024. https://doi.org/10.1097/QAD.0000000000003937.
34. Persaud D, Coletti C, Nelson BS, et al. ART-free HIV-1 remission in very early treated children: results from IMPAACT P1115. Denver CO: CROI; 2024.

UNITED STATES POSTAL SERVICE®

Statement of Ownership, Management, and Circulation (All Periodicals Publications Except Requester Publications)

1. Publication Title	2. Publication Number	3. Filing Date
CLINICS IN PERINATOLOGY	001 – 744	9/18/2024
4. Issue Frequency	5. Number of Issues Published Annually	6. Annual Subscription Price
MAR, JUN, SEP, DEC	4	$351.00

7. Complete Mailing Address of Known Office of Publication *(Not printer) (Street, city, county, state, and ZIP+4®)*
ELSEVIER INC.
230 Park Avenue, Suite 800
New York, NY 10169

Contact Person
Malathi Samayan
Telephone *(Include area code)*
91-44-4299-4507

8. Complete Mailing Address of Headquarters or General Business Office of Publisher *(Not printer)*
ELSEVIER INC.
230 Park Avenue, Suite 800
New York, NY 10169

9. Full Names and Complete Mailing Addresses of Publisher, Editor, and Managing Editor *(Do not leave blank)*

Publisher *(Name and complete mailing address)*
DOLORES MELONI, ELSEVIER INC.
1600 JOHN F KENNEDY BLVD. SUITE 1600
PHILADELPHIA, PA 19103-2899

Editor *(Name and complete mailing address)*
KERRY HOLLAND, ELSEVIER INC.
1600 JOHN F KENNEDY BLVD. SUITE 1600
PHILADELPHIA, PA 19103-2899

Managing Editor *(Name and complete mailing address)*
PATRICK MANLEY, ELSEVIER INC.
1600 JOHN F KENNEDY BLVD. SUITE 1600
PHILADELPHIA, PA 19103-2899

10. Owner *(Do not leave blank. If the publication is owned by a corporation, give the name and address of the corporation immediately followed by the names and addresses of all stockholders owning or holding 1 percent or more of the total amount of stock. If not owned by a corporation, give the names and addresses of the individual owners. If owned by a partnership or other unincorporated firm, give its name and address as well as those of each individual owner. If the publication is published by a nonprofit organization, give its name and address.)*

Full Name	Complete Mailing Address
WHOLLY OWNED SUBSIDIARY OF REED/ELSEVIER, US HOLDINGS	1600 JOHN F KENNEDY BLVD. SUITE 1600 PHILADELPHIA, PA 19103-2899

11. Known Bondholders, Mortgagees, and Other Security Holders Owning or Holding 1 Percent or More of Total Amount of Bonds, Mortgages, or Other Securities. If none, check box → ☐ None

Full Name	Complete Mailing Address
N/A	

12. Tax Status *(For completion by nonprofit organizations authorized to mail at nonprofit rates) (Check one)*
The purpose, function, and nonprofit status of this organization and the exempt status for federal income tax purposes:
☒ Has Not Changed During Preceding 12 Months
☐ Has Changed During Preceding 12 Months *(Publisher must submit explanation of change with this statement)*

13. Publication Title	14. Issue Date for Circulation Data Below
CLINICS IN PERINATOLOGY	JUNE 2024

15. Extent and Nature of Circulation	Average No. Copies Each Issue During Preceding 12 Months	No. Copies of Single Issue Published Nearest to Filing Date
a. Total Number of Copies *(Net press run)*	377	383
b. Paid Circulation *(By Mail and Outside the Mail)* (1) Mailed Outside-County Paid Subscriptions Stated on PS Form 3541 (Include paid distribution above nominal rate, advertiser's proof copies, and exchange copies)	289	287
(2) Mailed In-County Paid Subscriptions Stated on PS Form 3541 *(Include paid distribution above nominal rate, advertiser's proof copies, and exchange copies)*	0	0
(3) Paid Distribution Outside the Mails Including Sales Through Dealers and Carriers, Street Vendors, Counter Sales, and Other Paid Distribution Outside USPS®	73	74
(4) Paid Distribution by Other Classes of Mail Through the USPS (e.g., First-Class Mail®)	12	18
c. Total Paid Distribution *[Sum of 15b (1), (2), (3), and (4)]* ▶	374	379
d. Free or Nominal Rate Distribution *(By Mail and Outside the Mail)* (1) Free or Nominal Rate Outside-County Copies included on PS Form 3541	3	3
(2) Free or Nominal Rate In-County Copies Included on PS Form 3541	0	0
(3) Free or Nominal Rate Copies Mailed at Other Classes Through the USPS (e.g., First-Class Mail)	0	0
(4) Free or Nominal Rate Distribution Outside the Mail *(Carriers or other means)*	1	1
e. Total Free or Nominal Rate Distribution *(Sum of 15d (1), (2), (3) and (4))*	4	4
f. Total Distribution *(Sum of 15c and 15e)* ▶	377	383
g. Copies not Distributed *(See Instructions to Publishers #4 (page #3))* ▶	0	0
h. Total *(Sum of 15f and g)*	377	383
i. Percent Paid *(15c divided by 15f times 100)* ▶	99.03%	98.96%

* If you are claiming electronic copies, go to line 16 on page 3. If you are not claiming electronic copies, skip to line 17 on page 3.

16. Electronic Copy Circulation	Average No. Copies Each Issue During Preceding 12 Months	No. Copies of Single Issue Published Nearest to Filing Date
a. Paid Electronic Copies ▶		
b. Total Paid Print Copies (Line 15c) + Paid Electronic Copies (Line 16a) ▶		
c. Total Print Distribution (Line 15f) + Paid Electronic Copies (Line 16a) ▶		
d. Percent Paid (Both Print & Electronic Copies) (16b divided by 16c × 100) ▶		

☒ **I certify that 50% of all my distributed copies (electronic and print) are paid above a nominal price.**

17. Publication of Statement of Ownership
☒ If the publication is a general publication, publication of this statement is required. Will be printed in the DECEMBER 2024 issue of this publication. ☐ Publication not required.

18. Signature and Title of Editor, Publisher, Business Manager, or Owner
Malathi Samayan - Distribution Controller *Malathi Samayan*
Date 9/18/2024

I certify that all information furnished on this form is true and complete. I understand that anyone who furnishes false or misleading information on this form or who omits material or information requested on the form may be subject to criminal sanctions (including fines and imprisonment) and/or civil sanctions (including civil penalties).

Printed and bound by CPI Group (UK) Ltd, Croydon, CR0 4YY
16/12/2024
01807065-0001